Diagnostic Challenges in Liver Pathology

Guest Editor

JAY H. LEFKOWITCH, MD

CLINICS IN LIVER DISEASE

www.liver.theclinics.com

Consulting Editor
NORMAN GITLIN, MD

November 2010 • Volume 14 • Number 4

SAUNDERS an imprint of ELSEVIER, Inc.

W.B. SAUNDERS COMPANY

A Division of Elsevier Inc.

1600 John F. Kennedy Boulevard, Suite 1800 • Philadelphia, PA 19103-2899
http://www.theclinics.com

CLINICS IN LIVER DISEASE Volume 14, Number 4
November 2010 ISSN 1089-3261, ISBN-13: 978-1-4377-2533-9

Editor: Kerry Holland
Developmental Editor: Donald Mumford

Clinics in Liver Disease (ISSN 1089-3261) is published quarterly by Elsevier Inc., 360 Park Avenue South, New York, NY 10010-1710. Months of issue are February, May, August, and November. Business and Editorial Offices: 1600 John F. Kennedy Blvd., Ste. 1800, Philadelphia, PA 19103-2899. Customer Service Office: 3251 Riverport Lane, Maryland Heights, MO 63043. Periodicals postage paid at New York, NY and additional mailing offices. Subscription prices are $251.00 per year (U.S. individuals), $124.00 per year (U.S. student/resident), $343.00 per year (U.S. institutions), $333.00 per year (foreign individuals), $171.00 per year (foreign student/ resident), $413.00 per year (foreign instituitions), $290.00 per year (Canadian individuals), $171.00 per year (Canadian student/resident), and $413.00 per year (Canadian institutions). Foreign air speed delivery is included in all *Clinics* subscription prices. All prices are subject to change without notice. **POSTMASTER:** Send address changes to *Clinics in Liver Disease*, Elsevier Health Sciences Division, Subscription Customer Service, 3251 Riverport Lane, Maryland Heights, MO 63043. **Customer Service: Telephone: 1-800-654-2452 (U.S. and Canada); 314-447-8871 (outside U.S. and Canada). Fax: 314-447-8029.** E-mail: journalscustomer service-usa@elsevier.com (for print support); journalsonlinesupport-usa@elsevier.com (for online support).

Reprints. For copies of 100 or more of articles in this publication, please contact the Commercial Reprints Department, Elsevier Inc., 360 Park Avenue South, New York, NY 10010-1710. Tel.: 212-633-3812; Fax: 212-462-1935; E-mail: reprints@elsevier.com.

Clinics in Liver Disease is covered in *MEDLINE/PubMed (Index Medicus)*. Science Citation Index Expanded, Journal Citation Reports/Science Edition, and Current Contents/Clinical Medicine.

Printed and bound by CPI Group (UK) Ltd, Croydon, CR0 4YY

Transferred to Digital Print 2011

Contributors

CONSULTING EDITOR

NORMAN GITLIN, MD, FRCP(London), FRCPE(Edinburgh), FACG, FACP
Formerly, Professor of Medicine, Chief of Hepatology, Emory University; Currently,
Consultant, Atlanta Gastroenterology Associates, Atlanta, Georgia

GUEST EDITOR

JAY H. LEFKOWITCH, MD
Professor of Clinical Pathology, Department of Pathology, College of Physicians
and Surgeons of Columbia University, New York, New York

AUTHORS

ISAAC MORSE ABBOTT, MS
Electrical & Computer Engineering, University of Houston, Houston, Texas

ELIZABETH M. BRUNT, MD
Professor, Department of Pathology and Immunology, Washington University School
of Medicine, St Louis, Missouri

ELAINE S. CHAN, MD
Resident, Department of Pathology School of Medicine, University of Washington School
of Medicine, Seattle, Washington

NATASHA CORBITT, BS
Department of Pathology, Division of Transplantation, University of Pittsburgh Medical
Center, Pittsburgh, Pennsylvania

JAMES M. CRAWFORD, MD, PhD
Hofstra North Shore-Long Island Jewish School of Medicine, North Shore-Long Island
Jewish Health System, Manhasset, New York

A.J. DEMETRIS, MD
Department of Pathology, Division of Transplantation, University of Pittsburgh Medical
Center, Pittsburgh, Pennsylvania

M. ISABEL FIEL, MD
Professor, The Lillian and Henry M. Stratton-Hans Popper Department of Pathology,
The Mount Sinai Medical Center, Mount Sinai School of Medicine, New York, New York

MILTON J. FINEGOLD, MD
Professor of Pathology and Pediatrics, Department of Pathology, Baylor College
of Medicine, Texas Children's Hospital, Houston, Texas

PAUL GISSEN, MBChB, PhD
School of Clinical and Experimental Medicine, University of Birmingham; The Metabolic
Unit, Birmingham Children's Hospital, Birmingham, United Kingdom

KEDAR GRAMA, MS
Electrical & Computer Engineering, University of Houston, Houston, Texas

MAHA GUINDI, FRCPC
Associate Professor of Pathology, Department of Laboratory Medicine and Pathobiology, University of Toronto; Laboratory Medicine Program, University Health Network, Toronto, Canada

KUMIKO ISSE, MD, PhD
Department of Pathology, Division of Transplantation, University of Pittsburgh Medical Center, Pittsburgh, Pennsylvania

AEZAM KATOONIZADEH, MD
Liver Research Unit, Laboratory of Morphology and Molecular Pathology, University of Leuven, Minderbroederstraat, Leuven, Belgium

A.S. KNISELY, MD
Institute of Liver Studies, King's College Hospital, Denmark Hill, London, United Kingdom

MINA KOMUTA, MD, PhD
Liver Research Unit, Department of Morphology and Molecular Pathology, University of Leuven, Minderbroederstraat 12, Leuven, Belgium

STEPHEN M. LAGANA, MD
Postdoctoral Residency Fellow, Department of Pathology and Cell Biology, Columbia University Medical Center, New York, New York

KATHRYN LAW, MD
Instructor, Department of Pathology and Immunology, Washington University School of Medicine, St Louis, Missouri

WILLIAM M.F. LEE, MD, PhD
Department of Medicine, Abramson Cancer Center, University of Pennsylvania, Philadelphia, Pennsylvania

JAY H. LEFKOWITCH, MD
Professor of Clinical Pathology, Department of Pathology, College of Physicians and Surgeons of Columbia University, New York, New York

ANDREW LESNIAK
Department of Pathology, Division of Transplantation, University of Pittsburgh Medical Center, Pittsburgh, Pennsylvania

JOHN G. LUNZ, PhD
Department of Pathology, Division of Transplantation, University of Pittsburgh Medical Center, Pittsburgh, Pennsylvania

YOSHIAKI MIZUGUCHI, MD, PhD
Department of Pathology, Division of Transplantation, University of Pittsburgh Medical Center, Pittsburgh, Pennsylvania

ROGER K. MOREIRA, MD
Assistant Professor, Department of Pathology and Cell Biology, Columbia University Medical Center, New York, New York

VALÉRIE PARADIS, MD, PhD
Pathology Department, Beaujon Hospital, Clichy Cedex; INSERM, Paris, France

TANIA ROSKAMS, MD, PhD
Head, Liver Research Unit, Laboratory of Morphology and Molecular Pathology, University of Leuven, Minderbroederstraat, Leuven, Belgium

ANGSHUMOY ROY, MD, PhD
Department of Pathology, Baylor College of Medicine, Houston, Texas

BADRINATH ROYSAM, PhD
Hugh and Lillie Cranz Cullen University Professor; Chair, Electrical & Computer Engineering, University of Houston, Houston, Texas

LAURA RUBBIA-BRANDT, MD, PhD
Professor, Division of Clinical Pathology, University Hospital, Geneva, Switzerland

SUSAN SPECHT, MS
Department of Pathology, Division of Transplantation, University of Pittsburgh Medical Center, Pittsburgh, Pennsylvania

MATTHEW M. YEH, MD, PhD
Associate Professor, Department of Pathology, University of Washington School of Medicine, Seattle, Washington

Contents

Preface   xiii

Jay H. Lefkowitch

Pathology of Chronic Hepatitis B and Chronic Hepatitis C   555

M. Isabel Fiel

Histologic evaluation of the liver is a major component in the medical management and treatment algorithm of patients with chronic hepatitis B (HBV)
and chronic hepatitis C (HCV). Liver biopsy in these patients remains the
gold standard, and decisions on treatment are often predicated on the
degree of damage and stage of fibrosis. This article outlines the clinical
course and serologic diagnosis of HBV and HCV for the clinician and the
pathologist, who together have a close working relationship in managing
patients with acute and chronic liver disease. The salient histologic
features are elucidated in an attempt to provide the clinician with an understanding of the basic histopathology underlying chronic HCV and HBV.

Histology of Autoimmune Hepatitis and its Variants   577

Maha Guindi

Autoimmune hepatitis does not have a pathognomonic feature, and its laboratory, serologic, and histologic manifestations are shared with a variety
of acute and chronic liver diseases. The disease has active and quiescent
phases and thus variable histologic appearances. This article outlines the
many histologic faces of autoimmune hepatitis. It discusses the fulminant
and acute forms, as well as the chronic hepatitic forms. Overlap syndromes with primary biliary cirrhosis and primary sclerosing cholangitis
are described. The role of the pathologist in reporting the biopsies is
discussed.

Nonalcoholic Fatty Liver Disease   591

Kathryn Law and Elizabeth M. Brunt

Nonalcoholic fatty liver disease (NAFLD) significantly contributes to the
morbidity and mortality of large proportions of the population across all
age ranges, which will continue for the foreseeable future. Since NAFLD
and nonalcoholic steatohepatitis were originally described, understanding
of pathogenesis, relationships to insulin resistance and the metabolic syndrome, and histopathologic lesions has progressed. However, no clinical
or imaging parameters can yet accurately predict inflammatory activity
or fibrosis stage across the spectrum of disease. Liver needle biopsy interpretation remains essential in this role; liver biopsy evaluation is also
needed for recognition of concurrent (or alternate) liver disease processes.
Thus, an understanding of the histologic spectrum of findings in NAFLD
and the methods of semiquantitative evaluations used are required for
pathologists who sign out liver biopsies. This article describes histologic

findings, and provides insights into the pathologic processes and clinical implications across the spectrum of NAFLD.

Hepatic Granulomas: Pathogenesis and Differential Diagnosis   605

Stephen M. Lagana, Roger K. Moreira, and Jay H. Lefkowitch

Granulomatous liver disease constitutes a category of hepatic disorders and is at present diagnosed in approximately 4% of liver biopsies. Hepatic granulomas develop through the interactions of T lymphocytes and macrophages, with the integral involvement of T-helper (T_H) 1 or T_H2 pathways or both, depending on the specific granulomatous disease. Hepatic granulomas may be manifested clinically by elevated levels of serum alkaline phosphatase and g-glutamyltransferase enzymes, damage to specific structures (eg, intrahepatic bile ducts in primary biliary cirrhosis), or infrequently, progressive liver disease with portal hypertension and cirrhosis (eg, sarcoidosis). Systemic immunologic disorders, infectious diseases, drug hepatotoxicity, and reaction to neoplastic disease are the major causative factors responsible for granulomas in the liver. These causes and recent epidemiologic trends are covered in this discussion.

Trafficking and Transporter Disorders in Pediatric Cholestasis   619

A.S. Knisely and Paul Gissen

This article describes the uses of immunostaining in the diagnosis of cholestasis. To immunostain for bile salt export pump (BSEP) and multidrug resistance protein 3 in severe hepatobiliary disease manifest early in life can rapidly identify whether sequencing of ABCB11 or ABCB4 is likely to yield a genetic diagnosis. To immunostain for canalicular ectoenzymes as well as transporters, with transmission electron microscopy, can suggest whether sequencing of ATP8B1 is likely to yield a genetic diagnosis. Demonstrating BSEP expression can direct attention to bile acid synthesis disorders. Immunostaining for multidrug resistance-associated protein 2 serves principally as a control for adequacy of processing.

Vascular Disorders of the Liver   635

James M. Crawford

Hepatic vascular disorders are a set of conditions that may be acute, or may be insidious and subclinical for many years. They can be organized into 3 categories: obstruction to hepatic vascular inflow, obstruction to blood flow through the liver, and obstruction to hepatic vascular outflow. In the first category are portal vein thrombosis, hepatic artery thrombosis, and presinusoidal causes of vascular obstruction. In the second category are sickle cell disease, disseminated intravascular coagulation, intrasinusoidal malignancy, and infection. In the third category are macroscopic hepatic venous thrombosis, thrombosis of the retrohepatic inferior vena cava, and venoocclusive disease. There are 2 nodular conditions of the liver that are not neoplastic but the result of occlusion of hepatic vasculature with compensatory hyperplasia of well-vascularized parenchyma. Hepatic vascular disorders constitute a heterogeneous group of conditions that must be considered in the differential diagnosis of any patient with hepatic compromise.

Sinusoidal Obstruction Syndrome   651

Laura Rubbia-Brandt

Sinusoidal obstruction syndrome (SOS), formerly named venoocclusive disease, is a well-known complication of hematopoietic stem cell transplantation and ingestion of food or drinks contaminated by pyrrolizidine alkaloids. Many other drugs and toxins have been associated with SOS, including several chemotherapeutic agents and immunosuppressors. SOS contributes to significant morbidity and mortality in all these settings. This review describes the histologic lesions of SOS, details its pathogenesis as it is understood today, specifies the recent data on its causes and how it may influence clinical management of colorectal liver metastases, and discusses the current knowledge on diagnosis and preventive options.

Adding Value to Liver (and Allograft) Biopsy Evaluation Using a Combination of Multiplex Quantum Dot Immunostaining, High-Resolution Whole-Slide Digital Imaging, and Automated Image Analysis   669

Kumiko Isse, Kedar Grama, Isaac Morse Abbott, Andrew Lesniak, John G. Lunz, William M.F. Lee, Susan Specht, Natasha Corbitt, Yoshiaki Mizuguchi, Badrinath Roysam, and A.J. Demetris

Various technologies including nucleic acid, protein, and metabolic array analyses of blood, liver tissue, and bile are emerging as powerful tools in the study of hepatic pathophysiology. The entire lexicon of liver disease, however, has been written using classical hematoxylin-eosin staining and light microscopic examination. The authors' goal is to develop new tools to enhance histopathologic examination of liver tissue that would enrich the information gained from liver biopsy analysis, enable quantitative analysis, and bridge the gap between various "-omics" tools and interpretation of routine liver biopsy results. This article describes the progress achieved during the past 2 years in developing multiplex quantum dot (nanoparticle) staining and combining it with high-resolution whole-slide imaging using a slide scanner equipped with filters to capture 9 distinct fluorescent signals for multiple antigens. The authors first focused on precise characterization of leukocyte subsets, but soon realized that the data generated were beyond the practical limits that could be properly evaluated, analyzed, and interpreted visually by a pathologist. Therefore, the authors collaborated with the open source FARSIGHT image analysis project (http://www.farsight-toolkit.org). FARSIGHT's goal is to develop and disseminate the next-generation toolkit of automated image analysis methods to enable quantification of molecular biomarkers on a cell-by-cell basis from multiparameter images. The resulting data can be used for histocytometric studies of the complex and dynamic tissue microenvironments that are of biomedical interest. The authors envisage that these tools will eventually be incorporated into the routine practice of surgical pathology and precipitate a revolution in the specialty.

The Use of Immunohistochemistry in Liver Tumors   687

Elaine S. Chan and Matthew M. Yeh

A variety of benign and malignant neoplasms can be encountered in the liver. Hematoxylin and eosin–stained tissue sections alone may not yield sufficient information to definitively diagnose liver tumors; therefore, ancillary studies with immunohistochemical markers can play a crucial role in differentiating the different hepatic neoplasms. The recent development of oncofetoprotein glypican-3 has added to the value of immunohisto-chemistry in diagnosing liver cancer. This review discusses the immuno-histochemical markers used most often in the diagnosis of hepatic tumors.

Hepatic Progenitor Cells: An Update   705

Tania Roskams, Aezam Katoonizadeh, and Mina Komuta

Liver progenitor cells are activated in most human liver diseases. The dynamics, and therefore subpopulations, of progenitor cells are, however, different in acute versus chronic hepatocytic diseases and in biliary dis-eases. The role of Wnt and Notch signaling pathways in activation and dif-ferentiation of human hepatic progenitor cells holds great promise because they can be manipulated by drugs. Hepatocytic differentiation requires inhibition of Notch (numb switched on), whereas cholangiocytic differentiation requires Notch activation. In this way, the patients' own regenerative response could be supported, which could eventually even avoid the need for transplantation in several patients.

Benign Liver Tumors: An update   719

Valérie Paradis

One of the consequences of extensive use of abdominal imaging, and especially liver ultrasonography, is the detection of asymptomatic liver tumors. In the absence of underlying chronic liver disease, the vast major-ity of these lesions correspond to benign liver tumors including solid and cystic lesions. This article is dedicated to hepatocellular tumors and also addresses hemangiomas as the most common benign liver tumors, and angiomyolipomas as a rare tumor often misdiagnosed.

Hepatic Neoplasia and Metabolic Diseases in Children   731

Angshumoy Roy and Milton J. Finegold

Hepatic neoplasia is a rare but serious complication of metabolic diseases in children. The risk of developing neoplasia, the age at onset, and the measures to prevent it differ in various diseases. This article reviews the most common metabolic disorders in humans that are associated with neoplasms, with a special emphasis on the molecular etiopathogenesis of this process. The cellular pathways driving carcinogenesis are poorly understood, but best known in tyrosinemia.

Advances in Hepatobiliary Pathology: Update for 2010   747

Jay H. Lefkowitch

Recent publications on hepatology and hepatic pathology provide a wealth of new information on wideranging topics. Morphologic aspects of liver dis-ease associated with hepatitis B and C viruses, autoimmune hepatitis, and HIV infection were addressed, as was the prevalent problem of nonalco-holic fatty liver disease. Advances in diagnosis and pathogenesis of primary biliary cirrhosis, primary sclerosing cholangitis, and the increasingly complex spectrum of IgG4 hepatobiliary diseases were also reported.

The histologic and immunohistochemical features of the rare "calcifying nested stromal-epithelial tumor" of the liver were described in a 9-case series. For benign and malignant liver tumors, immunohistochemistry plays a major diagnostic role, and several recent studies demonstrate the value of immunostains in distinguishing between liver-cell adenoma and focal nodular hyperplasia.

Index   763

FORTHCOMING ISSUES

February 2011
Hepatobiliary Manifestations of Diseases Involving Other Organs and Systems
Ke-Qin Hu, MD, *Guest Editor*

May 2011
Hepatocellular Carcinoma
Adrian Reuben, MD, *Guest Editor*

August 2011
Hepatitis C Virus
Fred Poordad, MD, *Guest Editor*

RECENT ISSUES

August 2010
Chronic Hepatitis B: An Update
Naoky C.S. Tsai, MD, *Guest Editor*

May 2010
Endoscopy and Liver Disease
Andres Cardenas, MD, MMSC
and Paul J. Thuluvath, MD, FRCPC,
Guest Editors

February 2010
Health Care-Associated Transmission of Hepatitis B and C Viruses
Bandar Al Knawy, MD, FRCPC,
Guest Editor

THE CLINICS ARE NOW AVAILABLE ONLINE!

Access your subscription at:
www.theclinics.com

Preface

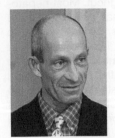

Jay H. Lefkowitch, MD
Guest Editor

This issue of *Clinics in Liver Disease* is a forum on liver pathology, with contributions by an expert panel of hepatic pathologists on many of the current diagnostic issues of hepatology, including assessment of biopsy changes in, as well as grading and staging of, chronic hepatitis B and C and autoimmune hepatitis, the spectrum of changes in nonalcoholic fatty liver disease (NAFLD), and manifestations of post-liver transplantation liver injury. Genomic and molecular diagnostics and immunohisto-chemistry have had a major impact on liver pathology practices, and these are also discussed in this issue.

Leading off the issue, Dr Fiel discusses chronic hepatitis B and C and provides a time capsule view of the various landmarks in scoring systems for chronic hepatitis since the 1960s. The photomicrographs included are classics in the histopathology of chronic hepatitis and Fig. 3 merits close attention since it beautifully illustrates and compares (with trichrome stain) the several staging systems which are currently in use for fibrosis in chronic hepatitis (ie, Ishak, METAVIR, Scheuer, and Batts and Ludwig). This article examines the general features of chronic hepatitis, including the portal, periportal interface, and lobular necroinflammatory components along with associated changes such as the ductular reaction, secondary iron deposition, and large and small cell dysplasia. For chronic hepatitis B, Dr Fiel provides a concise description of its immunologic phases (tolerance, activity, inactivity, and, last, the proposed "recovery" phase of hepatitis B surface antigen clearance). For chronic hepatitis C there are a number of histologic markers, including lymphoid aggregates/follicles, bile duct damage, and steatosis, and these are covered along with mention of the recognized 7 HCV genotypes.

The histologic features of autoimmune hepatitis (AIH) are dealt with next by Dr Guindi in the context of the diagnostic challenges encountered when classical serologic data (such as antinuclear and anti-smooth muscle antibodies) are present, absent, or confounded by other data (such as positive antimitochondrial antibodies). Scoring systems for AIH are reviewed, and the problems of AIH overlap with primary biliary cirrhosis or with primary sclerosing cholangitis, as well as transition from 1 condition to another, are covered. Dr Guindi also offers several possible explanations

Clin Liver Dis 14 (2010) xiii–xvi
doi:10.1016/j.cld.2010.07.010
1089-3261/10/$ – see front matter © 2010 Elsevier Inc. All rights reserved.

liver.theclinics.com

of autoimmune features in chronic hepatitis C (including positive serum autoantibodies and liver biopsy features of AIH). The importance of accurate histologic diagnosis for initiating appropriate therapeutic management is stressed throughout. Most hepato- logic clinical and pathologic practices now frequently must deal with NAFLD and the problems of abnormal serum liver tests and morphologic liver disease related to obesity, diabetes, hyperlipidemia, and the metabolic syndrome. Drs Law and Brunt detail all the histopathologic features, from the type and distribution of steatosis to hepatocyte ballooning and formation of Mallory-Denk bodies to the degree of portal inflammation in both adult and pediatric NAFLD. Grading and staging systems are described and the calculation and significance of the NAFLD activity score or NAS (steatosis, lobular inflammation, hepatocyte ballooning) are set forth with exceptional clarity.

Granulomas remain a common finding in liver biopsies, and an article from our center with my coauthors Drs Lagana and Moreira describes some of the changing epidemiologic data and causes. The revolutionary advances in and complexity of bile canalicular secretion of bile are nowhere better exemplified than in pediatric cholestatic disease, disorders that are frequently localized to bile salt transporter proteins and their genes, as superbly detailed in the article by Drs Knisely and Gis- sen. Beginning with an overview of bile acid synthesis, modifications, and intestinal transport, a consideration follows of the "low-serum GGT" syndromes (progressive familial intrahepatic cholestasis type 1, PFIC1, and benign recurrent intrahepatic cholestasis), which result from mutations in *ATP8B1* encoding the "floppase" (alter- natively termed "flippase") for phosphatidylserine localization to the inner leaflet of the canalicular membrane. Brief discussion is included of Dubin-Johnson and Rotor syndromes (conjugated hyperbilirubinemias), multidrug resistance 3 deficiencies (eg, PFIC-3), and the role of immunostaining for bile salt export pump, multidrug resistance 3, and other transporters in establishing the diagnosis in these chole- static diseases.

The vascular anatomy and microanatomy of the liver are succinctly reviewed by Dr Crawford, with coverage including impaired hepatic artery and portal vein flow, the morphologic and physiologic features of idiopathic portal hypertension, and altered vascular flow in cirrhosis. He also examines the problem of *parenchymal extinction*, whereby thrombotic obstruction of veins or sinusoids leads to contiguous hepatocyte loss, collapse, and eventual fibrosis. The reasons for considering focal nodular hyperplasia (FNH) and nodular regenerative hyperplasia to be inherently vascular lesions of the liver are also outlined. This article on vascular diseases sets the stage for the overview by Dr Rubbia-Brandt on *sinusoidal obstruction syndrome,* a term which subsumes the older term *veno-occlusive disease*. Utilizing gross, histologic, ultrastructural, and diagrammatic illustrations, Dr Rubbia-Brandt reviews the historical background of veno-occlusive disease (eg, senecio poisoning in South Africa and bush tea pyrrolizidine alkaloid toxicity in Jamaica) and brings us up to date by discussing animal models of sinusoidal obstruction syndrome and human disease associated with toxicity of the platinum derivative chemotherapy agent oxaliplatin.

An illuminating presentation by Dr Isse and colleagues looks at the interface of new technology with traditional histopathologic assessment. The authors discuss the potential uses of multiplex quantum dot immunostaining with whole slide digital imaging in assessing liver biopsies after liver transplantation. Some of the limitations of the "pure histology" assessment as well as its strengths in areas such as grading and staging chronic hepatitis and diagnosing liver allograft rejection are presented. Several diagnostic problem areas in the allograft are mentioned followed by a detailed report on the procedural aspects and multiple antigens (particularly leukocyte subsets) available for multiplex staining and software analysis, with illustrated examples. The challenges of incorporating these techniques into pathology practice are outlined and stress is placed on the valuable information to be gained concerning molecular signaling mechanisms.

Immunohistochemistry plays an essential role in diagnostic pathology and Drs Chan and Yeh provide essentially a "user's guide" to practical immunostaining in the diagnosis of liver tumors. They discuss the important immunostains for distinguishing between metastatic and primary tumors (the latter including hepatocellular carcinoma and cholangiocarcinoma, among several others) and address the specificity and sensitivity of the important trio of current immunostains, which includes glypican-3, glutamine synthetase, and heat shock protein 70. Immunohistochemistry of FNH, liver-cell adenoma, and angiomyolipoma are also discussed.

Drs Roskams and Katoonizadeh provide an update on hepatic progenitor cells and the roles of tumor necrosis factor-like weak inducer of apoptosis, other inflammatory cytokines and chemokines, Hedgehog signaling, and Wnt and Notch signaling in their activation. Comparison to rodent oval cells and immunohistochemical stains for identifying progenitor cells are reviewed and the potential role of progenitor cells in hepatocarcinogenesis is also cited. The authors' recent work on comparative progenitor cell signaling pathways in primary biliary cirrhosis vs chronic hepatitis C vs acute hepatitis will be of interest. The realm of benign liver tumors is detailed by Dr Paradis, including FNH, liver-cell adenoma, adenomatosis, hemangiomas, and angiomyolipoma. Of particular interest is Dr Paradis' discussion of the genomic-phenotype correlations now available for liver-cell adenoma. Biallelic mutation in the *TCF1* gene that inactivates hepatocyte nuclear factor 1α transcription factor results in adenomas with steatosis and without atypia. There is now an association of mono-allelic mutations of hepatocyte nuclear factor 1α with diabetes and adenomatosis ($\geq$10 hepatic adenomas). Further consideration is given to adenomas with atypia and β-catenin-activating mutations (which have risk of progression to hepatocellular carcinoma) and the telangiectatic/inflammatory adenoma (formerly telangiectatic FNH) with its associated mutations in the *IL6ST* gene that result in activation of the IL6 signaling pathway.

Hereditary tyrosinemia (fumarylacetoacetate hydrolase deficiency), alpha-1-antitrypsin deficiency, and glycogen storage diseases are important settings for the emergence of hepatocellular carcinoma in children, and these conditions, including their genomic abnormalities, are reviewed by Drs Roy and Finegold in the context of hepatic histopathology. Readers with only a passing familiarity with tyrosinemia will find especially intriguing the authors' discussion of the founder effect seen in a French Canadian population of Quebec as well as the treatment options for the disease. Hereditary hemochromatosis and Wilson disease and their risks of hepatic neoplasia are also briefly mentioned. The final article of this issue is a selective survey of publications from the past year, which impacts on the morphologic diagnosis and pathogenesis of a broad spectrum of hepatobiliary diseases.

The content of this issue provides further testimony to the ongoing role liver pathology plays in the diagnosis and management of individuals with liver disease and in elucidating basic mechanisms of liver disease. The contributors to the issue have provided outstanding contemporary updates on their respective topics and it has been a pleasure to serve as the Guest Editor for such a compilation. Many thanks are due to Dr Norman Gitlin, Consulting Editor for *Clinics in Liver Disease*, whose advocacy for a specific issue devoted to liver histopathology is greatly appreciated. The

Clinics editor, Kerry Holland, has, as usual, provided enthusiasm, momentum, and expert guidelines for keeping the production schedule on track.

Jay H. Lefkowitch, MD
Department of Pathology
College of Physicians and
Surgeons of Columbia University
630 West 168th Street–PH 15 West, Room 1574
New York, NY 10032, USA

E-mail address:
JHL3@columbia.edu

Pathology of Chronic Hepatitis B and Chronic Hepatitis C

M. Isabel Fiel, MD

KEYWORDS

- Liver pathology • Chronic hepatitis C • Chronic hepatitis B
- Grade • Stage of fibrosis • Inflammation

Chronic hepatitis is defined as inflammation of the liver, often in the setting of raised aminotransferase levels for a period of 6 months or longer.[1] The hepatotropic viruses responsible for chronic hepatitis are hepatitis B virus (HBV), hepatitis C virus (HCV), and hepatitis delta virus (HDV). Current medical practice requires staging and evaluation of the degree of fibrosis formation in the liver, and less importantly, the degree of necroinflammation. Because a liver biopsy has inherent risks, with the incidence of complications requiring hospitalization associated with percutaneous liver biopsy estimated to be 0.9%,[2] surrogate serum markers and various imaging techniques have been developed to assess the severity of liver fibrosis,[3–5] However, these noninvasive tests have limited ability to discriminate between the stages of fibrosis and, at best, are predictive in distinguishing minimal fibrosis from significant fibrosis.[6,7] The liver injury present in chronic hepatitis may be variable, but the basic morphologic changes in all types of chronic viral hepatitis are similar. In this regard, the liver biopsy remains the gold standard and is an important tool in the evaluation of patients with liver disease.[8]

APPROACH TO THE DIAGNOSIS OF CHRONIC HEPATITIS
Specimen Adequacy

Adequate tissue for evaluation is requisite for grading and staging of liver disease, because small biopsy specimen size can affect the accuracy of histologic interpretation.[9] Specimens obtained with cutting biopsy needles are superior to those obtained with suction needles.[10] Larger-gauge needles (14- to 16-gauge) and biopsy specimens at least 2 cm long are more likely to be adequate for assessing histologic changes.[9] The number of portal tracts required for an adequate liver needle biopsy is between 6 and 11, although 11 portal tracts are generally considered an optimal

No funding support is relevant to the article. The author has nothing to disclose.

The Lillian and Henry M. Stratton-Hans Popper Department of Pathology, The Mount Sinai Medical Center, Mount Sinai School of Medicine, Box 1194, 1468 Madison Avenue, New York, NY 10029, USA

E-mail address: mariaisabel.fiel@mountsinai.org

Clin Liver Dis 14 (2010) 555–575
doi:10.1016/j.cld.2010.07.001
1089-3261/10/$ – see front matter © 2010 Elsevier Inc. All rights reserved.

specimen.[9] Sampling error is also a major obstacle[11] regardless of the length or width of the core, because a needle core biopsy represents only one-fifty thousandth of the entire liver. Another pitfall is the experience of the pathologist.[11] Rousselet and colleagues[12] found that a pathologist with a subspecialty in hepatopathology and practicing at an academic center has better consistency and accuracy in interpretation of liver biopsies than pathologists in community practice.

THE SCORING SYSTEMS FOR GRADING AND STAGING CHRONIC HEPATITIS

Over the last few decades, several grading and staging schemes for chronic hepatitis have been proposed and developed. Before this, De Groote and colleagues[13] had described 2 types: chronic persistent hepatitis considered to have a benign course and chronic active hepatitis considered to have a worse outcome. In 1971, Popper and Schaffner[14] added lobular hepatitis. Knodell and colleagues[15] provided the first paper detailing a numerical scoring system for chronic hepatitis, the histologic activity index (HAI), which was the sum of periportal necrosis, intralobular necrosis, portal inflammation, and fibrosis. A higher total score indicated greater liver damage. Combining necroinflammation and fibrosis, which could be discordant, is a problem with the Knodell score. A simple scoring system that separates necroinflammation from fibrosis was developed by Scheuer.[16] Scores ranging from 0 to 4 based on increasing severity were each given to degree of portal inflammation and interface hepatitis and to degree of lobular inflammation. A separate score (range 0–4) was given to increasing stages of fibrosis, 4 being cirrhosis. A position paper by Desmet and colleagues[17] in further support of the Scheuer scheme was published. The authors placed emphasis on integrating the cause of the chronic hepatitis into the diagnosis. In 1995, Batts and Ludwig[18] created the modified Scheuer system with accompanying diagrams depicting the different grades and stages of chronic hepatitis (Table 1). In the same year, Ishak[19] and a group of hepatopathologists called the "Gnomes" published the modified Knodell HAI. In this landmark paper, grades for necroinflammation were separately categorized from the stage of fibrosis. The Ishak system contains more stages of fibrosis (0–6) than other systems. In recent years, the Ishak staging system has become widely used in clinical trials because of its ability to more clearly differentiate milder changes in fibrosis. Westin and colleagues[20] found that the Ishak system has fair-to-good reproducibility between observers. In the mid-1990s, a French group consisting of hepatologists and liver pathologists published an algorithm for grading necroinflammation and created a staging system for fibrosis (F0–F4).[21,22]

In investigative studies, particularly those involving antiviral therapies, semiquantitative methods may be needed. The choice of the classification scheme to be used is entirely up to the group of investigators. The Knodell scoring system and the Ishak fibrosis scores are more commonly used in such studies.[15,19]

Grade of Necroinflammation: Portal and Lobular Changes

In any of the classification and scoring schemes, grade is based on the degree of damage found in the liver for both portal and lobular areas.[23] Bridging necrosis and confluent necrosis may be present.[24] In general, the greater the degree of liver damage, the greater the elevation of the aminotransaminases.

Portal Changes

Inflammation in the portal tracts may be patchy or diffuse, involving all portal areas in the biopsy specimen. The inflammatory infiltrate consists of mature lymphocytes

Table 1
Commonly used staging systems for fibrosis

Fibrosis	Score
Ishak System	
No fibrosis	0
Fibrous expansion of some portal areas, with or without short fibrous septa	1
Fibrous expansion of most portal areas, with or without short fibrous septa	2
Fibrous expansion of most portal areas with occasional portal-to-portal (P-P) bridging	3
Fibrous expansion of portal areas with marked P-P bridging and portal-to-central (P-C) bridging	4
Marked bridging (P-P and/or P-C) with occasional nodules (incomplete cirrhosis)	5
Cirrhosis, probable or definite	6
METAVIR System	**Stage**
No fibrosis	F0
Portal fibrosis without septa	F1
Portal fibrosis with few septa	F2
Numerous septa without cirrhosis	F3
Cirrhosis	F4
Scheuer System	**Stage**
No fibrosis	0
Enlarged, fibrotic portal tracts	1
Periportal or portal-portal septa, but intact architecture	2
Fibrosis with architectural distortion, but no obvious cirrhosis	3
Probable or definite cirrhosis	4
Batts and Ludwig	**Score**
No fibrosis	0
Portal fibrosis	1
Periportal fibrosis	2
Septal fibrosis	3
Cirrhosis	4

Data from Scheuer PJ. Classification of chronic viral hepatitis: a need for reassessment. J Hepatol 1991;13(3):372–4; Batts KP, Ludwig J. Chronic hepatitis. An update on terminology and reporting. Am J Surg Pathol1995;19(12):1409–17; Ishak K, Baptista A, Bianchi L, et al. Histological grading and staging of chronic hepatitis. J Hepatol 1995;22(6):696–9; Intraobserver and interobserver variations in liver biopsy interpretation in patients with chronic hepatitis C. The French METAVIR cooperative study group.

admixed with a sprinkling of plasma cells and, rarely, some eosinophils. Lymphoid aggregates and follicles are more commonly seen in chronic HCV but may also be present in chronic HBV infection[25–27] In its mildest form, the inflammatory infiltrate is confined to the portal tracts, and the edges of the portal areas remain smooth. In its most severe form, the portal tract is expanded, with erosion of the limiting plate throughout its circumference.[17,24] Mild interface hepatitis and severe interface hepatitis are illustrated in **Fig. 1**. With spillage of inflammatory cells into the periportal area, the hepatocytes along the limiting plate and beyond are eroded, a process termed interface hepatitis (formerly called piecemeal necrosis), which is an immune-mediated

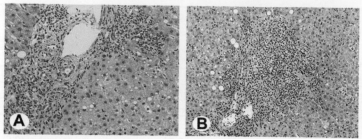

Fig. 1. Interface hepatitis. These 2 portal tracts show inflammatory cells spilling over into the periportal area, creating an irregular outline of the portal tract. (*A*) mild interface hepatitis with focal erosion of the limiting plate and (*B*) severe interface hepatitis that results in an irregular outline of the entire circumference of the portal tract.

type of inflammation that results in hepatocyte apoptosis.[28] The result is that of a portal tract with irregular borders and a loss of periportal hepatocytes.[29]

Lobular Changes

Different forms and degrees of parenchymal injury may be seen in chronic hepatitis. Apart from interface hepatitis, other types of injury include ballooning degeneration, apoptosis, and spotty, bridging, and confluent necrosis. Ballooning degeneration is a type of injury occurring when the hepatocyte loses its normal polygonal shape and becomes swollen and rounded. Apoptosis is seen as shrunken hepatocytes, with or without nuclear fragments, having a deeply eosinophilic cytoplasm (**Fig. 2**).[23] Early apoptosis within intact liver cell plates usually manifests as a single hepatocyte with eosinophilic cytoplasm surrounded by lymphocytes.[23] Later on in apoptosis, the nuclear component is extruded, and all that is left is an acidophilic body with or without accompanying inflammatory cells. Spotty necrosis, representing areas of hepatocyte loss, consists of small aggregates of inflammatory cells composed mostly of lymphocytes and macrophages (see **Fig. 2**). Hence, these foci are often referred to as "tombstones." Bridging necrosis occurs when 2 vascular structures are linked by a row of necrotic hepatocytes, whereas confluent necrosis occurs when several lobules lose hepatocytes and the parenchyma collapses.[14]

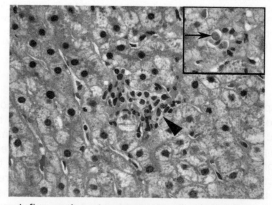

Fig. 2. Lobular necroinflammation. An aggregate of inflammatory cells (*arrowhead*) is shown. The inset shows 2 apoptotic bodies.

Stage of Fibrosis: Architectural Changes

In the evaluation of chronic hepatitis, one has to consider that fibrosis is a dynamic process occurring over time and that scarring results from chronic inflammation. Hepatic stellate cells and portal myofibroblasts contribute to the collagen formation. Trichrome or other connective tissue stains such as Sirius red should be used to fully characterize the degree of fibrosis. The initial damage consists of portal fibrosis with or without formation of fibrous septa extending into the lobular parenchyma.[25] This process constitutes the earliest forms of scarring in chronic HBV and HCV. Over time, fibrous septa extend from expanded portal tracts and link adjacent portal tracts. As fibrosis progresses, there is increasing distortion of the architecture. This is apparent when portal tracts that are linked by fibrous tissue have more pronounced fibrous bridges. Eventually, fibrous septa enclose nodules, which constitutes cirrhosis.[14] **Table 1** shows the different staging systems, with the descriptive term and corresponding fibrosis scores. The development of fibrosis in chronic hepatitis is illustrated in **Fig. 3**, which also provides a graphic portrayal of the staging schemes for fibrosis commonly used in clinical practice and investigative studies.

Other Features seen in Chronic Hepatitis

Ductular reaction is a process that is also called ductular proliferation, proliferation of bile ductules, or formation of neocholangioles. Ductular reaction results when hepatic progenitor cells proliferate in response to hepatocyte loss and because of an insufficient replicative capacity of the mature hepatocytes.[30] Severe ductular reaction in chronic liver injury indicates greater parenchymal damage, and the residual hepatocytes are unable to replicate through the normal pathway. The area of ductular reaction directly correlates with stage of fibrosis.[31]

Iron deposition, in Kupffer cells alone or in Kupffer cells and hepatocytes, is often seen in chronic hepatitis and has to be reported when present.[32,33] Depletion of iron has been shown to lower transaminases and affords better response to interferon and ribavirin therapy in chronic HCV.[33]

Liver cell dysplasia indicates a group of cytologic abnormalities found in specimens from patients with chronic hepatitis and cirrhosis.[34] It is more common in HBV-infected individuals. Large cell change (formerly called large cell dysplasia) is identified as a focus of hepatocytes that are enlarged and display nuclear pleomorphism, hyperchromasia, and multinucleation (**Fig. 4**).[34,35] Large cell change in chronic viral hepatitis has also been reported to depict hepatocyte senescence rather than being a precursor of hepatocellular carcinoma.[36] Small cell dysplasia is characterized by small

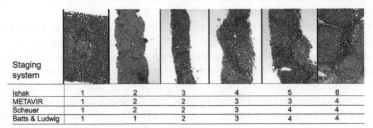

Staging system						
Ishak	1	2	3	4	5	6
METAVIR	1	2	2	3	3	4
Scheuer	1	2	2	3	4	4
Batts & Ludwig	1	1	2	3	4	4

Fig. 3. Fibrosis progression in chronic hepatitis. The initial damage is portal fibrosis (*from left to right*); as chronic injury progresses, there is gradual expansion of portal areas by fibrous tissue, with linking of portal tracts by septa followed by creation of more bridges of fibrous tissue, which eventually results in cirrhosis. The bottom panels show the corresponding fibrosis scores based on the different staging schema.

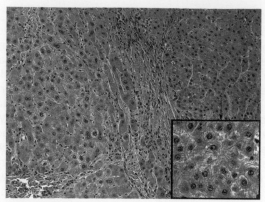

Fig. 4. Liver cell dysplasia in chronic hepatitis and cirrhosis. The left portion shows large cell changes as demonstrated by large pleomorphic nuclei; on the right is a focus of small cell dysplasia. The inset shows cytologic atypia with crowded and hyperchromatic nuclei and a high nuclear-cytoplasmic ratio.

hepatocytes with high nuclear-cytoplasmic ratio that closely resemble hepatocellular carcinoma (HCC; see **Fig. 4**).[37] This is considered to be the earliest morphologically recognizable precursor lesion of HCC.[38] On the other hand, in a recent study of patients with chronic HBV, Koo and colleagues[39] found that large cell dysplasia was associated with a threefold increased risk of developing HCC. They also found that there was no significant association between small cell dysplasia and the development of HCC when compared with patients without small cell dysplasia.

CHRONIC HEPATITIS B

The prevalence of chronic HBV infection worldwide is estimated to be 5%, which translates to about 350 million people.[40] The prevalence differs between regions; in high-prevalence areas (8%–20% of the population), such as in southeast Asia and sub-Saharan Africa, the infection mostly occurs from HBV early antigen (HBeAg)-positive mothers transmitting the virus to their offspring perinatally (vertical transmission) or during early childhood (horizontal transmission).[41,42] Currently in the United States, the highest incidence is seen between ages 25 and 44 years, and the lowest among children younger than 15 years. The prevalence of hepatitis B surface antigen (HBsAg)-positive individuals is estimated to be 0.30%, which projects to about 800,000 Americans with HBV infection.[43]

HBV is an enveloped double-stranded DNA virus of the Hepadnaviridae family and can cause acute or chronic liver disease.[44] HBV has been classified into 8 genotypes (A–H) and multiple subgenotypes,[45] with genotypes C and D reported to have a greater chance of progression.[46,47] HBV infection acquired in childhood is different from that acquired during adulthood. Among infants infected at birth, 90% have persistent infection. Among infected adults, up to 90% can clear the virus, and only 1% to 5% go on to become chronically infected.[48] In acute infection, clinical hepatitis B becomes apparent after an incubation period of 45 to 180 days.[49] Viral elimination begins several weeks before disease onset and is largely mediated by antiviral cytokines from cells of the innate and adaptive immune responses. After viral DNA declines, a cytolytic immune response seen as hepatocyte apoptosis and necrosis ensues, coincident with clinical hepatitis.[50] The main mechanism of necroinflammation results mainly from CD8 cytotoxic cells that recognize virus-infected hepatocytes and recruit other inflammatory cells, which is then followed by a cascade of immunologic damage.[19,51]

CLINICAL COURSE

The natural history of chronic HBV infection is complex and generally consists of 3 phases: immune-tolerant, immune-active, and inactive hepatitis B phases.[52] An infected person may pass through these phases or may stay in one phase for a long period of time. A fourth phase, recovery, has been proposed.[53] The immune-tolerant phase often occurs after perinatal infection from HBsAg/HBeAg-positive mothers. Serum alanine aminotransferase (ALT) levels are normal and HBV DNA, elevated (from 200,000 to>1 million copies international unit (IU)/mL). During this phase, the HBV integrates into the host's hepatocyte DNA. During the immune-active phase, called the chronic hepatitis B phase or immune-clearance phase, patients may be HBeAg-positive or HBeAg-negative[52,54] Those who are HBeAg-positive have elevated ALT levels and the HBV DNA level is greater than 20,000 IU/mL, whereas those patients who are HBeAg-negative but positive for anti-HBe usually have lower levels of HBV DNA (>2000 IU/mL) and mildly elevated ALT. The inactive hepatitis B phase is characterized by the absence of HBeAg and the presence of anti-HBe, normal ALT levels, and HBV DNA less than 2000 IU/mL. Individuals who clear HBsAg have been classified as being in the recovery phase. The clinical outcome after clearance of HBsAg is generally better than in people who continue to be HBsAg-positive.[52,55] Liver inflammation and fibrosis improve over time.[56] Undetectable serum HBsAg, however, does not prevent HCC from developing many years later, because low-titer serum HBV DNA may still be present, despite the HBsAg being negative, from the virus becoming integrated into the host genome. Studies have shown HBV DNA to be present in liver tissue in some of these individuals.[55,57]

CLINICAL DIAGNOSIS

Testing for HBV markers is necessary for the detection and diagnosis of HBV. The serologic markers are HBsAg and its antibody (anti-HBs), HBeAg and its antibody (anti-HBe), and immunoglobulins G and M antibody to hepatitis B virus core antigen (IgG anti-HBc and IgM anti-HBc). HBsAg seropositivity indicates infection; the presence of HBeAg indicates high HBV replication and infectivity.[52,58] Previous infection is diagnosed by the detection of anti-HBc and anti-HBs. Persistence of serum HBsAg for more than 6 months implies progression to chronic infection.[59]

HISTOLOGIC FEATURES OF CHRONIC HEPATITIS B

Acute HBV infection resembles any type of acute hepatitis and is characterized by lobular disarray, ballooning degeneration, apoptotic bodies, and lobular and portal inflammation. Similar histology is found in chronic HBV with acute flares, acute super-infection with hepatitis D, and concurrent drug-induced liver injury.[50] This type of histology is also seen in the presence of precore mutation that leads to HBeAg negativity and presents with relapsing disease.[60] In severe acute fulminant cases, confluent and bridging necrosis may occur, leading to massive or submassive hepatic necrosis.[61] HBV replicates in hepatocytes but is not directly cytopathic. The damage seems to be immune-mediated, with HBV-specific T cells playing a major role.[54,55] In immunocompetent people, HBV is not cytopathic, and hepatocellular damage is induced by the host immune system's efforts to eliminate HBV.[62]

Ongoing inflammation is the driving force that leads to fibrosis, and increasing grade is associated with more fibrosis.[14] There is usually no correlation with inflammatory activity and clinical, biochemical, or virological parameters, with 10% of patients with normal ALT having bridging fibrosis or even cirrhosis.[63] Furthermore, 30% of patients with persistently normal ALT may have significant fibrosis (stage 2–4). Also, no consistent relationship exists between serum HBV DNA levels and histology, especially in patients who are HBeAg-positive.[55,56]

A histopathologic hallmark of HBV infection is the presence of ground-glass hepatocytes (GGH) that represent HBsAg-containing liver cells. The hepatocytic cytoplasm exhibits a smooth almost homogeneous appearance, with accentuation of the cell membrane and, sometimes, with an artifactual "halo" caused by the retraction of the cytoplasm.[64] The nucleus is often pushed to the edge of the cell. GGH are usually highlighted by immunohistochemical staining (**Fig. 5**). Ultrastructurally, GGH are characterized by an abundance of smooth endoplasmic reticulum with an accumulation of HBV surface antigen.[64] Similar hepatocytic characteristics are seen in non-HBV-infected individuals and should be considered in the differential diagnoses. For example, Lafora bodies are seen in patients with myoclonus epilepsy[65]; polyglucosanlike inclusions, in patients on polypharmacotherapy[66]; GGH-like cells, in patients taking cyanamide as part of an alcohol aversion therapy; liver glycogen bodies, in transplanted patients[67]; and induction hepatocytes, in patients on certain medications.[68]

Immune-Tolerant Phase

The immune-tolerant phase can last from a few years to more than 30.[52,69] During this phase, liver inflammation and fibrosis are absent or minimal. Patients with chronic HBV who have remained in this phase have mild disease, with disease progression being minimal; whereas patients who progress to the immune-active phase often have disease progression.[69] In this setting, GGH are numerous. On immunostaining, there is a diffuse nuclear HBcAg (**Fig. 6**) and membranous pattern of HBsAg staining (**Fig. 7**). Furthermore, studies have shown that there is an inverse relationship between the degree of diffuse membranous staining and[70] inflammatory activity.[55,56,71]

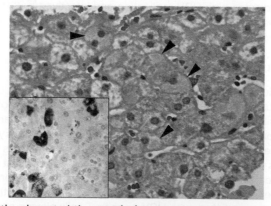

Fig. 5. GGH with the characteristic smooth, homogeneous, lightly eosinophilic cytoplasm with eccentric nuclei (*arrowheads*). Immunostain for HBsAg confirms the presence of HBV surface antigen (*inset*).

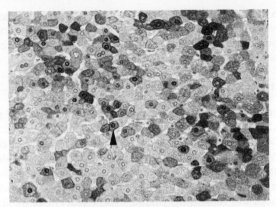

Fig. 6. Immunostain for HBcAg. Numerous hepatocytes have positive nuclear immunoreactivity; many of these demonstrate spillage of the antigen into the cytoplasm. The presence of positive cytoplasmic staining indicates active viral replication.

Immune-Active (-Clearance) Phase

In this phase, lymphocytic portal inflammation with interface hepatitis and spotty lobular inflammation are prominent. Sometimes, bridging and confluent necrosis may be identified. Ongoing necroinflammatory damage may lead to variable degrees of fibrosis or cirrhosis. On immunostaining, cytoplasmic and membranous expression of HBcAg correlates with liver damage (see **Fig. 6**).[70] The presence of HBcAg cytoplasmic staining has been shown to be a strong predictor of high hepatitis B viremia.[72] In both groups, inflammation is present in the liver, with or without fibrosis. The cumulative incidence of cirrhosis developing in patients who were HBsAg carriers positive for anti-HBe (inactive carriers) has been estimated to be 15% after 25 years follow-up.[55,56] Pure cytoplasmic staining may represent the presence of mutations that block the translocation of HBcAg, particularly in individuals with core and precore promoter mutations.

Immune-Inactive Phase

Liver histology in this and the immune-tolerant phase is similar, inflammation being minimal.[55,56] There is usually improvement in liver fibrosis and inflammation over

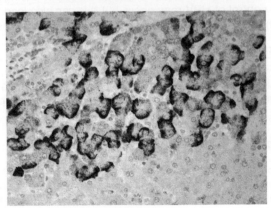

Fig. 7. HBsAg immunostain. A group of hepatocytes with positive staining for HBsAg (clonal pattern) is demonstrated. The staining is mainly submembranous, a finding which indicates active viral replication.

time. In those who remain in the inactive phase, the liver fibrosis is absent or minimal in degree and shows no evidence of progression over time. Immunostaining shows groups of hepatocytes that are positive for HBsAg; however, staining for HBcAg has negative results.[70]

IMMUNOHISTOCHEMICAL STAINING PATTERNS

Immunostaining using primary antibodies directed against the HBV surface and core antigens is routinely used in clinical practice.[73] Positive findings confirm HBV infection. Also, the pattern of expression may help determine the phase of infection. Two major types of GGH have been identified based on morphology and distribution.[70] The 2 types have different biologic significance, each one having specific pre-S deletion mutations.[74] Type I GGH are usually scattered randomly throughout the lobules and are found throughout the replicative phase. Type I GGH have eccentric nuclei, with ground-glass inclusions within the cytoplasm. Type II GGH are distributed in large groups called clonal patterns and are usually seen in the late nonreplicative stage or in the cirrhotic liver (see **Fig. 7**).[70] These Type II GGH exhibit a submembranous pattern of staining (see **Fig. 7**).[74] In any case, diffuse membranous staining for HBsAg suggests active viral replication.[70]

HBV CO-INFECTION WITH HDV, HIV AND HCV
HBV-HDV Co-infection

Chronic HBV and HDV co-infection leads to more severe liver disease than HBV monoinfection. The fibrosis progression is accelerated, and there is earlier hepatic decompensation, with an increased risk of developing HCC.[75] A positive immunostain result for HDV in the nucleus and sometimes in the cytoplasm is necessary to make a diagnosis of active infection, because serologic markers for HDV do not distinguish between ongoing or past HDV infection.[60]

HBV-Human Immunodeficiency Virus Co-infection

In chronic HBV infection, HBV replication is upregulated, particularly HBV protein X, which has been shown to hyperinduce human immunodeficiency virus (HIV)-1 replication. These findings indicate that HBV-X could promote faster progression of HIV in HBV-HIV co-infected individuals. With immune reconstitution during highly active anti-retroviral therapy, control of HBV may occur, but this can also lead to hepatitis reactivation. Most of the liver damage occurs because of the immune response to HBV.[76]

HBV-HCV Co-infection

HBV and HCV co-infection has been associated with more severe liver disease and frequent progression to cirrhosis and HCC than with monoinfection with either virus. Some studies have shown that there is a reciprocal replicative suppression between the 2 viruses.[77]

CHRONIC HEPATITIS C

Approximately 3% of the world population or 170 million individuals are infected with HCV[78] There are estimated to be some 3.2 million and 5 million infected people in the United States and Europe, respectively. The highest prevalence is found in Egypt at 15% to 20%.[79] Unlike other viral hepatitis infections which can clear, HCV establishes a persistent infection and has the propensity to cause chronic disease, with nearly 80% of new infections progressing to chronic infection.[80,81]

HCV infects only humans and chimpanzees, and the virus is transmitted mainly through injected drug use or other types of direct blood contact.[82] HCV is a member of the family Flaviviridae and consists of a 9.6-kilobase single-stranded, positive-sense RNA genome that encodes a single open reading frame. To date, there are 7 major HCV genotypes identified, with about 100 subtypes.[83] In the United States, Europe, and Australia, genotypes 1a or 1b are the most prevalent followed by genotypes 2 and 3. In contrast, most Japanese patients are infected by genotype 1b, followed by genotype 2. Genotype 1 is reported to have a more aggressive course and is less responsive to therapy. Some genotypes predominantly occur in locally restricted areas, such as genotype 4 in Egypt, genotype 5 in South Africa, and genotype 6 in East Asia.[79]

Diagnosis

Chronic HCV infection is diagnosed based on the presence of anti-HCV antibodies, HCV RNA, and abnormal liver enzymes.[80] To detect the presence of circulating HCV RNA, serum is used to test for the quantity of viral particles by the reverse transcriptase-polymerase chain reaction. The detection of HCV antibody is generally performed with commercially available enzyme-linked immunosorbent assay (ELISA) or enzyme immunoassay that incorporates various recombinant antigens derived from HCV (eg, core, NS3, NS4, and NS5). A positive ELISA result may be confirmed with a more specific supplementary test called recombinant immunoblot assay that tests for antibody response to these HCV antigens individually.[80] The antibody response to HCV can be detected within 7 to 8 weeks of inoculation using these assays.[82] Unlike HBV or hepatitis A virus, however, antibody response to HCV indicates ongoing infection rather than protective immunity.

CLINICAL COURSE

Acute hepatitis C is frequently asymptomatic or causes only a mild-to-moderate disease; fulminant acute hepatitis C is extremely rare.[84,85] Within days of infection, HCV RNA titers increase; however, the diagnosis is made only after the transaminase levels increase, approximately 8 to 12 weeks later. At this time, antibodies to HCV are also detectable. About 15% to 30% of patients with acute hepatitis C are able to achieve spontaneous viral clearance without treatment.[26] The Centers for Disease Control estimate that 75% to 80% of HCV infections become chronic, with 60% to 70% developing liver disease, 5% to 20% developing cirrhosis over a period of 20 to 30 years, and 1 to 5 dying of the consequences of viral infection.[78] Among immunocompetent people, HCV antibodies develop against several viral antigens, including the envelope proteins. The development of virus-specific antibodies, however, does not correlate with control of viremia or the outcome of acute hepatitis C.[86]

Chronic HCV infection may develop with or without ALT abnormalities and with or without chronic inflammation and increasing fibrosis in the liver. Studies conducted in patients who acquired HCV by blood transfusion 15 to 25 years previously indicate that 20% to 30% were found to have progressed to cirrhosis, including 5% to 10% with end-stage liver disease and 4% to 8% dying of liver-related causes.[87] Many studies suggest that there is a variable rate of disease progression to cirrhosis and its complications. Factors that lead to the progression of chronic HCV to cirrhosis are poorly understood.[88–90] The single most important factor known to contribute to the progression of liver damage in chronic HCV infection is persistent inflammation. Previous reports indicated transfusion-acquired HCV to be associated with more aggressive periportal necroinflammatory activity and fibrosis than was chronic hepatitis HCV resulting from intravenous drug abuse.[25] More recent reports have shown several variables that influence the natural course of HCV. Among these factors are age at acquisition of infection, male sex, race, duration of infection, viral genotype, and host genetic factors.[91] Acquired infection after age 40 years, male sex, excessive alcohol-consumption, HBV or HIV co-infection, steatosis, and immunosuppressed state have been identified as cofactors associated with progression of fibrosis and development of cirrhosis.[91–96]

Several studies have shown that patients with chronic HCV tend to have more severe liver disease if they are obese or diabetic.[89,90] Weight gain and insulin resistance were shown to be associated with worse outcome in patients.[90] Ogawa and colleagues[97] noted that HCV uses lipid droplets for the production of infectious virus particles. Substantial steatosis on liver biopsy was associated with worse outcomes in noncirrhotic patients; however, it was shown that when the liver reaches the cirrhotic state, the presence of steatosis diminishes.[90] Lok and colleagues[98] demonstrated in serial liver biopsies that steatosis diminishes in patients with chronic HCV as the progression of advanced fibrosis to cirrhosis develops. HCV and alcohol also act synergistically in the progression of chronic hepatitis. Also, the combination of alcohol and HCV leads to greater than a 100-fold risk of the development of HCC.[95] The presence of iron can also worsen necroinflammation and fibrosis in chronic HCV.[33] The prevalence of increased iron stores (ferritin and transferrin saturation) in HCV patients is 28%.[99] These patients were found to have more active chronic hepatitis and more fibrosis when compared with those without increased iron stores.[100]

HISTOPATHOLOGIC FEATURES OF CHRONIC HEPATITIS C

Three characteristic features of chronic HCV, although not pathognomonic, were originally described as (1) epithelial damage of small bile ducts, (2) formation of lymphoid aggregates and sometimes lymphoid follicles with germinal centers in portal tracts and, (3) steatosis (**Fig. 8**).[26,87,101] This histologic triad rarely is seen in chronic HBV or autoimmune hepatitis and therefore strongly suggests the diagnosis of chronic HCV.[102] The pathogenesis of these characteristic changes has not been elucidated. In addition to these 3 features, some reports have been made regarding Kupffer cell hyperplasia as a feature of HCV infection.[103] Also, ductular reaction and an increased number of hepatic progenitor cells are associated with a greater degree of fibrosis.[31]

Bile Duct Lesions

The prevalence of bile duct damage in HCV patients ranges from 15% to 91%.[104] This histologic feature is seen more frequently in livers having more severe necroinflammation and is also associated with lymphoid follicle formation (see **Fig. 8C**). The presence of hepatic bile duct injuries in Chinese patients with chronic HCV was significantly correlated with HCV genotype 1b infection, and the patients with these injuries had more severe portal inflammation and formation of lymphoid aggregates/follicles. The pathogenesis and clinical significance remain unclear. Reports indicate that these bile duct lesions mimic the chronic nonsuppurative destructive cholangitis of primary biliary cirrhosis.

Lymphoid Follicles and Lymphoid Aggregates

These are discrete and densely packed collections of small mature lymphocytes within the portal connective tissue with or without the formation of germinal centers, and they are located near or surrounding bile ducts (see **Fig. 8**A, B). The prevalence

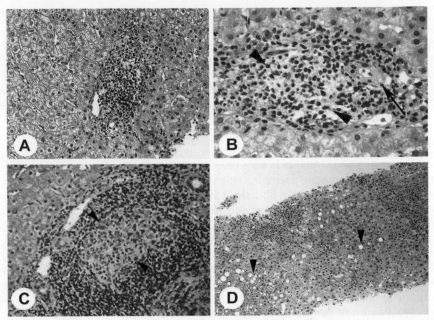

Fig. 8. The classic histologic triad of chronic hepatitis C. (*A*) a portal tract with a lymphoid aggregate. (*B*) another lymphoid aggregate (*arrowheads*) with a damaged bile duct (*arrow*). (*C*) a portal tract containing a lymphoid follicle with arrowheads delineating the germinal center. Lymphoid follicles are not as commonly seen as lymphoid aggregates. (*D*) steatosis (*arrowheads*) associated with lobular and portal inflammation.

of lymphoid aggregates and follicles ranges from 17% to 85% in patients with chronic HCV.[27] The pathogenesis of lymphoid collections remains unclear; however, lymphoid aggregates in chronic HCV may play a role in liver injury as an immune mechanism similar to that of autoimmune hepatitis. Lymphoid aggregates in portal tracts and lymphocyte infiltration of lobules and bile ducts suggest that immune mechanisms play a role in the mediation of cell injury.[26,81,86]

Steatosis

Steatosis is a well-documented feature of HCV and is typically a mixture of small- and large-droplet fat (see **Fig. 8**D). Steatosis has been found to be present in 74% of patients with genotype 3 and in 50% of patients with nongenotype 3 HCV. HCV genotype 3 directly induces development of steatosis and correlates directly with viral load,[105,106] whereas in patients with nongenotype 3 chronic HCV infection, insulin resistance plays a key role in its pathophysiology.[106] The high prevalence of steatosis is 2- to 3-fold what can be expected by chance alone and higher than that observed in the general population. A few studies have documented that baseline steatosis was an independent predictor of fibrosis progression.[88,92,96,105] HCV core protein can induce accumulation of triglyceride-rich droplets in hepatocytes and also damage mitochondria, with subsequent impairment in lipid oxidation leading to steatosis[107]; HCV core protein can inhibit microsomal triglyceride transfer protein, which inhibits the assembly of very low-density lipoprotein leading to accumulation of triglycerides.[108] Also, HCV uses lipid droplets for the production of infectious viral particles.[97]

Inflammation/Degree of Injury

The degree of hepatocellular injury in chronic HCV is variable, but most cases have only mild inflammatory changes. Apoptotic bodies are almost readily identifiable in the lobules in chronic HCV.[109] Degeneration and spotty necrosis of hepatocytes and mixed inflammatory cell infiltration of the lobular parenchyma and portal tracts are found, similar to the findings in other types of chronic hepatitis.[101] In chronic HCV, interface hepatitis may have minor foci or be severe, encircling the entire portal tract (see **Fig. 1**).[26]

Fibrosis/Architectural Changes

End-stage liver disease/cirrhosis from chronic HCV evolves over a long period of time. Some patients may remain asymptomatic throughout the course of infection and may have a far-advanced degree of fibrosis at initial presentation. In 4 large trials involving a total of 4493 adults, 19.6% presented with bridging fibrosis and 4.9% already had cirrhosis.[110–113] There is an inherent assumption that fibrosis progression occurs at a linear rate over time, but evidence indicates that the rate seems to accelerate with time, even after controlling for age.[113] With image analysis, Goodman and colleagues[114] have demonstrated the nonlinear changes in fibrosis over time. In this study, 1269 unfragmented biopsies were assessed via morphometry. Although there was correlation between the fibrosis stage and collagen content, a considerable overlap in the amount of fibrous tissue among the various stages was found.

In addition to inflammation, other factors, such as ductular reaction, may promote fibrosis. Ductular reaction at the portal interface was noted by Clouston and colleagues,[31] and they noted that there was a highly significant correlation between the area of ductular reaction and the fibrosis stage. They also found that the number of hepatic progenitor cells also correlated with fibrosis development. Their findings suggest that in HCV, there is impaired hepatocyte replication leading to an altered regeneration pathway, which then drives the ductular reaction that subsequently triggers fibrosis.[31]

OTHER ENTITIES ASSOCIATED WITH CHRONIC HEPATITIS C
Overlap Syndrome of Hepatitis C and Autoimmune Hepatitis

The overlap syndrome of autoimmune hepatitis (AIH) and chronic HCV constitutes the presence of high-titer ($\geq$1:320) autoantibodies, hypergammaglobulinemia, concurrent HCV RNA in serum, and histologic features that suggest autoimmune hepatitis, such as diffuse portal, interface, and panacinar hepatitis with significant plasma cell infiltrates.[115,116] Although no single histologic feature is pathognomonic of HCV or AIH, distinct composite histologic patterns have been described for each entity. In a study by Bach and colleagues[102] in which biopsy specimens from patients with HCV and AIH were compared, patients with AIH were more likely to have severe lobular necrosis and inflammation, piecemeal necrosis, multinucleated hepatocytes, and broad areas of parenchymal collapse, whereas patients with HCV were more likely to have bile duct damage, bile duct loss, steatosis, and lymphoid cell follicles within portal tracts. According to Carpenter and Czaja,[116] the combination of portal lymphoid aggregates and steatosis was found to have 91% specificity for HCV, whereas the pattern of lymphoplasmacytic portal, interface, and acinar hepatitis had 81% specificity for AIH. Corticosteroids are used as first-line therapy in some patients with the HCV-AIH overlap syndrome, resulting in normalization of serum ALT and γ-globulin levels, with significant improvement in modified HAI scores on serial liver biopsies despite the absence of viral eradication.[115]

Hepatitis C with Autoimmune Features

This entity constitutes a challenge among pathologists and clinicians alike. The diagnosis of chronic HCV with autoimmune features is made when HCV patients test positive for autoantibodies and mainly have portal lymphoid aggregates and macrovesicular steatosis. No histologic features of autoimmune hepatitis, such as plasma cell infiltrates or bridging or confluent necrosis, are present.[116]

Fibrosing Cholestatic Hepatitis

Fibrosing Cholestatic Hepatitis (FCH) is a severe form of hepatitis originally described in HBV patients. FCH cases have been described in HCV individuals post-liver transplantation, in HCV-positive patients who underwent renal, cardiac, or bone marrow transplantation, in those with acquired immunodeficiency syndrome, and in those who underwent cytotoxic chemotherapy.[117,118] The most characteristic pathologic findings are extensive dense portal fibrosis with immature fibrous bands extending into sinusoidal spaces, ductular proliferation and hypercellularity, marked canalicular and cellular cholestasis, and moderate mononuclear inflammation.[119]

PRACTICAL APPROACH TO DIAGNOSIS

Adequate clinical information must be provided by the clinician in order for a pathologist to render the most complete diagnosis. A statement regarding viral serologic markers, whether positive or negative, has to be indicated in the requisition slip. In cases of HCV and HBV, knowledge of HCV RNA viral load and HBV DNA is helpful. Also, information that may not be directly related to HCV or HBV may be important, such as being overweight or morbidly obese, drinking alcohol, or family history of metabolic liver disease. This information aids the pathologist in closely assessing certain features that may be subtle or even masked by the chronic hepatitis histology. The pathologist has to be informed if the patient has received antiviral therapy and whether a previous biopsy was performed. If available, a comment as to the interval changes in degree of fibrosis and inflammation should be made part of the diagnosis. This interval change helps guide the clinician in patient management during or after receiving antiviral therapy.

For pathologists, the components to be covered in a report should include (1) a comment on the cause, (2) the grade of necroinflammation, (3) the stage of fibrosis and staging system used. As an example, the report may read as follows: "Chronic hepatitis C with mild activity in transition to cirrhosis, grade 2 of 4, stage 3 of 4, modified Scheuer." Close and ongoing communication between pathologist and clinician is essential.

ACKNOWLEDGMENTS

The author would like to thank Joseph Samet for his technical assistance in the preparation of the photomicrographs and illustrations.

REFERENCES

1. Terminology of chronic hepatitis. International working party. Am J Gastroenterol 1995;90(2):181–9.
2. Firpi RJ, Soldevila-Pico C, Abdelmalek MF, et al. Short recovery time after percutaneous liver biopsy: should we change our current practices? Clin Gastroenterol Hepatol 2005;3(9):926–9.

3. Cross TJ, Rizzi P, Berry PA, et al. King's score: an accurate marker of cirrhosis in chronic hepatitis C. Eur J Gastroenterol Hepatol 2009;21(7):730–8.
4. Denzer UW, Luth S. Non-invasive diagnosis and monitoring of liver fibrosis and cirrhosis. Best Pract Res Clin Gastroenterol 2009;23(3):453–60.
5. Leroy V, Hilleret MN, Sturm N, et al. Prospective comparison of six non-invasive scores for the diagnosis of liver fibrosis in chronic hepatitis C. J Hepatol 2007; 46(5):775–82.
6. Cross TJ, Calvaruso V, Maimone S, et al. Prospective comparison of fibroscan, king's score and liver biopsy for the assessment of cirrhosis in chronic hepatitis C infection. J Viral Hepat 2010;17(8):546–54.
7. Shire NJ, Rao MB, Succop P, et al. Improving noninvasive methods of assessing liver fibrosis in patients with hepatitis C virus/human immunodeficiency virus co-infection. Clin Gastroenterol Hepatol 2009;7(4):471–80, 480.e1–2.
8. Lefkowitch JH. Liver biopsy assessment in chronic hepatitis. Arch Med Res 2007;38(6):634–43.
9. Colloredo G, Guido M, Sonzogni A, et al. Impact of liver biopsy size on histological evaluation of chronic viral hepatitis: the smaller the sample, the milder the disease. J Hepatol 2003;39(2):239–44.
10. Sherman KE, Goodman ZD, Sullivan ST, et al. Liver biopsy in cirrhotic patients. Am J Gastroenterol 2007;102(4):789–93.
11. Regev A, Berho M, Jeffers LJ, et al. Sampling error and intraobserver variation in liver biopsy in patients with chronic HCV infection. Am J Gastroenterol 2002; 97(10):2614–8.
12. Rousselet MC, Michalak S, Dupre F, et al. Sources of variability in histological scoring of chronic viral hepatitis. Hepatology 2005;41(2):257–64.
13. De Groote J, Desmet VJ, Gedigk P, et al. A classification of chronic hepatitis. Lancet 1968;2(7568):626–8.
14. Popper H, Schaffner F. The vocabulary of chronic hepatitis. N Engl J Med 1971; 284(20):1154–6.
15. Knodell RG, Ishak KG, Black WC, et al. Formulation and application of a numerical scoring system for assessing histological activity in asymptomatic chronic active hepatitis. Hepatology 1981;1(5):431–5.
16. Scheuer PJ. Classification of chronic viral hepatitis: a need for reassessment. J Hepatol 1991;13(3):372–4.
17. Desmet VJ, Gerber M, Hoofnagle JH, et al. Classification of chronic hepatitis: diagnosis, grading and staging. Hepatology 1994;19(6):1513–20.
18. Batts KP, Ludwig J. Chronic hepatitis. An update on terminology and reporting. Am J Surg Pathol 1995;19(12):1409–17.
19. Ishak K, Baptista A, Bianchi L, et al. Histological grading and staging of chronic hepatitis. J Hepatol 1995;22(6):696–9.
20. Westin J, Lagging LM, Wejstal R, et al. Interobserver study of liver histopathology using the Ishak score in patients with chronic hepatitis C virus infection. Liver 1999;19(3):183–7.
21. Bedossa P, Poynard T. An algorithm for the grading of activity in chronic hepatitis C. The METAVIR cooperative study group. Hepatology 1996;24(2): 289–93.
22. Intraobserver and interobserver variations in liver biopsy interpretation in patients with chronic hepatitis C. The French METAVIR cooperative study group. Hepatology 1994;20(1 Pt 1):15–20.
23. Scheuer PJ. Chronic hepatitis: what is activity and how should it be assessed? Histopathology 1997;30(2):103–5.

24. Hubscher SG. Histological grading and staging in chronic hepatitis: clinical applications and problems. J Hepatol 1998;29(6):1015–22.
25. Gerber MA. Histopathology of HCV infection. Clin Liver Dis 1997;1(3):529–41, vi.
26. Lauer GM, Walker BD. Hepatitis C virus infection. N Engl J Med 2001;345(1): 41–52.
27. Luo JC, Hwang SJ, Lai CR, et al. Clinical significance of portal lymphoid aggregates/follicles in Chinese patients with chronic hepatitis C. Am J Gastroenterol 1999;94(4):1006–11.
28. Kerr JF, Cooksley WG, Searle J, et al. The nature of piecemeal necrosis in chronic active hepatitis. Lancet 1979;2(8147):827–8.
29. Saitou Y, Shiraki K, Fuke H, et al. Involvement of tumor necrosis factor-related apoptosis-inducing ligand and tumor necrosis factor-related apoptosis-inducing ligand receptors in viral hepatic diseases. Hum Pathol 2005;36(10):1066–73.
30. Roskams T, Desmet V. Ductular reaction and its diagnostic significance. Semin Diagn Pathol 1998;15(4):259–69.
31. Clouston AD, Powell EE, Walsh MJ, et al. Fibrosis correlates with a ductular reaction in hepatitis C: roles of impaired replication, progenitor cells and steatosis. Hepatology 2005;41(4):809–18.
32. Theise ND. Liver biopsy assessment in chronic viral hepatitis: a personal, practical approach. Mod Pathol 2007;20(Suppl 1):S3–14.
33. Batts KP. Iron overload syndromes and the liver. Mod Pathol 2007;20(Suppl 1): S31–9.
34. Anthony PP. Liver cell dysplasia: a premalignant condition. J Pathol 1973;109(1): Pxvii.
35. Park YN, Roncalli M. Large liver cell dysplasia: a controversial entity. J Hepatol 2006;45(5):734–43.
36. Ikeda H, Sasaki M, Sato Y, et al. Large cell change of hepatocytes in chronic viral hepatitis represents a senescent-related lesion. Hum Pathol 2009;40(12): 1774–82.
37. Watanabe S, Okita K, Harada T, et al. Morphologic studies of the liver cell dysplasia. Cancer 1983;51(12):2197–205.
38. Libbrecht L, Desmet V, Roskams T. Preneoplastic lesions in human hepatocarcinogenesis. Liver Int 2005;25(1):16–27.
39. Koo JS, Kim H, Park BK, et al. Predictive value of liver cell dysplasia for development of hepatocellular carcinoma in patients with chronic hepatitis B. J Clin Gastroenterol 2008;42(6):738–43.
40. Lavanchy D. Worldwide epidemiology of HBV infection, disease burden, and vaccine prevention. J Clin Virol 2005;34(Suppl 1):S1–3.
41. Okada K, Kamiyama I, Inomata M, et al. e antigen and anti-e in the serum of asymptomatic carrier mothers as indicators of positive and negative transmission of hepatitis B virus to their infants. N Engl J Med 1976;294(14):746–9.
42. Botha JF, Ritchie MJ, Dusheiko GM, et al. Hepatitis B virus carrier state in black children in Ovamboland: role of perinatal and horizontal infection. Lancet 1984; 1(8388):1210–2.
43. Weinbaum CM, Williams I, Mast EE, et al. Recommendations for identification and public health management of persons with chronic hepatitis B virus infection. MMWR Recomm Rep 2008;57(RR-8):1–20.
44. Summers J, Mason WS. Replication of the genome of a hepatitis B–like virus by reverse transcription of an RNA intermediate. Cell 1982;29(2):403–15.
45. Chotiyaputta W, Lok AS. Hepatitis B virus variants. Nat Rev Gastroenterol Hepatol 2009;6(8):453–62.

46. Sumi H, Yokosuka O, Seki N, et al. Influence of hepatitis B virus genotypes on the progression of chronic type B liver disease. Hepatology 2003;37(1):19–26.

47. Chan HL, Wong GL, Tse CH, et al. Hepatitis B virus genotype C is associated with more severe liver fibrosis than genotype B. Clin Gastroenterol Hepatol 2009;7(12):1361–6.

48. Seeff LB, Beebe GW, Hoofnagle JH, et al. A serologic follow-up of the 1942 epidemic of post-vaccination hepatitis in the United States army. N Engl J Med 1987;316(16):965–70.

49. Villeneuve JP. The natural history of chronic hepatitis B virus infection. J Clin Virol 2005;34(Suppl 1):S139–42.

50. Visvanathan K, Lewin SR. Immunopathogenesis: role of innate and adaptive immune responses. Semin Liver Dis 2006;26(2):104–15.

51. Ito Y, Kakumu S, Yoshioka K, et al. Cytotoxic T lymphocyte activity to hepatitis B virus DNA-transfected HepG2 cells in patients with chronic hepatitis B. Gastroenterol Jpn 1993;28(5):657–65.

52. Liaw YF, Chu CM. Hepatitis B virus infection. Lancet 2009;373(9663):582–92.

53. McMahon BJ. The natural history of chronic hepatitis B virus infection. Hepatology 2009;49(Suppl 5):S45–55.

54. Lok AS, McMahon BJ. Chronic hepatitis B: update 2009. Hepatology 2009;50(3):661–2.

55. Chu CM, Liaw YF. Incidence and risk factors of progression to cirrhosis in inactive carriers of hepatitis B virus. Am J Gastroenterol 2009;104(7):1693–9.

56. Chu CM. Natural history of chronic hepatitis B virus infection in adults with emphasis on the occurrence of cirrhosis and hepatocellular carcinoma. J Gastroenterol Hepatol 2000;15(Suppl):E25–30.

57. Bruix J, Sherman M. Diagnosis of Small HCC. Gastroenterology 2005;129(4):1364.

58. Liang TJ, Ghany M. Hepatitis B e antigen–the dangerous endgame of hepatitis B. N Engl J Med 2002;347(3):208–10.

59. Kao JH. Diagnosis of hepatitis B virus infection through serological and virological markers. Expert Rev Gastroenterol Hepatol 2008;2(4):553–62.

60. Mani H, Kleiner DE. Liver biopsy findings in chronic hepatitis B. Hepatology 2009;49(Suppl 5):S61–71.

61. Hytiroglou P, Dash S, Haruna Y, et al. Detection of hepatitis B and hepatitis C viral sequences in fulminant hepatic failure of unknown etiology. Am J Clin Pathol 1995;104(5):588–93.

62. Dunn C, Peppa D, Khanna P, et al. Temporal analysis of early immune responses in patients with acute hepatitis B virus infection. Gastroenterology 2009;137(4):1289–300.

63. Sigal SH, Ala A, Ivanov K, et al. Histopathology and clinical correlates of end-stage hepatitis B cirrhosis: a possible mechanism to explain the response to antiviral therapy. Liver Transpl 2005;11(1):82–8.

64. Vazquez JJ. Ground-glass hepatocytes: light and electron microscopy. Characterization of the different types. Histol Histopathol 1990;5(3):379–86.

65. Ng IO, Sturgess RP, Williams R, et al. Ground-glass hepatocytes with Lafora body like inclusions–histochemical, immunohistochemical and electronmicroscopic characterization. Histopathology 1990;17(2):109–15.

66. Lefkowitch JH, Lobritto SJ, Brown RS Jr, et al. Ground-glass, polyglucosan-like hepatocellular inclusions: a "new" diagnostic entity. Gastroenterology 2006;131(3):713–8.

67. Bejarano PA, Garcia MT, Rodriguez MM, et al. Liver glycogen bodies: ground-glass hepatocytes in transplanted patients. Virchows Arch 2006;449(5):539–45.

68. Soars MG, McGinnity DF, Grime K, et al. The pivotal role of hepatocytes in drug discovery. Chem Biol Interact 2007;168(1):2–15.
69. Hui CK, Leung N, Yuen ST, et al. Natural history and disease progression in Chinese chronic hepatitis B patients in immune-tolerant phase. Hepatology 2007;46(2):395–401.
70. Chu CM, Liaw YF. Membrane staining for hepatitis B surface antigen on hepatocytes: a sensitive and specific marker of active viral replication in hepatitis B. J Clin Pathol 1995;48(5):470–3.
71. Naoumov NV, Portmann BC, Tedder RS, et al. Detection of hepatitis B virus antigens in liver tissue. A relation to viral replication and histology in chronic hepatitis B infection. Gastroenterology 1990;99(4):1248–53.
72. ter Borg F, ten Kate FJ, Cuypers HT, et al. A survey of liver pathology in needle biopsies from HBsAg and anti-HBe positive individuals. J Clin Pathol 2000; 53(7):541–8.
73. Roskams T. The role of immunohistochemistry in diagnosis. Clin Liver Dis 2002; 6(2):571–89, x.
74. Wang HC, Wu HC, Chen CF, et al. Different types of ground glass hepatocytes in chronic hepatitis B virus infection contain specific pre-S mutants that may induce endoplasmic reticulum stress. Am J Pathol 2003;163(6):2441–9.
75. Wedemeyer H, Manns MP. Epidemiology, pathogenesis and management of hepatitis D: update and challenges ahead. Nat Rev Gastroenterol Hepatol 2010;7(1):31–40.
76. Benhamou Y. Hepatitis B in the HIV-coinfected patient. J Acquir Immune Defic Syndr 2007;45(Suppl 2):S57–65 [discussion: S66–7].
77. Bellecave P, Gouttenoire J, Gajer M, et al. Hepatitis B and C virus coinfection: a novel model system reveals the absence of direct viral interference. Hepatology 2009;50(1):46–55.
78. Lavanchy D. The global burden of hepatitis C. Liver Int 2009;29(Suppl 1):74–81.
79. Te HS, Jensen DM. Epidemiology of hepatitis B and C viruses: a global overview. Clin Liver Dis 2010;14(1):1–21, vii.
80. Chou R, Clark EC, Helfand M, et al. Screening for hepatitis C virus infection: a review of the evidence for the U.S. Preventive services task force. Ann Intern Med 2004;140(6):465–79.
81. Diepolder HM. New insights into the immunopathogenesis of chronic hepatitis C. Antiviral Res 2009;82(3):103–9.
82. Rehermann B. Hepatitis C virus versus innate and adaptive immune responses: a tale of coevolution and coexistence. J Clin Invest 2009;119(7):1745–54.
83. Nainan OV, Alter MJ, Kruszon-Moran D, et al. Hepatitis C virus genotypes and viral concentrations in participants of a general population survey in the United States. Gastroenterology 2006;131(2):478–84.
84. Kanda T, Yokosuka O, Imazeki F, et al. Acute hepatitis C virus infection, 1986-2001: a rare cause of fulminant hepatitis in Chiba, Japan. Hepatogastroenterology 2004;51(56):556–8.
85. Funaoka M, Kato K, Komatsu M, et al. Fulminant hepatitis caused by hepatitis C virus during treatment for multiple sclerosis. J Gastroenterol 1996;31(1):119–22.
86. Chang KM. Immunopathogenesis of hepatitis C virus infection. Clin Liver Dis 2003;7(1):89–105.
87. Alberti A, Chemello L, Benvegnu L. Natural history of hepatitis C. J Hepatol 1999;31(Suppl 1):17–24.
88. Castera L, Pawlotsky JM, Dhumeaux D. Worsening of steatosis and fibrosis progression in hepatitis C. Gut 2003;52(10):1531.

89. Charlton MR, Pockros PJ, Harrison SA. Impact of obesity on treatment of chronic hepatitis C. Hepatology 2006;43(6):1177–86.

90. Everhart JE, Lok AS, Kim HY, et al. Weight-related effects on disease progression in the hepatitis C antiviral long-term treatment against cirrhosis trial. Gastroenterology 2009;137(2):549–57.

91. Missiha SB, Ostrowski M, Heathcote EJ. Disease progression in chronic hepatitis C: modifiable and nonmodifiable factors. Gastroenterology 2008;134(6):1699–714.

92. Kurosaki M, Matsunaga K, Hirayama I, et al. The presence of steatosis and elevation of alanine aminotransferase levels are associated with fibrosis progression in chronic hepatitis C with non-response to interferon therapy. J Hepatol 2008;48(5):736–42.

93. Meriden Z, Forde KA, Pasha TL, et al. Histologic predictors of fibrosis progression in liver allografts in patients with hepatitis C virus infection. Clin Gastroenterol Hepatol 2010;8(3):289–96 296.e1–8.

94. Moriishi K, Matsuura Y. Host factors involved in the replication of hepatitis C virus. Rev Med Virol 2007;17(5):343–54.

95. Mueller S, Millonig G, Seitz HK. Alcoholic liver disease and hepatitis C: a frequently underestimated combination. World J Gastroenterol 2009;15(28):3462–71.

96. Nieminen U, Arkkila PE, Karkkainen P, et al. Effect of steatosis and inflammation on liver fibrosis in chronic hepatitis C. Liver Int 2009;29(2):153–8.

97. Ogawa K, Hishiki T, Shimizu Y, et al. Hepatitis C virus Utilizes lipid droplet for production of infectious virus. Proc Jpn Acad Ser B Phys Biol Sci 2009;85(7):217–28.

98. Lok AS, Everhart JE, Chung RT, et al. Evolution of hepatic steatosis in patients with advanced hepatitis C: results from the hepatitis C antiviral long-term treatment against cirrhosis (HALT-C) trial. Hepatology 2009;49(6):1828–37.

99. Gattoni A, Parlato A, Vangieri B, et al. Role of hemochromatosis genes in chronic hepatitis C. Clin Ter 2006;157(1):61–8.

100. Price L, Kowdley KV. The role of iron in the pathophysiology and treatment of chronic hepatitis C. Can J Gastroenterol 2009;23(12):822–8.

101. Scheuer PJ, Ashrafzadeh P, Sherlock S, et al. The pathology of hepatitis C. Hepatology 1992;15(4):567–71.

102. Bach N, Thung SN, Schaffner F. The histological features of chronic hepatitis C and autoimmune chronic hepatitis: a comparative analysis. Hepatology 1992;15(4):572–7.

103. Tu Z, Pierce RH, Kurtis J, et al. Hepatitis C virus core protein subverts the antiviral activities of human Kupffer cells. Gastroenterology 2010;138(1):305–14.

104. Hwang SJ, Luo JC, Chu CW, et al. Hepatic steatosis in chronic hepatitis C virus infection: prevalence and clinical correlation. J Gastroenterol Hepatol 2001;16(2):190–5.

105. Westin J, Nordlinder H, Lagging M, et al. Steatosis accelerates fibrosis development over time in hepatitis C virus genotype 3 infected patients. J Hepatol 2002;37(6):837–42.

106. Bjornsson E, Angulo P. Hepatitis C and steatosis. Arch Med Res 2007;38(6):621–7.

107. Moriya K, Shintani Y, Fujie H, et al. Serum lipid profile of patients with genotype 1b hepatitis C viral infection in Japan. Hepatol Res 2003;25(4):371–6.

108. Perlemuter G, Sabile A, Letteron P, et al. Hepatitis C virus core protein inhibits microsomal triglyceride transfer protein activity and very low density lipoprotein secretion: a model of viral-related steatosis. FASEB J 2002;16(2):185–94.

109. Wertheimer AM, Polyak SJ, Leistikow R, et al. Engulfment of apoptotic cells expressing HCV proteins leads to differential chemokine expression and STAT signaling in human dendritic cells. Hepatology 2007;45(6):1422–32.
110. McHutchison JG, Gordon SC, Schiff ER, et al. Interferon alfa-2b alone or in combination with ribavirin as initial treatment for chronic hepatitis C. Hepatitis Interventional Therapy Group. N Engl J Med 1998;339(21):1485–92.
111. Lindsay KL, Trepo C, Heintges T, et al. A randomized, double-blind trial comparing pegylated interferon alfa-2b to interferon alfa-2b as initial treatment for chronic hepatitis C. Hepatology 2001;34(2):395–403.
112. Manns MP, McHutchison JG, Gordon SC, et al. Peginterferon alfa-2b plus ribavirin compared with interferon alfa-2b plus ribavirin for initial treatment of chronic hepatitis C: a randomised trial. Lancet 2001;358(9286):958–65.
113. Poynard T, McHutchison J, Manns M, et al. Impact of pegylated interferon alfa-2b and ribavirin on liver fibrosis in patients with chronic hepatitis C. Gastroenterology 2002;122(5):1303–13.
114. Goodman ZD, Stoddard AM, Bonkovsky HL, et al. Fibrosis progression in chronic hepatitis C: morphometric image analysis in the HALT-C trial. Hepatology 2009;50(6):1738–49.
115. Schiano TD, Te HS, Thomas RM, et al. Results of steroid-based therapy for the hepatitis C-autoimmune hepatitis overlap syndrome. Am J Gastroenterol 2001; 96(10):2984–91.
116. Carpenter HA, Czaja AJ. The role of histologic evaluation in the diagnosis and management of autoimmune hepatitis and its variants. Clin Liver Dis 2002; 6(3):685–705.
117. Dickson RC, Caldwell SH, Ishitani MB, et al. Clinical and histologic patterns of early graft failure due to recurrnet hepatitis C in four patients after liver transplantation. Transplantation 1996;61(5):701–5.
118. Ceballos-Viro J, Lopez-Picazo JM, Perez-Gracia JL, et al. Fibrosing cholestatic hepatitis following cytotoxic chemotherapy for small-cell lung cancer. World J Gastroenterol 2009;15(18):2290–2.
119. Dixon LR, Crawford JM. Early histologic changes in fibrosing cholestatic hepatitis C. Liver Transpl 2007;13(2):219–26.

Histology of Autoimmune Hepatitis and its Variants

Maha Guindi, FRCPC[a,b,*]

KEYWORDS

- Autoimmune hepatitis • Overlap syndrome • Chronic hepatitis
- Autoimmune liver disease • Histology • Biopsy

Autoimmune hepatitis (AIH) does not have a pathognomonic feature, and its laboratory, serologic, and histologic manifestations are found in acute and chronic liver disease of diverse causes.[1,2] Consequently, the diagnosis of AIH requires confident exclusion of other causative factors. Difficulties in distinguishing toxic, drug-related, virus-induced, and autoimmune causes of severe acute liver injury can result in misclassification.[3]

OVERVIEW OF AIH DIAGNOSTIC SCORING SYSTEMS

In 1992, the International Autoimmune Hepatitis Group (IAIHG) devised a diagnostic scoring system.[4] The aim was to categorize patients as having either "definite" or "probable" AIH in an objective manner. A positive weighting was given to female gender, hepatocellular rather than cholestatic damage, and the presence of autoantibodies. Because there was no definite evidence that autoantibodies were directly involved in the pathogenesis of AIH, this working classification did not exclude a diagnosis of AIH in the absence of antinuclear antibodies (ANA), anti-smooth muscle antibodies (SMA), or liver kidney microsomal 1 antibodies (LKM-1) at presentation. The diagnosis of definite AIH required a liver biopsy. Several studies showed the scoring system had very high sensitivity, ranging from 97% to 100%, for diagnosis of AIH in different populations: North America, Europe, and Japan.[5–7] The overall diagnostic accuracy of the scoring system was 89.8%.[8]

This scoring system was complex; its criteria were devised by expert consensus but were insufficiently validated, and did not adequately distinguish "probable" AIH from other liver, especially autoimmune biliary diseases. The IAIHG decided to

[a] Department of Laboratory Medicine and Pathobiology, Faculty of Medicine, University of Toronto, Medical Sciences Building, 1 King's College Circle, Toronto, ON M5S 1A8, Canada
[b] Toronto General Hospital, 200 Elizabeth Street, Eaton 11- 444, Toronto, ON M5G 2C4, Canada
* Corresponding author. Department of Pathology, Toronto General Hospital, 200 Elizabeth Street, Toronto, Ontario, Canada M5G 2C4.
E-mail address: maha.guindi@uhn.on.ca

Clin Liver Dis 14 (2010) 577–590
doi:10.1016/j.cld.2010.07.003
1089-3261/10/$ – see front matter © 2010 Elsevier Inc. All rights reserved.

revise it and developed a simplified scoring system for wider applicability in routine clinical practice based on the data of patients with well-established diagnoses.[8] In this version, biopsy remained crucial, with five points deducted for absence of characteristic histologic evidence of AIH. Weighting against biliary disease was increased (**Table 1**).

These changes, when used to reanalyze a group of previously reported primary sclerosing cholangitis (PSC) patients for exclusion of AIH from these PSC patients, increased specificity from 64.9% to 89.5%.[9,10]

Hennes and colleagues[11] introduced a new scoring system for the diagnosis of AIH. Their simplified scoring system is intended for routine clinical practice, whereas the original criteria of the IAIHG[4] were designed with research purposes in mind to enable comparison between different studies. The new system condenses the liver histology criteria into three categories (**Table 2**). In this new system by Hennes and colleagues,[11] the presence of histologic evidence of hepatitis is a necessary finding.

Interface hepatitis is a pathologic hallmark of active AIH It is especially prominent during disease flares.[12,13] Whereas this lesion is characteristic of AIH, it is not specific; interface hepatitis is also common in various forms of chronic liver disease including chronic hepatitis due to viral or drug-induced reactions[12–14] among others. Interface activity may occur even in biliary disease such as primary biliary cirrhosis (PBC).[13] Interface hepatitis in AIH is characterized by a prominent lymphohistiocytic infiltrate at the portal tract mesenchymal-parenchymal junction with accompanying histologic evidence of liver cell damage. CD8-positive T cells are a dominant subset of lymphocytes within areas of interface hepatitis, and CD4-positive T cells predominate within the portal tracts.[15]

Histologically, AIH has many faces depending on the course of the disease, the form of its initial presentation, its evolution, and effects of treatment. Thus the histologic features described in the various diagnostic disease scoring systems may not be present or may be modified in a given biopsy due to histologic variants, presence of overlap syndromes, or dampening by previous therapy or remission. The pattern that the pathologist encounters depends on the stage of disease in a given patient at the time of obtaining material for histologic examination, diagnosis or follow up. This article discusses the variable histologic features of AIH as they present themselves in biopsies and on occasion in resected material.

ACUTE AIH

Long-standing but indolent AIH may have a spontaneous exacerbation that can be mistaken for de novo severe acute or fulminant disease.[16,17] In these patients, the

Table 1
Increased weighting against biliary diseases in revised scoring system in 1999

Feature	Modification in the 1999 Revised Scoring System
ALP:AST Ratio Cutoff	No points for ALP:AST ratios between 1.5 and 3.0 deduct 2 points for ratios over 3.0
Negative Score for AMA Seropositivity	Raised from −2 to −4
Negative Scoring for Histologic Evidence of Bile Duct Damage	Increased from −1 to −3

Abbreviation: ALP, alkaline phosphatase.
Data from Alvarez F, Berg PA, Bianchi FB, et al. International autoimmune hepatitis group report: review of criteria for diagnosis of autoimmune hepatitis. J Hepatol 1999;31:929–38.

Table 2
Histologic component of the simplified criteria for the diagnosis of AIH

Histologic Category	Description	Points
Typical	Includes interface hepatitis, lymphocytic or lymphoplasmacytic infiltrates in portal tracts extending into the lobule, emperipolesis,[a] and hepatocyte rosette formation	2
Compatible	Chronic hepatitis with lymphocytic infiltration without all the features considered typical	1
Atypical	Includes evidence of another diagnosis	0[b]

[a] Emperipolesis: active penetration by one cell into and through a larger cell, uncertain value.
[b] Earlier systems deducted points for histologic features consistent with other diseases.
   Data from Hennes EM, Zeniya M, Czaja AJ, et al. Simplified criteria for the diagnosis of autoimmune hepatitis. Hepatol 2008;48:169–76.

chronic nature of the illness may be overlooked, and the failure to institute corticosteroid therapy may jeopardize survival.[3] Acute and fulminant forms of AIH were recognized by the IAIHG in 1992 when it codified diagnostic criteria and waived the requirement for 6 months of disease activity to establish the diagnosis.[18] Liver histology in patients with recent-onset AIH hepatitis shows evidence of chronic liver disease in many patients despite the lack of correlating clinical chronicity. The histologic evidence of chronicity includes septal fibrosis and overt cirrhosis.[17]

Superimposed on this are features of brisk, recent, ongoing immune-mediated hepatitic activity. There is portal inflammation and diffuse lobular necroinflammation (**Fig. 1**). Hepatitis activity may show zone 3 accentuation or predominance (**Fig. 2**). Bridging necrosis may occur. Evidence of hepatocellular injury and necrosis (ballooning degeneration, spotty hepatocyte necrosis, and apoptotic bodies) are common but not specific. Lobular disarray is present (see **Fig. 1**). Interface hepatitis may be extensive. Plasma cells typically predominate (**Fig. 3**) at the interface and throughout the lobules and portal areas. Injury may be followed by regeneration in the form of thickened hepatic plates and hepatic rosette formation.

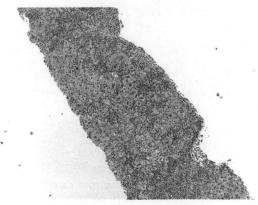

Fig. 1. Low power view of typical acute AIH liver biopsy core. Brisk diffuse parenchymal mononuclear, as well as portal, inflammation (hematoxylin and eosin, 25× magnification).

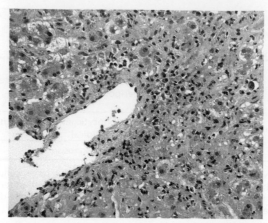

Fig. 2. Hepatic vein with surrounding centrilobular zone 3 hepatic parenchyma showing a lymphoid inflammatory infiltrate with plasma cells as part of lobular necroinflammation (hematoxylin and eosin, 100× magnification).

Most of these patients probably have a lobular "flare" in disease activity, which likely precipitated the clinical presentation as an acute hepatitis. Few patients may not have evidence of underlying fibrosis or present with a truly acute hepatitis as a first presentation of what is to become chronic disease. Thus, AIH is by definition a chronic disease and the term "chronic" is redundant and may be eliminated from AIH lexicon.

Variations on the Histologic Theme

Zone 3 necrosis with or without portal inflammation

This can also occur in viral and drug-induced hepatitis (**Fig. 4**). Zone 3 necrosis has not been formally included in the histologic spectrum of AIH. Many of the patients who were described in the initial reports of AIH as showing this histologic finding lacked

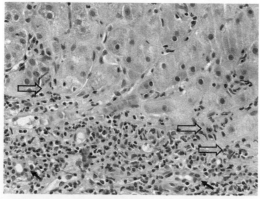

Fig. 3. Edge of portal tact and adjacent periportal liver parenchyma. Typical features with dense portal lymphoplasmacytic infiltrate with interface activity (*hollow arrows*). Mild bile duct injury with minimal infiltration by lymphocytes (*solid arrows*) (hematoxylin and eosin, 400× magnification).

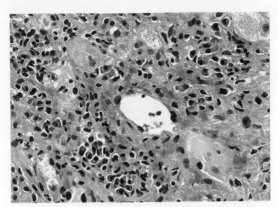

Fig. 4. Predominantly zone 3 involvement with plasma cell rich infiltrate and hepatocyte drop out and necrosis (hematoxylin and eosin, 200× magnification).

autoantibodies and hypergammaglobulinemia, and the true autoimmune nature of their disease remains unknown.[19]

Sparsity or absence of plasma cells in the inflammatory infiltrate
Predominance of plasma cell infiltration is not specific for AIH and does not occur in all patients with the disease. Its presence supports the diagnosis and the finding is more common in this condition (66%) than in chronic hepatitis B (40%) or chronic hepatitis C (21%).[20,21] Thirty-four percent of patients with AIH have few or no plasma cells (**Fig. 5**), and their absence does not preclude the diagnosis.[22,23]

Giant syncytial multinucleated hepatocytes
Giant syncytial multinucleated hepatocytes may be a dominant feature in AIH ("syncytial giant cell hepatitis") (**Fig. 6**); however, they are also associated with drug toxicity and viral infection, especially with the paramyxovirus.[24,25] Other causes should be sought before concluding that they represent an autoimmune process.

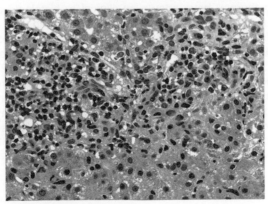

Fig. 5. Portal tract with dense lymphoid infiltrate and only rare plasma cells (hematoxylin and eosin, 400× magnification).

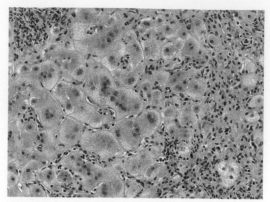

Fig. 6. Liver parenchyma showing lymphoplasmacytic inflammation and several large multinucleated hepatocytes in the center of the field (hematoxylin and eosin, 400× magnification).

Duct injury in AIH

Bile duct destruction is generally not prominent in AIH, but up to 12% of biopsies may show duct destruction. Lymphocytic infiltration of bile duct epithelium (see **Fig. 3**) without duct loss can be seen in another 12%.[26]

Variations on the Serologic Theme

Seronegative AIH

Approximately 10% to 15% of AIH is marker negative.[27,28] Data suggest that seronegative AIH s similar to seropositive AIH with respect to demographics, aminotransferase levels at diagnosis or after treatment, response to therapy, and histologic parameters, including portal and lobular inflammation, interface activity, and centrilobular necrosis.[29] The author's personal observations suggest that seronegative AIH may or may not show a preponderance of plasma cells.

Antimitochondrial antibody-M2 positive AIH

Antimitochondrial antibody (AMA) can be found in AIH, for example, and the significance of this requires further study. In a study from the author's institution, some patients with overt AIH who test positive for AMA at initial presentation and are treated with corticosteroid therapy have shown no clinical or histologic evidence of PBC despite the continued detection of AMA over a follow-up of up to 27 years.[30] Possible explanations for this phenomenon include (1) this group of patients may represent another subtype of AIH (ie, AMA-positive AIH), which, nevertheless, responds well to corticosteroids and is not associated with features of PBC; (2) early treatment with high-dose prednisone given to patients with circulating AMA prevents the development of subsequent PBC; or (3) the introduction of immunosuppressive therapy in patients presenting with AIH and treated as such at presentation may have prevented any subsequent progression to PBC. The long-term follow-up of these cases suggests that patients with overt AIH who also have circulating AMA may not have coexistent PBC and should be managed as is appropriate for AIH.[30]

FULMINANT AIH

Fulminant AIH was recognized by the IAIHG in 1992, as mentioned above. Numerous clinical descriptions of severe acute or fulminant AIH have emerged from small retrospective analyses within single institutions before and after that decision. These limited experiences have attested mainly to the uncommon nature of fulminant presentation of AIH and the difficulty in developing a confident management algorithm for this manifestation. The features are similar to but more severe than acute AIH. In addition to lobular necrosis, some patients with AIH exhibit bridging, zonal, and multi-lobular necrosis. Massive hepatocyte necrosis and drop out, parenchymal extinction (**Fig. 7**), and stromal collapse may be present.[23,31] Regenerative foci of hepatocytes may be present and mimicking parenchymal nodules of established cirrhosis.

CHRONIC "GRUMBLING" HEPATITIS

AIH can assume a chronic hepatitis pattern of injury, with portal and periportal lympho-plasmacytic infiltrates and interface hepatitis. Plasma cells are often, but not always, prominent, and are sometimes seen singly and in clusters in the lobule. The severity of necroinflammatory activity is quite variable. Ballooning degeneration, spotty hepato-cyte necrosis, and apoptotic bodies are common but not specific.[13] Hepatocytes may form regenerating rosette-like structures.

AIH, Hepatitis C Virus, or Both?

Worthy of special note is the issue of concurrent AIH and hepatitis C (HCV). Both give rise to a pattern of chronic hepatitis in the liver biopsy. The three potential scenarios are summarized as follows[13]: (1) patients with true AIH and false-positive HCV serology (anti-HCV antibody testing falsely positive but HCV-RNA undetectable); (2) patients with true HCV and autoantibodies at low titers, with no other features of AIH; and (3) patients with true HCV and clinical and serologic features of AIH. HCV infection appears to induce a genetic susceptibility to autoimmune processes, including in the liver.[32–34]

When differentiating HCV from AIH or determining whether AIH is coexistent with HCV clinically and histologically, the difficulty stems from the fact that HCV infection by itself in the nontransplant setting can be associated with multiple immune-mediated extrahepatic manifestations and chronic HCV liver disease can be associated with AIH-like features in native liver.[35,36] Czaja and Carpenter[35] reported higher serum

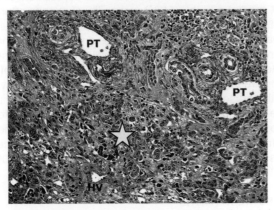

Fig. 7. Fulminant hepatitis with severe hepatocyte drop out from lobule (*star*). Lobular parenchyma replaced by ductular reaction and inflammation. Hepatic architecture is preserved with normal spatial organization of portal tracts (PT) and hepatic vein (HV) (elastic trichrome, 50× magnification).

levels of gamma globulin and immunoglobulin G, higher frequency of cirrhosis, a higher mean Knodell score, a higher frequency of human leukocyte antigens (HLA)-DR3, and a high titer of smooth muscle antibodies associated with the AIH-like pattern of HCV-induced liver injury in the general population.

The distinction of AIH from HCV and determination as to whether they are coexistent is not a pure histologic one but requires correlation with presence or absence of HCV RNA, history and clinical signs of hepatic and extrahepatic autoimmune manifestations, and autoimmune serology. The finding of prominent plasma cells in a biopsy for HCV—although not diagnostic—should be noted in the pathology report and thus prompt appropriate investigation for AIH and an informed discussion with the clinician.

AIH POST TREATMENT (INACTIVE CHRONIC LIVER DISEASE OR CHRONIC HEPATITIS WITH RESIDUAL ACTIVITY)

The findings are those of chronic liver disease with fibrosis, without or with mild lobular, portal, or interface necroinflammatory activity or a combination of these. This scenario is typically seen on biopsies of AIH post treatment. However, they may be encountered in the setting of subclinical AIH where elevated transaminases are incidentally discovered at a time when underlying AIH may be inactive or minimally active. In this scenario, it may be difficult to determine that AIH is the cause of liver disease given the lack of specificity of findings. In biopsies obtained after therapy, there is reduction in all parameters of hepatitic activity.[22,37–40]

After treatment, the pathologist is key in evaluation of treatment response. The histologic interpretation may affect treatment duration. The goals of corticosteroid therapy are to resolve symptoms, normalize laboratory tests, and improve histologic findings to normal, quiescent portal hepatitis, or inactive cirrhosis. Liver biopsy is the only means of confirming remission and it should be performed before drug withdrawal. Histologic improvement lags behind clinical and laboratory improvement by 3 to 6 months and, in 55% of instances, liver biopsy examination at the time of clinical and laboratory normality discloses residual interface hepatitis.[22]

What is the Pathologist's Approach in this Setting?

The key issue is not diagnosis of disease but rather assessment of response. Histologic findings that predict a high (>50%) probability of relapse after drug withdrawal must be documented so that premature withdrawal of medication can be averted.[37,41] The degree and nature of residual inflammation and whether there has been progression to cirrhosis are important as they predict the likelihood of relapse after drug withdrawal and define the next step in management. Restoration of normal hepatic architecture during treatment is associated with a 20% frequency of relapse after drug withdrawal; the presence of portal hepatitis is associated with a 50% frequency of relapse; and the presence of interface hepatitis of any degree or progression to 20% frequency of relapse after drug withdrawal; the presence of portal hepatitis is associated with a 50% frequency of relapse; and the presence of interface hepatitis of any degree or progression to cirrhosis is associated with an 87% to 100% frequency of relapse.[22,37,38,42–45]

CRYPTOGENIC CHRONIC HEPATITIS

Fig. 8 shows the histologic features of chronic hepatitis in a patient with clinical and laboratory findings of AIH but with no detectable autoantibodies.[21,22,27,46] It is a diagnosis of exclusion. Interface hepatitis or panacinar hepatitis are present.

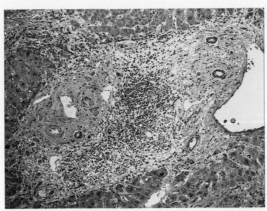

Fig. 8. Portal area with mild lymphoid infiltrate, minimally active. Appearance is nonspecific (hematoxylin and eosin, 100× magnification).

CRYPTOGENIC CIRRHOSIS, REGRESSED OR OTHERWISE

Fig. 9 shows inactive cirrhosis of a nonspecific appearance in a patient awaiting liver transplantation.[47] Obvious causes of cirrhosis have been excluded by a combination of laboratory tests and absence of characteristic histologic features such as biliary disease, alpha-1-antitrypsin deficiency, or iron overload. Remaining possibilities include burnt-out processes without specific laboratory findings and absent disease activity to allow characterization of the process. Burnt-out AIH and steatohepatitis are usually at the top of the list. Rojkind and Dunn,[48] Wanless,[49] Cotler and colleagues,[50] and Czaja and Carpenter[51] reported fibrosis or cirrhosis regression in patients with AIH subjected to immunosuppressive treatment (**Fig. 10**). In addition to regression of cirrhosis, immunosuppressive treatment improved the fibrosis scores in children, with an arrest in its progression and no development into cirrhosis. Fibrosis control is mainly associated with regression of necroinflammatory activity.[52]

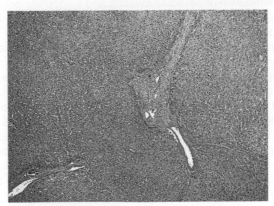

Fig. 9. Low-power view of liver explant from a patient with treated AIH in remission. Liver transplantation performed for portal hypertension. No evidence of active immune-mediated inflammation and no activity to the cirrhosis, thus diagnosis of AIH not feasible with past history or previous biopsy (hematoxylin and EOSIN, 25× magnification).

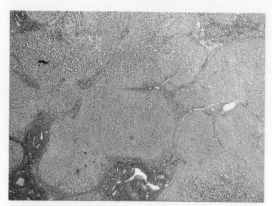

Fig. 10. Low-power view of liver explant with regressed cirrhosis. Boundaries of parenchymal cirrhotic nodules are subtle and surrounding septa appear as delicate, incomplete black lines (Gordon and sweet reticulin stain, 25× magnification).

AIH AS PART OF AN OVERLAP SYNDROME
AIH-PBC Overlap

PBC is a chronic cholestatic liver disease that is characterized by gradual destruction of the interlobular bile ducts that leads to damage of the hepatocytes. Approximately 10% of patients who have all the features of PBC—positive antimitochondrial antibodies and cholestatic biochemical findings—present with additional features of AIH. These features include other autoantibodies such as smooth muscle antibodies, hypergammaglobulinemia with a fivefold elevation of aspartate aminotransferase (AST) or alanine aminotransferase (ALT), or a 10-fold elevation of the AST. Histologically, these patients may have lymphoplasmacytic interface hepatitis in addition to the typical florid duct lesions present in PBC. In addition to AIH-PBC overlap that is present at the time of diagnosis, a "sequential" overlap syndrome of AIH with PBC can occur. There are several reports of cases where AIH occurred during the course of PBC. In AIH-PBC overlap the histologic features includes a variable combination of inflammatory lymphoplasmacytic infiltrates directed at biliary epithelium and hepatocytes producing duct injury, interface hepatitis, and parenchymal necroinflammation. The latter is associated with hepatocyte swelling and acidophilic bodies. Stage 2 PBC is characterized by portal lymphoplasmacytic inflammation and interface hepatitis, and it may be impossible to distinguish from AIH (AIH as the main disease process or as an overlapping component) if diffuse lobular hepatitis is not present. Distinction requires correlation with other clinical and laboratory parameters.[13,23,53,54]

When embarking on a diagnosis of AIH-PBC overlap syndrome, the pathologist needs to take into account that overlap syndromes are a clinical pathologic diagnosis. ANA can be found in high rates in PBC patients,[55,56] this autoantibody is not considered a helpful marker of overlap syndrome. Classification of patients with AIH overlap syndromes may change with time depending on the prevalent disease and transitioning from one component to the other; that is, cholestatic to hepatitic enzymes. PBC alone can demonstrate interface hepatitis; the latter has been implicated in progression of PBC to cirrhosis.[57] An AIH overlap should not be applied to otherwise typical cases of PBC with prominent interface.

AIH-PSC Overlap

AIH-PSC overlap is not uncommon in young patients with autoimmune liver disease and may comprise 6% of patients with AIH and 8% of PSC patients. Similarly in adults with PSC, an overlap with AIH may be seen. In the Kings cohort of pediatric AIH, "auto-immune sclerosing cholangitis," as they called it, and AIH were even more prevalent in childhood (50%). Histology can reflect features of both conditions synchronously or sequentially. Histologic examination may show duct lesions of PSC, fibrous oblitera-tion of bile ducts (fibrous knots), or concentric periductal fibrosis. However, the char-acteristic duct lesions of PSC are uncommon in biopsies in general and rare in biopsies from children. Biopsies may show portal inflammation with piecemeal necrosis resembling AIH. There may be loss of interlobular bile ducts. Variation in the intensity of the ductal lesions and variability between affected portal tracts are noted in PSC. Because biliary epithelium is not easily identified in the inflammatory infiltrate, immunohistochemistry for keratins 7 and 19 can be useful. The inflammatory infiltrate is variable both in intensity and composition, and ranges from a mixture of lymphocytes and polymorphonuclear cells to a lymphoplasmacytic infiltrate as is usually observed in patients who have AIH. Discordance between clinical, laboratory, and radiologic findings resulting from sampling limitations and errors are frequently reported, in part because the bile duct injury is not homogenously distributed in the liver.[9,58]

In study from the author's center shows that when using dedicated liver MRI and liver histology, 12% of adult patients with AIH will have detectable subtle biliary changes. Two patients with a normal magnetic resonance cholangiography (MRC) had distinct bile duct changes suggestive of the concentric periductal onion-skin fibrosis seen in PSC, raising the possibility of small-duct PSC in these two patients.[59] The presence of PSC detected by MRC and from liver histology in adult patients with AIH may not be clinically overt, and thus the prevalence of this AIH-PSC overlap may be higher than previously recognized. The author's data suggests that routine radio-logical evaluation of the biliary tree should be performed in adults given a diagnosis of AIH.

SUMMARY

The histologic findings of AIH are limited by the overlap between AIH, viral-related, drug-induced, immune-mediated liver injury, and often do not otherwise discriminate between them. AIH has many histologic faces depending on the course of the disease, the form of its initial presentation, its evolution, and effects of treatment. Atypical morphologic features must be sought because they may indicate an overlap syndrome or explain an unexpected clinical behavior or treatment response. The clas-sification of an autoimmune liver disease in the setting of an overlap syndrome may change over time as enzymes, clinical features, and histology transition from one pattern to another. Communication between the pathologist and the clinician is crucial in AIH, beginning with a proper clinical history accompanying the biopsy and a clinical pathologic correlation discussion upon review of the biopsy. The liver biopsy can yield important prognostic information, including stage of fibrosis and response to therapy in post treatment biopsies.

REFERENCES

1. Czaja AJ, Freese DK. Diagnosis and treatment of autoimmune hepatitis. Hepato-logy 2002;36:479–97.
2. Krawitt EL. Autoimmune hepatitis. N Engl J Med 2006;354:54–66.
3. Czaja. Corticosteroids or not in severe acute or fulminant autoimmune hepatitis: therapeutic brinksmanship and the point beyond salvation. Liver Transpl 2007;13:953–5.

4. Johnson PJ, McFarlane IG. Meeting report: International Autoimmune Hepatitis Group. Hepatology 1993;18:998–1005.
5. Czaja A, Carpenter HA. Validation of scoring system for diagnosis of autoimmune hepatitis. Dig Dis Sci 1996;41:305–14.
6. Bianchi FB, Cassani F, Lenzi M, et al. Impact of International Autoimmune Hepatitis Group scoring system in definition of autoimmune hepatitis—An Italian experience. Dig Dis Sci 1996;41:166–71.
7. Toda G, Zeniya M, Watanabe F, et al. Present status of autoimmune hepatitis in Japan—correlating the characteristics with international criteria in an area with a high rate of HCV infection. Japanese National Study Group of Autoimmune Hepatitis. J Hepatol 1997;26:1207–12.
8. Alvarez F, Berg PA, Bianchi FB, et al. International Autoimmune Hepatitis Group report: review of criteria for diagnosis of autoimmune hepatitis. J Hepatol 1999; 31:929–38.
9. Boberg KM, Fausa O, Haaland T, et al. Features of autoimmune hepatitis in primary sclerosing cholangitis: an evaluation of 114 primary sclerosing cholangitis patients according to a scoring system for the diagnosis of autoimmune hepatitis. Hepatology 1996;23:1369–76.
10. Choi G, Peters MG. The challenge of diagnosing autoimmune hepatitis: less is more. Hepatology 2008;48(1):10–2.
11. Hennes EM, Zeniya M, Czaja AJ, et al. Simplified criteria for the diagnosis of autoimmune hepatitis. Hepatology 2008;48:169–76.
12. Dienes HP. Viral and autoimmune hepatitis. Morphologic and pathogenetic aspects of cell damage in hepatitis with potential chronicity. Veroff Pathol 1989; 132:1–107.
13. Washington KM. Autoimmune liver disease: overlap and outliers. Mod Pathol 2007;20:S15–30.
14. Theise ND, Bodenheimer HC Jr, Ferrell LD. Acute and chronic viral hepatitis. In: Burt AD, Porman BC, Ferrell LD, editors. Ween's pathology of the liver. 5th edition. Edinburgh (UK): Churchill Livingstone; 2007. p. 399–441.
15. Ichiki Y, Aoki CA, Bowlus CL, et al. T-cell immunity in autoimmune hepatitis. Autoimmun Rev 2005;4:315–21.
16. Nikias GA, Batts KP, Czaja AJ. The nature and prognostic implications of autoimmune hepatitis with an acute presentation. J Hepatol 1994;21:866–71.
17. Burgart LJ, Batts KP, Ludwig J, et al. Recent onset autoimmune hepatitis: biopsy findings and clinical correlations. Am J Surg Pathol 1995;19:699–708.
18. Johnson PJ, McFarlane IG, Alvarez F, et al. Meeting report. International Autoimmune Hepatitis Group. Hepatology 1993;18:998–1005.
19. Pratt DS, Fawaz KA, Rabson A, et al. A novel histological lesion in glucocorticoid-responsive chronic hepatitis. Gastroenterology 1997;113:664–8.
20. Bach N, Thung SN, Schaffner F. The histological features of chronic hepatitis C and autoimmune chronic hepatitis: a comparative analysis. Hepatology 1992; 15:572–7.
21. Czaja AJ, Carpenter HA. Sensitivity, specificity and predictability of biopsy interpretations in chronic hepatitis. Gastroenterology 1993;105:1824–32.
22. Carpenter HA, Czaja AJ. The role of histologic evaluation in the diagnosis and management of autoimmune hepatitis and its variants. Clin Liver Dis 2002;6: 397–417.
23. Czaja AJ, Carpenter HA. Autoimmune hepatitis. In: Burt AD, Porman BC, Ferrell LD, editors. Macsween's pathology of the liver. 5th edition. Edinburgh (UK): Churchill Livingstone; 2007. p. 493–515.

24. Devaney K, Goodman ZD, Ishak KG. Postinfantile giant-cell transformation in hepatitis. Hepatology 1992;16:327–33.
25. Phillips MJ, Blendis LM, Poucell S, et al. Syncytial giant-cell hepatitis. Sporadic hepatitis with distinctive pathological features, a severe clinical course, and paramyxoviral features. N Engl J Med 1991;324:455–60.
26. Czaja AJ, Carpenter HA. Autoimmune hepatitis with incidental histologic features of bile duct injury. Hepatology 2001;34:659–65.
27. Czaja AJ, Carpenter HA, Santrach PJ, et al. The nature and prognosis of severe cryptogenic chronic active hepatitis. Gastroenterology 1993;104(6):1755–61.
28. Czaja AJ. The variant forms of autoimmune hepatitis. Ann Intern Med 1996; 125(7):588–98.
29. Mehendiratta V, Mitroo P, Bombonati A, et al. Serologic markers do not predict histologic severity or response to treatment in patients with autoimmune hepatitis. Clin Gastroenterol Hepatol 2009;7(1):98–103.
30. O'Brien C, Joshi S, Feld JJ, et al. Long-term follow-up of antimitochondrial antibody-positive autoimmune hepatitis. Hepatology 2008;48(2):550–6.
31. Abe M, Onji M, Kawai–Ninomiya K, et al. Clinicopathologic features of the severe form of acute type 1 autoimmune hepatitis. Clin Gastroenterol Hepatol 2007;5: 255–8.
32. Dai YD, Carayanniotis G, Sercarz E. Antigen processing by autoreactive B cells promotes determinant spreading. Cell Mol Immunol 2005;2:169–75.
33. Vanderlugt CL, Miller SD. Epitope spreading in immune-mediated diseases: implications for immunotherapy. Nat Rev Immunol 2002;2:85–95.
34. Demetris AJ, Sebagh M. Plasma cell hepatitis in liver allografts: variant of rejection or autoimmune hepatitis? Liver Transpl 2008;14:750–5.
35. Czaja AJ, Carpenter HA. Histological findings in chronic hepatitis C with autoimmune features. Hepatology 1997;26:459–66.
36. Kessel A, Toubi E. Chronic HCV-related autoimmunity: a consequence of viral persistence and lymphotropism. Curr Med Chem 2007;14:547–54.
37. Czaja AJ, Davis GL, Ludwig J, et al. Complete resolution of inflammatory activity following corticosteroid treatment of HBsAg-negative chronic active hepatitis. Hepatology 1984;4:622–7.
38. Czaja AJ, Ludwig J, Baggenstoss AH, et al. Corticosteroid treated chronic active hepatitis in remission. Uncertain prognosis of chronic persistent hepatitis. N Engl J Med 1981;304:5–9.
39. Czaja AJ. Therapy of autoimmune hepatitis—state of the art. In: Manns MP, Paumgartner G, Leuschner U, editors. Immunology and liver, Falk Symposium 114. Dordrecht (The Netherlands): Kluwer Academic Publishers, BV; 2000. p. 311–24.
40. Czaja AJ. Treatment of autoimmune hepatitis. In: Krawitt EL, Wiesner RH, editors. Autoimmune liver disease. Amsterdam (The Netherlands): Elsevier Science Publishers; 1998. p. 399–415.
41. Stellon AJ, Keating JJ, Johnson PJ, et al. Maintenance of remission in autoimmune chronic active hepatitis with azathioprine after corticosteroid withdrawal. Hepatology 1988;8:781–4.
42. Czaja AJ, Beaver SJ, Shiels MT. Sustained remission following corticosteroid therapy of severe HBsAg-negative chronic active hepatitis. Gastroenterology 1987;92:215–9.
43. Davis GL, Czaja AJ. Immediate and long-term results of corticosteroid therapy for severe idiopathic chronic active hepatitis. In: Czaja AJ, Dickson ER, editors. Chronic active hepatitis. The mayo clinic experience. New York: Marcel Dekker; 1986. p. 269–83.

44. Hegarty JE, Nouri-Aria KT, Portmann B, et al. Relapse following treatment withdrawal in patients with autoimmune chronic active hepatitis. Hepatology 1983; 13:685–9.
45. Johnson PJ, McFarlane IG, Williams R. Azathioprine for long-term maintenance of remission in autoimmune hepatitis. N Engl J Med 1995;333:958–63.
46. Kaymakoglu S, Cakaloglu Y, Demir K, et al. Is severe cryptogenic chronic hepatitis similar to autoimmune hepatitis? J Hepatol 1998;28:78–83.
47. Greeve M, Ferrell L, Kim M, et al. Cirrhosis of undefined pathogenesis: absence of evidence for unknown viruses or autoimmune processes. Hepatology 1993;17: 593–8.
48. Rojkind M, Dunn M. Hepatic fibrosis. Gastroenterology 1979;76:849–63.
49. Wanless IR. Use of corticosteroid therapy in autoimmune hepatitis resulting in the resolution of cirrhosis. J Clin Gastroenterol 2001;32:371–2.
50. Cotler SJ, Jakate S, Jensen DM. Resolution of cirrhosis in autoimmune hepatitis with corticosteroid therapy. J Clin Gastroenterol 2001;32:428–30.
51. Czaja AJ, Carpenter HA. Decreased fibrosis during corticosteroid therapy of autoimmune hepatitis. J Hepatol 2004;40:646–52.
52. Ferreira AR, Roquete ML, Toppa NH, et al. Effect of treatment of hepatic histopathology in children and adolescents with autoimmune hepatitis. J Pediatr Gastroenterol Nutr 2008;46:65–70.
53. Gossard AA, Lindor KD. Development of autoimmune hepatitis in primary biliary cirrhosis. Liver Int 2007;27:1086–90.
54. Twaddell WS, Lefkowitch J, Ber PD. Evolution from primary biliary cirrhosis to primary biliary cirrhosis/autoimmune hepatitis overlap syndrome. Semin Liver Dis 2008;28(1):128–34.
55. Muratori P, Muratori L, Ferrari R, et al. Characterization and clinical impact of antinuclear antibodies in primary biliary cirrhosis. Am J Gastroenterol 2003;98(2): 431–7.
56. Rigopoulou EI, Davies ET, Pares A, et al. Prevalence and clinical significance of isotype specific antinuclear antibodies in primary biliary cirrhosis. Gut 2005; 54(4):528–32.
57. Corpechot C, Carrat F, Poupon R, et al. Primary biliary cirrhosis: incidence and predictive factors of cirrhosis development in ursodiol-treated patients. Gastroenterology 2002;122:652–8.
58. Gregorio GV, Portmann B, Karani J, et al. Autoimmune hepatitis/sclerosing cholangitis overlap syndrome in childhood: a 16-year prospective study. Hepatology 2001;33:544–53.
59. Abdalian R, Dhar P, Jhaveri K, et al. Prevalence of sclerosing cholangitis in adults with autoimmune hepatitis: evaluating the role of routine magnetic resonance imaging. Hepatology 2008;47:949–57.

Nonalcoholic Fatty Liver Disease

Kathryn Law, MD, Elizabeth M. Brunt, MD*

KEYWORDS

- Nonalcoholic fatty liver disease • Nonalcoholic steatohepatitis
- Steatosis • Fibrosis • Cirrhosis

In spite of recent encouraging information that the upward obesity trends of the past 2 decades in the United States are showing signs of leveling out in adults[1] but not heavy adolescents and children,[2] up to two-thirds of adults and 11.9% of children (2–19 yrs) are overweight and/or obese.[2] Many of the physical and metabolic complications from obesity are by now well-known; the most significant in terms of morbidity and mortality relate to cardiovascular diseases, diabetes mellitus, and malignancy. Fatty liver, which is estimated to affect 33% of US adults,[3] is a marker of cardiovascular risk (in adults and children),[4–6] and the ectopic fat itself may not be the harmful component of the process. In fact, studies have shown that formation of triglycerides (TG) is a protective mechanism, when a liver is overwhelmed with free fatty acid influx from insulin-resistant adipose tissue and cannot form or secrete TG[7,8] or oxidize fatty acids to keep pace with delivery or increased de novo lipogenesis induced by exposure to high fructose loads.[9,10] Aberrant lipid partitioning between potentially toxic and neutral lipids may result in the lipotoxicity of fatty liver.[11] Although mechanisms of lipid accumulation are becoming increasingly delineated, recent work has highlighted the roles of endoplasmic reticulum stress[12] and autophagy in fatty liver disease.[13,14]

Several long-term studies have shown increased morbidity and mortality in subjects with nonalcoholic fatty liver disease (NAFLD) compared with baseline populations; most have also shown that NAFLD is associated with increased risk of cardiovascular disease[15] and malignancy and that those with steatohepatitis have worse outcomes than those with steatosis.[16–18] Investigations have also shed light on actual hepatitic damage known to occur in a minority of subjects with steatosis.

It is estimated that only 3% to 5% of subjects with NAFLD have the progressive form, nonalcoholic steatohepatitis (NASH),[19] and cirrhosis develops in only 5% and 15% of those with NAFLD and NASH, respectively.[20] Immune[21]and genetic underpinnings are certainly present along many steps of the activated pathways, because of lipid accumulation, lipotoxicity, inflammation, fibrosis and cirrhosis, and ultimately

Department of Pathology and Immunology, Washington University School of Medicine, 660 South Euclid Avenue, Box 8118, St Louis, MO 63110, USA
* Corresponding author.
E-mail address: ebrunt@wustl.edu

Clin Liver Dis 14 (2010) 591–604
doi:10.1016/j.cld.2010.07.006
1089-3261/10/$ – see front matter © 2010 Elsevier Inc. All rights reserved.

liver.theclinics.com

and potentially, hepatocellular carcinoma. Ethnic differences, such as higher risk in Hispanic Americans than in African Americans, are well-recognized clinically[22,23]and in genetic studies,[24,25] and work has begun to highlight various single-nucleotide polymorphisms[26] and gene associations or alterations correlated with obesity, insulin and leptin signaling,[27] and/or fatty liver disease.[28,29] Environmental alterations (diet, television, and computer time), physical activity's multifaceted advantages,[30,31] and life-altering bariatric surgery[32] are all being actively studied as potentially effective therapeutic considerations for obesity and fatty liver.

Although the field has literally exploded with information and publications, histologic evaluation continues to play a significant role in clinical care, therapeutic studies, and experimental work. Fibrosis and cirrhotic remodeling have been shown to correspond closely with outcomes in longitudinal studies.[33] Multimodality noninvasive testing algorithms to predict fibrosis and steatohepatitis are progressing but, to date, remain best at the ends of the spectrum of disease.[34–36] Thus, for the foreseeable future, practicing pathologists require experience with the histologic manifestations of this common process.

MORPHOLOGY: OVERVIEW

NAFLD is characterized histologically by a spectrum of findings (**Fig. 1**). In the noncirrhotic liver, these include some degree of steatosis and, variably, the presence of (1) ballooning with or without Mallory-Denk bodies (MDB), (2) lobular and/or portal inflammation, and (3) fibrosis. Other findings that may occur are glycogenated nuclei, Kupffer cell aggregates, acidophil bodies, megamitochondria, and iron. A combination of these findings, as further discussed, leads to a diagnosis of steatohepatitis.

STEATOSIS

Steatosis, not specific to NAFLD, can be found in several disorders, some of which share a common underlying component of insulin resistance or disordered lipoprotein metabolism. The most commonly associated diseases characterized by steatosis include drug-/toxin-induced injury, viral hepatitis C, inherited disorders of lipoprotein metabolism, nutritional disorders on both ends of the spectrum, and various systemic, metabolic and endocrine disorders, including heat stroke. Steatosis is minimal criteria for the diagnosis of NAFLD in a noncirrhotic liver. In NAFLD, the predominant type is macrovesicular, and in most adults, shows acinar zone 3 (perivenular) predominance. This type of steatosis is characterized by intracytoplasmic large fat droplets and eccentric displacement of the nucleus. There may be a single large fat droplet or smaller fat droplets surrounding larger fat droplets. Studies have shown that up to 5.5% of the liver is lipid in otherwise normal individuals[37]; thus, NAFLD is minimally defined as more than 5% of hepatocytes with steatosis. The large-droplet steatosis can be seen with routine stains; thus, special stains for lipid (eg, oil red O) are not necessary for identification. Characterizing the degree of steatosis in NAFLD is commonly done by semiquantitation of the surface area of involvement, which can be organized using the acinar architecture into thirds, as discussed later in grading and staging.

Although zone 3 predominance of steatosis is characteristic in adults, individual cases may show irregular (nonzonal), pan-acinar distribution, and in children, zone 1 predominance.[38] Other liver diseases with zone 3 predominance include alcoholic fatty liver disease, whereas zone 1 predominance is common in hepatitis C, cachexia, heat stroke, AIDS, total parenteral nutrition, cystic fibrosis, phosphorous poisoning,

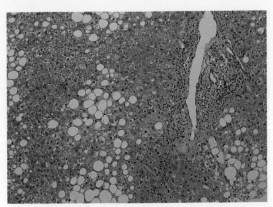

Fig. 1. The constellation of lesions of NASH: there is zone 1 sparing and zone 3 predominant steatosis, mild ballooning, and focal lobular inflammation. Portal inflammation is moderate in this portal tract. Scattered glycogenated nuclei are also seen throughout the lobules (hematoxylin-eosin, original magnification 20×).

and corticosteroid- and amiodarone-induced liver injury.[39] As yet not well understood, cirrhosis secondary to NASH may harbor minimal to no residual steatosis.[39]

Occasionally, nonzonal clusters of hepatocytes with purely microvesicular steatosis occur, composed of cells with central nuclei and foamy cytoplasm with intracytoplasmic delicate septations. This type of steatosis is typically related to mitochondrial injury with defects in β-oxidation, but in NAFLD, the significance is unknown. Microvesicular steatosis is uncommon in pediatric NAFLD. An association, such as that shown in alcoholic fatty liver, with increased risk of progression[40] has not been shown in NAFLD.

HEPATOCYTE BALLOONING

One of the markers of liver cell injury in NAFLD is hepatocyte ballooning (**Figs. 2–4**), which is characterized by hepatocytes that appear swollen and round with reticulated cytoplasm, enlarged nuclei, and prominent nucleoli. Often poorly formed MDB are

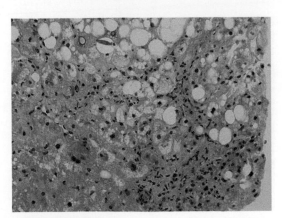

Fig. 2. Hepatocytes undergoing ballooning degeneration are demonstrated in the center of this field. Some of the hepatocytes also show ropy condensations consistent with poorly formed MDB (hematoxylin-eosin, original magnification 40×).

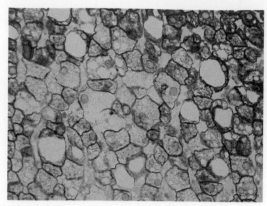

Fig. 3. In the center of this field are 2 hepatocytes showing ballooning degeneration. Note the delicately staining reticulated cytoplasm compared with the more darkly staining surrounding hepatocytes and the optically clear fat droplets. Densely stained MDB are also noted in one of the cells in this field (antikeratin 8/18 immunohistochemical stain, original magnification 60×).

observed in ballooned hepatocytes. Ballooned hepatocytes may be difficult to distinguish from microvesicular steatosis, and in some cases, they may contain small droplets of fat.[41] The histologic change may be related to increased intracellular fluid as in viral hepatitis.[42] Studies have shown that in NASH, ballooning is the manifestation of loss of normal cytoskeletal structure.[43] The hepatocyte cytoskeleton is derived from keratins 8 and 18 (K8/18). These keratins have been shown to be decreased to absent in ballooned hepatocytes in NASH[44]; also, K8/18 immunohistochemical stains highlight aggregates in MDB. In adult NASH, ballooned hepatocytes are zone 3 predominant. In pediatric NAFLD, ballooning may be absent.[38] As a marker of liver cell injury in NASH, many pathologists have suggested ballooning as a required criterion for steatohepatitis. Ballooned hepatocytes may occur in conjunction with perisinusoidal fibrosis. Matteoni and colleagues[45] found ballooning to be a feature associated with clinically progressive NAFLD. In a biopsy study of NAFLD, ballooning correlated with increased serum cholesterol, with a trend toward abnormal glycemic control,

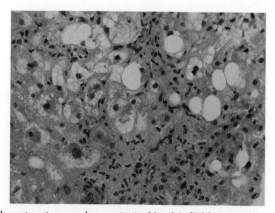

Fig. 4. Ballooned hepatocytes are demonstrated in this field. Note the delicate, reticulated cytoplasm, the enlarged nuclei, and the presence of poorly formed MDB in some of the cells (hematoxylin-eosin, original magnification 60×).

and with insulin resistance.[46] Ballooning has been associated with increased serum markers of necroinflammation.[47]

LOBULAR INFLAMMATION

Lobular inflammation in NAFLD is usually mild and is an important contributor to the diagnosis of NASH. In most cases, lobular inflammation is composed of mixed chronic inflammatory cells, small Kupffer cell aggregates (microgranulomas), and occasionally, interspersed neutrophils. Lobular inflammation can be found throughout the lobule. Neutrophils clustered around hepatocytes containing MDB are referred to as satellitosis; this is less common in NASH than in alcoholic steatohepatitis (ASH). At times, the central inflammation can be associated with fibrosis, with the presence of an artery,[48] and even with ductular reaction (DR)[49]; this may lead to misidentification as a portal tract, but the lack of a bona fide bile duct is key to identification. Such an area is illustrated in **Fig. 5**.

PORTAL INFLAMMATION

Portal inflammation is often present in NAFLD but is usually mild and less conspicuous than the zone 3 findings and lobular inflammation. More pronounced portal inflammation has been noted in pediatric NAFLD,[38] post-treatment biopsies with resolution after treatment,[50] and biopsies in adults and children with clinically and histologically severe NASH.[51] The last study, however, showed no association of portal inflammation with lobular inflammation, autoimmune markers, or serum ALT.[51]

Lymphocytes predominate in portal inflammation in NAFLD; if neutrophils are present and associated with DR, alternate causes of alcoholic hepatitis, pancreatitis, or biliary obstruction are suggested. Also, if the portal inflammation is *significant*, concomitant or even alternate liver diseases, such as hepatitis C, should be considered.[52] Overall, approximately 5% of NASH is associated with another concurrent liver disease[53,54]; considering this when evaluating liver biopsies for NAFLD is not inappropriate.

MDB

MDB are *ropy* aggregates of cytoskeletal material found within hepatocytes in ASH and NASH. Compared with MDB in ASH, those in NASH are often less well formed, are in

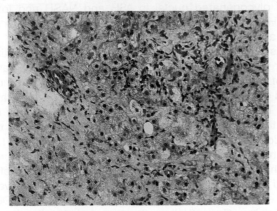

Fig. 5. A patient with stage 3 bridging fibrosis. The central inflammation in NASH can be associated with the presence of an artery and even DR. Therefore portal tracts must be identified by the presence of a true bile duct (trichrome, original magnification 40×).

ballooned hepatocytes, and require trichrome staining or immunohistochemistry (IHC) to identify. IHC that can be used for identification of MDB detects the antigens of the MDB K8 or K8/18 or the antigens of the proteosome/sequestosome that result in their formation, ubiquitin, and p62.[55] MDB are chemotactic and attract neutrophils, that is, the lesion recognized as satellitosis.[56] MDB themselves are not unique to steatohepatitis and can be found in various liver diseases; zonality may aid in the differential diagnosis. In chronic cholestatic conditions, in copper toxicity, and through treatment with certain drugs (eg, amiodarone, perhexiline maleate), MDB develop in zone 1; in focal nodular hyperplasia, hepatic adenomas, and hepatocellular carcinoma, they are nonzonal; their presence in zone 3 is associated with ASH and NASH.[39] MDB appear to be less common in pediatric NASH, particularly *type 2* pediatric NASH.[38,57] In one study of pediatric NAFLD, MDB were found in 19 of 100 biopsies; this included 41% of *type 1* (zone 3) pattern cases and 10% of *type 2* (zone 1) cases.[38]

MDB may be more commonly found in higher inflammatory grades of NASH,[47,58] and were one of the characteristics that Matteoni and colleagues[45] used to differentiate types 1 and 2 NAFLD that were less likely to progress from types 3 and 4 NAFLD that did progress to cirrhosis or death. Despite these associations, MDB are known to occur by metabolically active processes, rather than passive aggregation of damaged cytoskeletal filaments, and may have a protective role for the hepatocyte.[55,56]

ACIDOPHIL BODIES/APOPTOSIS

Although apoptosis is not a defining characteristic of NASH and not required for diagnosis, individual acidophil bodies are often present. Studies have shown that in NASH, compared with steatosis (NAFLD), controls, and ASH, apoptosis is increased.[59] Apoptosis correlates with fibrosis and inflammatory activity.[60] Because of these associations, an apoptotic index has been proposed in biopsy studies,[61] and serum assays of apoptotic fragments have been proposed for diagnosis of NASH.[62]

GLYCOGENATED NUCLEI, MICROGRANULOMAS, LIPOGRANULOMAS, IRON

Centrally cleared out, vacuolated nuclei in groups of hepatocytes are common in NAFLD.[63] However, this is not a diagnostic criterion for NAFLD. Glycogenated nuclei can also be found in any pediatric liver biopsies and are common in Wilson disease and diabetes-associated liver disease.[64] Cortez-Pinto and colleagues[65] compared the incidence of glycogenated nuclei in ASH and NASH and found them to be uncommon in ASH (10%–15%) compared with NASH (75%). In their study, glycogenated nuclei were associated with diabetes and obesity.

Lipogranulomas are common but are diagnostic of steatohepatitis. They can be lobular, portal, or perivenular in location. Lobular lipogranulomas are typically small and composed of as little as one lipid vacuole with surrounding mononuclear cells, Kupffer cells, and occasionally eosinophils. Lipogranulomas in portal tracts and perivenular locations may be large and surrounded by collagen. It is important not to include this with the stage of fibrosis, discussed later. Although a common finding, lipogranulomas do not seem to correlate with disease severity. Microgranulomas and single pigmented Kupffer cells may also be found. Lefkowitch and colleagues[66] used antimacrophage marker CD68 to demonstrate aggregates of Kupffer cells in zone 3 in ASH and NASH where the highest concentrations of reactive oxygen species are also found. The Kupffer cells were enlarged and rounded and CD68 showed granular, lysosomal staining. These findings were compared to the normal and steatotic controls, which showed individual, tapering Kupffer cells distributed in sinusoids throughout the hepatic lobule around portal tracts and central veins. It was noted that without CD68, the Kupffer cells might be confused with lymphocytes or endothelial cells; furthermore, the study demonstrated that some of them had phagocytosed intracytoplasmic hepatocyte lipid.

Iron deposition detectable by histochemical staining, if found in NAFLD, is usually mild (grade 1–2+ of 4) and has been described within hepatocytes and reticuloendothelial cells. Although conflicting studies can be found in the literature related to iron studies, HFE genotypes, and tissue deposition, a recent study of more than 580 subjects with NAFLD and 184 controls showed parenchymal deposition, but not reticuloendothelial system iron, was associated with severe liver damage (fibrosis) and was more prevalent in subjects with HFE mutations.[67] Although studies are ongoing related to significance, reviews of literature show iron staining from 10% to 95% of cases of NAFLD.[50]

Megamitochondria are eosinophilic, round or needle-shaped (cigar shaped), intracytoplasmic inclusions. In NAFLD, zonal accentuation has not been identified.[68] In ultrastructural studies, paracrystalline mitochondrial inclusions were found in 8 of 10 cases of NASH versus only 1 of 7 cases of ASH.[69] However, unlike ASH, mitochondrial gene deletion is not common in NASH.[70] Although the significance of megamitochondria in NASH has yet to be clarified, Caldwell and colleagues[71] speculate that they may represent a manifestation of cell injury or hepatocyte adaptation.

DISTINCTION BETWEEN NASH AND ASH

This can be a challenge at the mild end of disease activity; however, the presence of certain lesions are more strongly suggestive of ASH than NASH.[72] These entities may share similar inflammatory and fibrogenic pathways[39]; also, there are patients who may be at risk of both. Briefly, the fibro-occlusive venous lesions seen with ASH,[73] marked bile stasis, and dense ropy MDB are more common in ASH than NASH. Glycogenated nuclei seem to be more common in NASH. Use of a clinically derived alcoholic liver disease/NAFLD Index as well as IHC to detect insulin down-regulation have been proposed,[74,75] but the final diagnosis relies on careful clinical input.[39]

FIBROSIS AND CIRRHOSIS

Fibrosis is not considered a necessary criterion for establishing a diagnosis of NASH. In adults, the initial deposition of collagen is in zone 3 perisinusoidal space of Disse; at times, a pericellular ("chicken wire") fibrosis can be seen (see **Fig. 5; Fig. 6**). This early fibrosis may be quite delicate and appreciated best with special stains or may be dense and visible on routine hematoxylin-eosin (H&E) stains. Reticulin condensation due to cell injury and dropout cannot be distinguished from true collagen deposition by reticulin stain; the Masson's trichrome or picrosirius red stain highlights collagen. Elastic fiber deposition in newly forming fibrosis can be demonstrated by stains such as Shikata orcein.[76]

Following the initial zone 3 deposition, portal tract expansion and periportal fibrosis may be seen; in some cases, central-central, central-portal, or portal-portal bridging fibrosis occurs and cirrhosis may occur. At any of these stages, perisinusoidal fibrosis may or may not persist. In pediatric NAFLD and possibly in the bariatric population, portal fibrosis occurs in the absence of central fibrosis.[38,77,78] The significance of these differing patterns of disease is not well understood, but the localization of the early fibrosis does correlate with steatosis and damage in adults and children and suggests possible differences in etiopathogenesis. Bariatric subjects may be unique; the distribution of adipose tissue and weight cycling in the morbidly obese may result in differing histopathologic features of NAFLD, as noted in some early studies.[77]

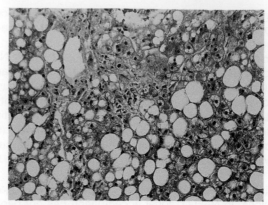

Fig. 6. The zone 3 perisinusoidal fibrosis characteristic of NAFLD is demonstrated. (trichrome stain, original magnification 40×).

Various studies have reported somewhat conflicting results with hepatic stellate cells (HSC) in NAFLD.[79,80] Although both studies showed increased HSC activation in NASH by increased alpha smooth muscle antigen detection in zone 3, the former found that activated HSC correlated with fibrosis stage but not with inflammatory activity or severity of steatosis, whereas the latter showed correlation with inflammation. Feldstein and colleagues[81] proposed a score and suggested a cut-off of 5 as an indicator of future progression based on a study in a cohort of NAFLD patients who, on initial biopsy, has stage 0 to 2 fibrosis. The results showed excellent specificity and positive predictive value at high levels; levels lower than 5 had very little predictive value; the authors ultimately concluded that measurement of HSC activation combined with clinical parameters, such as age, gender, ALT, and diabetes, proposed in many studies[82–84] may be combined to attempt more reliable prediction of which NAFLD patients are at risk of progression.

PROGENITOR CELLS IN NASH

Several studies have looked into the presence and significance of hepatic progenitor cells (HPC) in NAFLD. HPC can occur as single cells, strings of cells, cells lining the periportal canals of Hering, and small intralobular ductules.[85] Immunohistochemically, they can be identified by strong K7 or K19 reactivity. Activation results in proliferation of HPC, and the fibro-inflammatory process referred to as the DR. Roskams and colleagues[49] noted the presence and extent of HPC in mice and humans with ASH and NASH related to oxidative stress and hepatocyte senescence. Richardson and colleagues[86] further noted the correlation with portal fibrosis in chronic hepatitis C[87] and NASH. The Australian group has demonstrated DR concurrently with impaired hepatocyte regeneration (as measured by p21 immunohistochemistry) and has shown correlations with activity and fibrosis stage as well as clinical insulin resistance. The most recent work has shown activation of the hedgehog pathway in correlation with DR.[88,89] The relationships of activated HPC with resolution of NASH and with hepatocarcinogenesis continue to be under investigation.

GRADING AND STAGING THE HISTOPATHOLOGIC LESIONS OF NAFLD

Grading and staging schemes developed for use in clinical trials of chronic liver diseases are not applicable to NAFLD/NASH because of the differing nature of the necroinflammatory lesions and fibrosis as detailed earlier. The first classification scheme specifically for NAFLD was published in 1999.[45] This study, however, did not give semiquantitative assessments. Brunt and colleagues[58] proposed a semiquantitative scheme to assign a histologic grade (global assessment of necroinflammatory activity) and stage (extent of fibrosis) to cases of NASH. The authors looked at 10 histologic variables commonly associated with NASH in 51 liver biopsies from adult patients clinically characterized as having NASH to determine which were most significantly associated with increasing severity. These features included macrovesicular steatosis, hepatocellular ballooning, intra-acinar (lobular) inflammation, portal tract inflammation, MDB, acidophil bodies, periodic acid-Schiff with diastase-stained Kupffer cells, glycogenated nuclei, lipogranulomas, and hepatocellular iron. Steatosis, ballooning, and inflammation (lobular and portal) were found to be the significant variables; steatosis amount, however, had the least affect on global grade. Steatosis is graded as 0, no involvement of hepatocytes; 1, less than 33% involvement; 2, 33% to 66%; and 3, greater than 66%. Ballooning is graded from mild to marked based on the number of hepatocytes showing the changes. The number of inflammatory foci per 200x field (0; 1: 1–2; 2: ≤4; 3: >4) is used to grade the lobular inflammation. Portal inflammation is graded as 0, none; 1, mild; 2, moderate; and 3, severe. The combined findings are used to assign a overall grade of mild (grade 1), moderate (grade 2), or severe (grade 3). The proposed staging system was designed to reflect the observation that fibrosis is often first seen in zone 3 in NASH. Stage 1 indicates zone 3 perisinusoidal/pericellular fibrosis; Stage 2, zone 3 and portal periportal fibrosis; Stage 3, bridging fibrosis; and Stage 4, cirrhosis. In 2005, the National Institute of Healh sponsored the National Institute of Diabetes and Digestive Kidney Disease.; the NASH Clinical Research Network Pathology Committee published the results of a validated histologic scoring system that encompassed the full spectrum of NAFLD (with and without steatohepatitis) for adult and pediatric NAFLD. The stated purpose was to be able to detect changes in disease activity with therapy, not form the basis of diagnosis.[90] To facilitate using this system, it was designed to only require H&E- and Masson's trichrome-stained slides. The committee recognized that steatohepatitis is a pattern of injury, and defining exact criteria to discriminate between NASH and non-NASH is difficult. A NAFLD activity score (NAS) is composed of steatosis, lobular inflammation, and ballooning. The steatosis scoring system of Brunt is modified to allow for the small amount of steatosis (<5%) that can be seen in the unaffected population (score 0: 5%; score 1: 5%–33%; score 2: 33%–66%; score 3: >66%). For simplification, ballooning scores are reduced to categories of none(0), few(1), or many(2). The lobular inflammation score is the same as that proposed by Brunt (scores 0–3). The NAS is then defined as the unweighted sum of the scores for steatosis, ballooning, and lobular inflammation (NAS 0–8). In analyzing the responses, cases with NAS of 0 to 2 were predominantly not diagnosed as having NASH, whereas scores of 5 or greater were often diagnosed as having NASH. Scores of 3 and 4 were divided nearly evenly between NASH and non-NASH and are therefore considered borderline for NASH. The fibrosis scoring system of Brunt and colleagues was modified to consider that in pediatric NAFLD, portal-based fibrosis can be seen in the absence of perisinusoidal fibrosis (stage 1C), as well as to formally differentiate delicate perisinusoidal fibrosis (1A) from dense (1B).

DRAWBACKS OF LIVER BIOPSY IN NAFLD/NASH

Attention to the challenges of liver biopsy in this burgeoning disease population has included the potential drawbacks of liver biopsy evaluation. Included are the potential of sampling differences in bariatric patients within or between lobes[91,92]; many of these can be overcome with large-bore needles.[93] Another concern is morbidity and mortality from liver biopsy itself. Although not specifically studied in NAFLD/NASH, in general, risk of morbidity is around 0.06% to 0.35% and risk of mortality, 0.01% to 0.1%.[94] Finally, pathologist interobserver variability is a concern raised in clinical reviews. In fact, pathologists with a focus on liver pathology have shown quite good interobserver agreements with steatosis amounts, fibrosis, and ballooning[90,95] but generally poor agreement for inflammation.[96] As in chronic hepatitis,[97] specialists tend to perform better in scoring NAFLD.[98]

REFERENCES

1. Flegal KM, Carroll MD, Ogden CL, et al. Prevalence and trends in obesity among US adults, 1999–2008. JAMA 2010;303(3):235–41.
2. Ogden CL, Carroll MD, Curtin LR, et al. Prevalence of high body mass index in US children and adolescents, 2007–2008. JAMA 2010;303:242–9.
3. Browning JD, Szczepaniak LS, Dobbins R, et al. Prevalence of hepatic steatosis in an urban population in the United States: impact of ethnicity. Hepatology 2004; 40:1387–95.
4. Fabbrini E, Magkos F, Mohammed BS, et al. Intrahepatic fat, not visceral fat, is linked with metabolic complications of obesity. Proc Natl Acad Sci U S A 2009; 106:15430–5.
5. Korenblat KM, Fabbrini E, Mohammed BS, et al. Liver, muscle, and adipose tissue insulin action is directly related to intrahepatic triglyceride content in obese subjects. Gastroenterology 2008;134:1369–75.
6. Schwimmer JB, Pardee PE, Lavine JE, et al. Cardiovascular risk factors and the metabolic syndrome in pediatric nonalcoholic fatty liver disease. Circulation 2008;118:277–83.
7. Yamaguchi K, Yang L, McCall S, et al. Inhibiting triglyceride synthesis improves hepatic steatosis but exacerbates liver damage and fibrosis in obese mice with nonalcoholic steatohepatitis. Hepatology 2007;45:1366–74.
8. Fujita K, Nozaki Y, Wada K, et al. Dysfunctional very-low-density lipoprotein synthesis and release is a key factor in nonalcoholic steatohepatitis pathogenesis. Hepatology 2009;50:772–80.
9. Li Z, Berk M, McIntyre TM, et al. Hepatic lipid partitioning and liver damage in nonalcoholic fatty liver disease: role of stearoyl-CoA desaturase. J Biol Chem 2009;284:5637–44.
10. Collison KS, Saleh SM, Bakheet RH, et al. Diabetes of the liver: the link between nonalcoholic fatty liver disease and HFCS-55. Obesity (Silver Spring) 2009;17: 2003–13.
11. Alkhouri N, Dixon LJ, Feldstein AE. Lipotoxicity in nonalcoholic fatty liver disease: not all lipids are created equal. Expert Rev Gastroenterol Hepatol 2009;3:445–51.
12. Gregor MF, Yang L, Fabbrini E, et al. Endoplasmic reticulum stress is reduced in tissues of obese subjects after weight loss. Diabetes 2009;58:693–700.
13. Singh R, Kaushik S, Wang Y, et al. Autophagy regulates lipid metabolism. Nature 2009;458(7242):1131–5.
14. Singh R, Xiang Y, Wang Y, et al. Autophagy regulates adipose mass and differentiation in mice. J Clin Invest 2009;119(11):3329–39.
15. Gastaldelli A, Kozakova M, Hojlund K, et al. Fatty liver is associated with insulin resistance, risk of coronary heart disease, and early atherosclerosis in a large European population. Hepatology 2009;49:1537–44.

16. Sorderberg C, Stal P, Askling J, et al. Decreased survival of subjects with elevated liver function tests during a 28 year follow-up. Hepatology 2010;51:595–602.
17. Ekstedt M, Franzen LE, Mathiesen UL, et al. Long-term follow-up of patients with NAFLD and elevated liver enzymes. Hepatology 2006;44:865–73.
18. Adams LA, Lymp JF, St. Sauver J, et al. The natural history of nonalcoholic fatty liver disease: a population-based cohort study. Gastroenterology 2005;129:113–21.
19. Wanless IR, Lentz JS. Fatty liver hepatitis (steatohepatitis) and obesity: an autopsy study with analysis of risk factors. Hepatology 1990;12(5):1106–10.
20. Adams LA, Angulo P. Insulin resistance, auto-antibodies, and nonalcoholic fatty liver disease. Response to Letter. Am J Gastroenterol 2005;100:1201–2.
21. Maher JJ, Leon P, Ryan JC. Beyond insulin resistance: innate immunity in NASH. Hepatology 2008;48:670–8.
22. Weston SR, Leyden W, Murphy R, et al. Racial and ethnic distribution of nonalcoholic fatty liver in persons with newly diagnosed chronic liver disease. Hepatology 2005;41:372–9.
23. Browning JD, Kumar KS, Saboorian H, et al. Ethnic differences in the prevalence of cryptogenic cirrhosis. Am J Gastroenterol 2004;99(2):292–8.
24. Wagenknecht LE, Scherzinger A, Stamm E, et al. Correlates and heritability of nonalcoholic fatty liver disease in a minority cohort. Obesity 2009;17:1240–6.
25. Guerrero R, Vega GL, Grundy SM, et al. Ethnic differences in hepatic steatosis: an insulin resistance paradox? Hepatology 2009;49:791–801.
26. Miele L, Beale G, Patman G, et al. The kruppel-like factor 6 genotype is associated with fibrosis in nonalcoholic fatty liver disease. Gastroenterology 2008;135:282–91.
27. Bochukova EG, Huang N, Keogh J, et al. Large, rare chromosomal deletions associated with severe early-onset obesity. Nature 2010;463(7281):666–70.
28. Romeo S, Kozlitina J, Xing C, et al. Genetic variation in PNPLA3 confers susceptibility to nonalcoholic fatty liver disease. Nat Genet 2008;40(12):1461–5.
29. Stepanova M, Hossain N, Afendy A, et al. Hepatic gene expression of Caucasian and African-American Patients with obesity-related non-alcoholic fatty liver disease. Obes Surg 2010;20(5):640–50.
30. Zelber-Sagi S, Nitzan-Kaluski D, Goldsmith R, et al. Role of leisure-time physical activity in nonalcoholic fatty liver disease: a population-based study. Hepatology 2008;48(6):179 1–8.
31. Neuschwander-Tetri BA. Lifestyle modification as the primary treatment of NASH. Clin Liver Dis 2009;13:649–66.
32. Pillai AA, Rinella ME. Nonalcoholic fatty liver disease: is bariatric surgery the answer? Clin Liver Dis 2009;13:689–710.
33. Angulo P. Long-term mortality in nonalcoholic fatty liver disease: is liver histology of any prognostic significance? [editorial comment]. Hepatology 2010;51:373–5.
34. Guha IN, Parkes J, Roderick P, et al. Noninvasive markers of fibrosis in nonalcoholic fatty liver disease: Validating the European Liver Fibrosis Panel and exploring simple markers. Hepatology 2008;47(2):455–60.
35. Harrison SA, Oliver D, Arnold HL, et al. Development and validation of a simple NAFLD clinical scoring system for identifying patients without advanced disease. Gut 2008;57(10):1441–7.
36. Wieckowska A, Feldstein AE. Diagnosis of nonalcoholic fatty liver disease: invasive versus noninvasive. Semin Liver Dis 2008;28:386–95.
37. Browning JD, Szczepaniak LS, Dobbins R, et al. Prevalence of hepatic steatosis in an urban population in the United States: impact of ethnicity. Hepatology 2004;40:1387–95.

38. Schwimmer JB, Behling C, Newbury R, et al. Histopathology of pediatric nonalcoholic fatty liver disease. Hepatology 2005;42:641–9.
39. Brunt EM, Tiniakos DG. Alcoholic and nonalcoholic fatty liver disease. In: Odze RD, Goldblum JR, editors. Surgical pathology of the GI tract, liver, biliary tract and pancreas. 2nd edition. Philadelphia: Elsevier; 2009. p. 1007–14.
40. Teli MR, Day CP, Burt AD, et al. Determinants of progression to cirrhosis or fibrosis in pure alcoholic fatty liver. Lancet 1995;346:987–90.
41. Fuji H, Ikura Y, Arimoto J, et al. Expression of perilipin and adipophilin in nonalcoholic fatty liver disease; relevance to oxidative injury and hepatocyte ballooning. J Atheroscler Thromb 2009;16:893–901.
42. Ishak KG. Light microscopic morphology of viral hepatitis. Am J Clin Pathol 1976; 65:787–827.
43. Ku NO, Strnad P, Zhong BH, et al. Keratins let liver live: Mutations predispose to liver disease and crosslinking generates Mallory-Denk bodies. Hepatology 2007; 46:1639–49.
44. Lackner C, Zatloukal K, Stumptner C, et al. Keratin immunostaining as objective marker of hepatocyte ballooning in steatohepatitis. J Hepatol 2007;46(Suppl 1): S266A.
45. Matteoni CA, Younossi ZM, Gramlich T, et al. Nonalcoholic fatty liver disease: A spectrum of clinical and pathological severity. Gastroenterology 1999;116(6): 1413–9.
46. Brunt EM. Nonalcoholic steatohepatitis. Semin Liver Dis 2004;24:3–20.
47. Brunt EM, Neuschwander-Tetri BA, Oliver D, et al. Nonalcoholic steatohepatitis: histologic features and clinical correlations with 30 blinded biopsy specimens. Hum Pathol 2004;35(9):1070–82.
48. Ferrell L, Belt P, Bass N. Arterialization of central zones in nonalcoholic steatohepatitis. Hepatology 2007;46:732A.
49. Roskams T, Yang SQ, Koteish A, et al. Oxidative stress and oval cell accumulation in mice and humans with alcoholic and nonalcoholic fatty liver disease. Am J Pathol 2003;163:1301–11.
50. Brunt EM. Nonalcoholic fatty liver disease. In: Burt AD, Portmann BG, Ferrell LD, editors. MacSween's pathology of the liver. 5th edition. Edinburgh (UK): Churchill Livingstone; 2007. p. 367–98.
51. Brunt EM, Kleiner DE, Wilson LA, et al. Portal chronic inflammation in nonalcoholic fatty liver disease (NAFLD): A histologic marker of advanced NAFLD-Clinicopathologic correlations from the nonalcoholic steatohepatitis clinical research network. Hepatology 2009;46:809–20.
52. Brunt EM, Clouston AD. Histologic features of fatty liver disease. In: Bataller R, Caballeria J, editors. Nonalcoholic steatohepatitis (NASH). Barcelona (Spain): Permanyer; 2007. p. 95–110.
53. Brunt EM, Ramrakhiani S, Cordes BG, et al. Concurrence of histologic features of steatohepatitis with other forms of chronic liver disease. Mod Pathol 2003;16: 49–56.
54. Ramesh S, Sanyal AJ. Hepatitis C and nonalcoholic fatty liver disease. Semin Liver Dis 2004;24(4):399–413.
55. Stumptner C, Fuchsbichler A, Heid H, et al. Mallory Body - A disease-associated type of sequestosome. Hepatology 2002;35:1053–62.
56. Denk H, Stumptner C, Zatloukal K. Mallory bodies revisited. J Hepatol 2000;32: 689–702.
57. Carter-Kent CA, Yerian LM, Brunt EM, et al. Nonalcoholic Steatohepatitis in children: a multicenter clinicopathological study. Hepatology 2008;48:804A.

58. Brunt EM, Janney CG, Di Bisceglie AM, et al. Nonalcoholic steatohepatitis: a proposal for grading and staging the histological lesions. Am J Gastroenterol 1999;94(9):2467–74.
59. Feldstein AE, Gores GJ. Apoptosis in alcoholic and nonalcoholic steatohepatitis. Front Biosci 2005;10:3093–9.
60. Wieckowska A, Zein NN, Yerian LM, et al. In vivo assessment of liver cell apoptosis as a novel biomarker of disease severity in nonalcoholic fatty liver disease. Hepatology 2006;44:27–33.
61. Yeh M, Belt P, Brunt EM, et al. Acidophil body index may help diagnosing nonalcoholic steatohepatitis. Mod Pathol 2009;22:326A.
62. Feldstein AE, Wieckowska A, Lopez AR, et al. Cytokeratin-18 fragment levels as noninvasive biomarkers for nonalcoholic steatohepatitis: a multicenter validation study. Hepatology 2009;50(4):1072–8.
63. Brunt EM. Nonalcoholic steatohepatitis: Definition and pathology. Semin Liver Dis 2001;21(1):3–16.
64. Burt AD. Liver pathology associated with diseases of other organs or systems. In: Burt AD, Portmann BG, Ferrell LD, editors. MacSween's pathology of the liver. 5th edition. Edinburgh (UK): Churchill Livingstone; 2007. p. 811–932.
65. Cortez-Pinto H, Baptista A, Camilo ME, et al. Nonalcoholic steatohepatitis - clinicopathological comparison with alcoholic hepatitis in ambulatory and hospitalized patients. Dig Dis Sci 1996;41(1):172–9.
66. Lefkowitch JH, Haythe J, Regent N. Kupffer cell aggregation and perivenular distribution in steatohepatitis. Mod Pathol 2002;15:699–704.
67. Luca V, Ludovica FA, Elisabetta B, et al. HFE genotype, parenchymal iron accumulation, and liver fibrosis in patients with nonalcoholic fatty liver disease. Gastroenterology 2010;138(3):905–12.
68. Le TH, Caldwell SH, Redick JA, et al. The zonal distribution of megamitochondria with crystalline inclusions in nonalcoholic steatohepatitis. Hepatology 2004;39:1423–9.
69. Caldwell SH, Swerdlow RH, Khan EM, et al. Mitochondrial abnormalities in nonalcoholic steatohepatitis. J Hepatol 1999;31(3):430–4.
70. Sanyal AJ, Campbell-Sargent C, Mirshahi F, et al. Nonalcoholic steatohepatitis: association of insulin resistance and mitochondrial abnormalities. Gastroenterology 2001;120(5):1183–92.
71. Caldwell SH, Chang CY, Nakamoto RK, et al. Mitochondria in nonalcoholic fatty liver disease. Clin Liver Dis 2004;8:595–617.
72. Brunt EM. Alcoholic and nonalcoholic steatohepatitis. Clin Liver Dis 2002;6: 399–420.
73. Goodman ZD, Ishak KG. Occlusive venous lesions in alcoholic liver disease. Gastroenterology 1982;83:786–96.
74. Sanderson S, Smyrk TC. The use of protein tyrosine phosphatase 1B and insulin receptor immunostains to differentiate nonalcoholic from alcoholic steatohepatitis in liver biopsy specimens. Am J Clin Pathol 2005;123:503–9.
75. Dunn W, Angulo P, Sanderson S, et al. Utility of a new model to diagnose an alcoholic basis for steatohepatitis. Gastroenterology 2006;131:1057–63.
76. Nakayama H, Itoh H, Kunita S, et al. Presence of perivenular elastic fibers in nonalcoholic steatohepatitis fibrosis stage III. Histol Histopathol 2008;23:407–9.
77. Abrams GA, Kunde SS, Lazenby AJ, et al. Portal fibrosis and hepatic steatosis in morbidly obese subjects: a spectrum of nonalcoholic fatty liver disease. Hepatology 2004;40:475–83.
78. Patton HM, Lavine JE, Van Natta ML, et al. Clinical correlates of histopathology in pediatric nonalcoholic steatohepatitis. Gastroenterology 2008;135:1961–71.

79. Washington K, Wright K, Shyr Y, et al. Hepatic stellate cell activation in nonalcoholic steatohepatitis and fatty liver. Hum Pathol 2000;31(7):822–8.
80. Cortez-Pinto H, Baptista A, Camilo ME, et al. Hepatic stellate cell activation occurs in nonalcoholic steatohepatitis. Hepatogastroenterology 2001;48(37):87–90.
81. Feldstein AE, Papouchado BG, Angulo P, et al. Hepatic stellate cells and fibrosis progression in patients with nonalcoholic fatty liver disease. Clin Gastroenterol Hepatol 2005;3:384–9.
82. Angulo P, Keach JC, Batts KP, et al. Independent predictors of liver fibrosis in patients with nonalcoholic steatohepatitis. Hepatology 1999;30(6):1356–62.
83. Ratziu V, Giral P, Charlotte F, et al. Liver fibrosis in overweight patients. Gastroenterology 2000;118(6):1117–23.
84. Dixon JB, Bhatal PS, O'Brien PE. Nonalcoholic fatty liver disease: predictors of nonalcoholic steatohepatitis and liver fibrosis in the severely obese. Gastroenterology 2001;121:91–100.
85. Roskams TA, Theise ND, Balabaud C, et al. Nomenclature of the finer branches of the biliary tree: canals, ductules and ductular reactions in human livers. Hepatology 2004;39:1739–45.
86. Richardson MM, Jonsson JR, Powell EE, et al. Progressive fibrosis in nonalcoholic steatohepatitis: association with altered regeneration and the ductular reaction. Gastroenterology 2007;133:80–90.
87. Clouston AD, Powell EE, Walsh MJ, et al. Fibrosis correlates with a ductular reaction in hepatitis C: roles of impaired replication, progenitor cells and steatosis. Hepatology 2005;41:809–19.
88. Omenetti A, Porrello A, Jung Y, et al. Hedgehog signaling regulates epithelial-mesenchymal transition during biliary fibrosis in rodents and humans. J Clin Invest 2008;118:3331–42.
89. Syn W-K, Jung Y, Omenetti A, et al. Hedgehog-mediated epithelial-to-mesenchymal transition and fibrogenic repair in nonalcoholic fatty liver disease. Gastroenterology 2009;137(4):1478–88, e1478.
90. Kleiner DE, Brunt EM, Van Natta M, et al. Design and validation of a histological scoring system for nonalcoholic fatty liver disease. Hepatology 2005;41(6):1313–21.
91. Ratziu V, Charlotte F, Heurtier A, et al. Sampling variability of liver biopsy in nonalcoholic fatty liver disease. Gastroenterology 2005;128:1898–906.
92. Merriman RB, Ferrell LD, Patti MG, et al. Histologic correlation of paired right lobe and left lobe liver biopsies in morbidly obese individuals with suspected nonalcoholic fatty liver disease. Hepatology 2003;39:232A.
93. Larson SP, Bowers SP, Palekar NA, et al. Histopathologic variability between the right and left lobes of the liver in morbidly obese patients undergoing roux-en-Y bypass. Clin Gastroenterol Hepatol 2007;5:1329–32.
94. Brown KE, Washington K, Brunt EM. Liver biopsy: indications, technique, complications and interpretation. In: Bacon BR, O'Grady JG, Di Bisceglie AM, et al, editors. Comprehensive clinical hepatology. China: Mosby/Elsevier; 2006. p. 101–21.
95. Younossi ZM, Gramlich T, Liu YC, et al. Nonalcoholic fatty liver disease - assessment of variability in pathologic interpretations. Mod Pathol 1998;11(6):560–5.
96. Brunt EM. Pathology of fatty liver disease. Mod Pathol 2007;20:S40–8.
97. Rousselet M-C, Michalak S, Dupre F, et al. Sources of variability in histological scoring of chronic viral hepatitis. Hepatology 2005;41:257–64.
98. Vuppalanchi R, Unalp A, Van Natta ML, et al. Effects of liver biopsy sample length and number of readings on histologic yield for nonalcoholic fatty liver disease. Clin Gastroenterol Hepatol 2009;7:481–6.

Hepatic Granulomas: Pathogenesis and Differential Diagnosis

Stephen M. Lagana, MD[a],*, Roger K. Moreira, MD[a],
Jay H. Lefkowitch, MD[b]

KEYWORDS

• Hepatic granuloma • Granulomatous hepatitis • Sarcoidosis
• Primary biliary cirrhosis

Granulomas are rounded microscopic aggregates of macrophages and lymphocytes with or without other features, such as necrosis, organisms, inclusions, foreign materials, fibrosis, or multinucleated giant cells. Granulomas form as responses to a variety of exogenous and/or endogenous chronic antigenic stimuli. Hepatic granulomas may be a local response to a specific causative agent (eg, bacterial or fungal infections) or may reflect a more generalized systemic granulomatous disease (eg, sarcoidosis).

Although the specific cause of granulomas in individual cases is often unclear, they are thought to originate as a response to chronic exposure to antigens that are either foreign or native. Granulomas may be present in a wide range of conditions, and the search for a specific cause is frequently challenging.

This article summarizes the current principles concerning the biology of granuloma formation in different diseases and examines the histomorphology and causes of hepatic granulomas. The practical issues in the histopathologic differential diagnosis and workup of hepatic granulomas are also presented.

GRANULOMA BIOLOGY

Granulomas are formed through the interaction of a variety of immune cells, chiefly between CD4$^+$ helper T (T$_H$) lymphocytes and macrophages. The most basic immune-type granuloma is formed when antigen-presenting cells (APCs) engulf antigenic material that is presented to T lymphocytes. These APCs are frequently macrophages, but in some diseases, specifically sarcoidosis, there is an evolving literature concerning dendritic cells as APCs. Dendritic cells have more antigen-presenting

[a] Department of Pathology and Cell Biology, Columbia University Medical Center, New York, NY 10032, USA
[b] Department of Pathology, College of Physicians and Surgeons, Columbia University, 630 West 168th Street–PH 15 West, Room 1574, New York, NY 10032, USA
* Corresponding author. Department of Pathology and Cell Biology, Columbia University College of Physicians and Surgeons, 630 West 168th Street, VC14-239, New York, NY 10032.
E-mail address: sml9012@nyp.org

Clin Liver Dis 14 (2010) 605–617
doi:10.1016/j.cld.2010.07.005
1089-3261/10/$ – see front matter © 2010 Elsevier Inc. All rights reserved.

capacity than macrophages, although in sarcoidosis, they may have less than the dendritic cells of healthy controls.[1] In bronchoalveolar lavage fluid, patients with sarcoidosis displayed a 2-fold increase in dendritic cell count (with an immature phenotype) when compared with other inflammatory conditions of lung.[1] Regardless of the type of APC, the T lymphocytes then commonly produce a reaction through the T_H1 or T_H2 pathway. Each pathway is classically associated with various granulomatous disorders (T_H1 with tuberculosis and early sarcoidosis, T_H2 with parasitic infections),[2] although there are numerous examples of T_H phenotype switching throughout the course of disease. In the T_H1 pathway, the $CD4^+$ T lymphocytes produce IL-2 and interferon gamma (IFN-γ) which are cytokines that recruit additional $CD4^+$ T lymphocytes and macrophages, respectively, thus creating a positive feedback loop.[3] IFN-γ generally induces macrophage activity through the Jak/STAT1-α pathway.[2] These stages comprise what is referred to as the initiation and accumulation stages of the granulomatous reaction.[4] These 2 formative stages of granuloma development rely on a lengthy and nonspecific list of chemokines; however, it is thought that the most important chemical mediators of the formative process are osteopontin derived from macrophages and T lymphocytes, T-lymphocyte–derived tumor necrosis factor (TNF) and chemokine (C-C motif) ligand 2 and its receptors.[4] The role of TNF is further supported by the increased risk of infection with organisms commonly known to cause granulomatous disease in patients receiving TNF-inhibitor therapy. These same properties likely underlie the partial therapeutic efficacy of these drugs in patients with autoimmune (or possibly/partially autoimmune) disorders such as sarcoidosis, rheumatoid arthritis, and Wegener granulomatosis.[5] The next phase of granuloma development (effector phase) is the source of much of the variability in composition, because it is possible to have lymphocytic (with $CD8^+$ and $CD4^+$ T lymphocytes with either T_H1 or T_H2 phenotypes) and/or granulocytic effectors.[4] The T_H1 type is traditionally characterized by IFN-γ and TNF, whereas T_H2 is classically marked by IL-4, IL-5, and IL-13.[4]

The final stage is resolution in which T lymphocytes (possibly regulatory T lymphocytes) again play a vital role. A recent study was performed by serial tissue examination of the myocardium of a patient with cardiac sarcoidosis. This study demonstrated that early in the course of the disease, the cytokine milieu represented a T_H1-type response (high levels of IFN-γ, IL-2, IL-12) associated with numerous granulomas on endomyocardial biopsy. One year later, a shift to a T_H2-type (thought to be antiinflammatory) response had occurred (IL-4, IL-5, IL-10, IL-13). This shift coincided with the absence of granulomas on biopsy and the development of fibrosis.[6]

TRENDS IN THE INCIDENCE OF HEPATIC GRANULOMAS

The epidemiology of hepatic granulomas over the past several decades has shifted due to several factors including (1) the identification of the hepatitis C virus (HCV) and its recognition as a potential cause of hepatic granulomas; (2) the declining incidence of opportunistic agent–related granulomas in patients with human immunodeficiency virus or AIDS since the introduction of antiretroviral therapy; (3) the worldwide growth in liver transplantation, with possible associated granulomatous liver disease (discussed later); and (4) the growing list of therapeutic, alternative, and herbal agents, which may cause hepatic granulomas because of a hypersensitivity response.

The reported prevalence of granulomas in unselected liver biopsy samples is approximately 4% as summarized in several studies in **Table 1**. Noninfectious immunologic insults, infection, foreign body reactions, drugs, and neoplasia represent the 5 main underlying categories of conditions associated with hepatic granulomas.[7]

Table 1
Causative categories of granulomas as described in recent Western series

First Author	Country	Year	Number of Cases	Granuloma, Number (%)	Immune	Infectious	Drug	Foreign Body	Neoplastic	Idiopathic
Gaya[10,a]	Scotland	2003	1662	63(3.8)	31 (PBC 15, sarcoid 7, AIH 3)	9	6	0	5	12
Sartin[53,b]	United States	1991	Not provided	88 (NA)	24 (sarcoid 19, PBC 4)	9	5	0	3	47
McCluggage[11,c]	Ireland	1994	4075	163 (4)	129 (PBC 90, sarcoid 30)	6	2	1	3	22
Drebber[12,d]	Germany	2008	12,161	442 (3.6)	253 (PBC 215, sarcoid 37)	9	11	0	3	146
Dourakis[13]	Greece	2007	1768	66 (3.7)	51 (PBC 41, sarcoid 5)	8	2	0	1	4
Martin-Blondel[14]	France	2010	471	21 (4.5)	13 (PBC 5, sarcoid 2)	3	0	0	2	3

Certain cases in individual series are reclassified here for the purpose of tabulation.

Abbreviations: AIH, autoimmune hepatitis; NA, not available; PBC, primary biliary cirrhosis.
[a] Two cases of biliary obstruction cited in this report are shown here under idiopathic. Treatment with BCG vaccine was included under drug related.
[b] HCV cases are included under infectious.
[c] Gout, cryptogenic cirrhosis, and biliary obstruction are included under idiopathic.
[d] Cases of HCV, hepatitis B virus, syphilis, and *Bartonella henselae* are included under infectious. Ulcerative colitis is included under immune.

The commonality of possible causes varies depending on study, but some basic trends apply. Studies from the Western world show a striking preponderance of noninfectious immune-type insults, whereas those from the developing world skew heavily toward infection.[8,9] Some articles cite incidence rates as high as 15%, as described in an older study from Saudi Arabia,[8] with findings not generalizable to developed Western countries (such as high rates of schistosomiasis, tuberculosis, and other diseases). In fact, recent studies from Saudi Arabia have shown a markedly reduced rate of granulomatous inflammation (1.2%) in unselected liver biopsy samples.[9]

NONINFECTIOUS IMMUNOLOGIC DISEASES AND HEPATIC GRANULOMAS

Noninfectious immunologic insults are the most common cause of hepatic granulomas in the developed world and include primary biliary cirrhosis (PBC) and sarcoidosis. Morphologically, most hepatic granulomas in this category are epithelioid (**Fig. 1**), featuring enlarged macrophages with abundant cytoplasm and other constituents, including variable numbers of lymphocytes, neutrophils, and eosinophils, sometimes with necrosis.

PBC

PBC is the most common cause of hepatic granulomas in the developed world.[10–14] PBC causes chronic cholestasis because of autoimmune destruction of intrahepatic biliary epithelium and can lead to cirrhosis and liver failure. The hallmark serologic test is the M2 antimitochondrial antibody (AMA).[15] As with many rare diseases, the incidence of PBC is variable. A study of PBC in Canada found the incidence to be

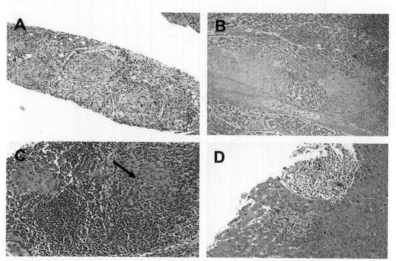

Fig. 1. (A) Multiple, large, epithelioid granulomas in a patient with sarcoidosis (hematoxylin-eosin, original magnification ×10). (B) Two large granulomas involving a branch of the portal vein in sarcoidosis (hematoxylin-eosin, original magnification ×4). (C) Two granulomas with a robust lymphoid infiltrate in a patient with primary biliary cirrhosis. The arrow demonstrates a native bile duct that is highly involved by inflammatory cells (hematoxylin-eosin, original magnification ×40). (D) A large periportal granuloma in a patient with acute rejection of an allograft (note the inflammatory infiltrate in the nearby portal tract) (hematoxylin-eosin, original magnification ×20). The patient originally underwent a transplant for acetaminophen overdose.

near to 30 per million persons, with a strong female predominance, as in most studies.[16]

PBC is caused by autoreactive lymphoid cells (primarily CD4$^+$ T lymphocytes) that target the E2 component of the pyruvate hydrogenase (PDC-E2) molecule on bile duct epithelium. There are strong genetic predisposing factors in PBC, with first-degree relatives having a 50- to 100-fold increased incidence. These genetic factors are likely those that interfere with proper immune tolerance because PBC-affected families also display a higher incidence of other autoimmune diseases.[15] Environmental factors likely play a role as well. AMA is known to react with prokaryotic antigens (PDC-E2 is widely conserved), and so, molecular mimicry may be a possible initiating event.[17]

Microscopically, the pathognomonic lesion of PBC is the florid bile duct lesion (segmental destructive cholangitis), which is characterized by portal inflammation composed of lymphocytes, plasma cells, and often, prominent eosinophils.

A recent study correlated histopathologic features with biochemical findings in more than 250 patients with suspected PBC or PBC-autoimmune hepatitis overlap syndrome. Granulomas were found in about half of biopsies of the PBC group, almost 75% showed fibrosis (usually mild), and 20% showed ductopenia. Almost 20% of these cases showed concentric periductal fibrosis (onion skinning), a feature that may create confusion with primary sclerosing cholangitis. Granulomas in PBC are typically situated within portal tracts surrounding, or near to, damaged bile ducts. However, as pointed out by Drebber and colleagues,[18] lobular granulomas may also be seen. When present, these granulomas are usually small and composed solely of macrophages.

Sarcoidosis

The incidence of sarcoidosis varies greatly by ethnic group and region and is high in African American and Scandinavian populations.[19,20] Hepatic involvement is uncommonly detected clinically (5%–21% of known cases have hepatomegaly), but involvement is often found microscopically (50%–80% prevalence in liver biopsies in known cases).[21,22] Notably, autopsy series tend not to show significantly greater sensitivity than biopsy in the detection of granulomas in patients with known sarcoidosis, suggesting that when present, hepatic involvement by sarcoid is fairly widespread.[22] This is in contrast to other organs (such as the heart) in which biopsy is a relatively insensitive diagnostic technique, as evidenced by higher levels of involvement at autopsy.[23] Indeed, biopsy is even more sensitive than laboratory testing, although about 35% of patients with sarcoidosis will have elevations in alkaline phosphatase and γ-glutamyltransferase levels.[22] Clinical consequences of liver disease are rare in patients with sarcoidosis, but in approximately 1% of the patients, severe complications such as cirrhosis, Budd-Chiari syndrome, and portal hypertension can develop.[21] It has been suggested that the pathogenesis of cirrhosis in sarcoid involves ischemia secondary to granulomatous phlebitis of portal and hepatic veins (see **Fig. 1B**).[24] Symptoms of liver disease (including cholestasis) have been reported as the only manifestation of sarcoid.[25]

The pathologic condition of hepatic sarcoidosis is characterized by nonnecrotizing portal tract–based granulomas, although sarcoid granulomas may be seen in any location (including the lobular parenchyma). The tendency of sarcoid granulomas to cluster in periportal regions and produce hyaline fibrosis is well recognized. Progression of the fibrosis may result in cirrhosis. Over time, sarcoid granulomas become more compact and have fewer lymphocytes.[26] The macrophages are usually epithelioid and form multinucleated giant cells. The giant cells can be foreign body type, or the more classic Langhan type and often contain Schaumann or asteroid bodies.

Schaumann bodies are irregular, concentrically laminated, intracellular inclusion bodies consisting of calcified proteins not very dissimilar to small psammoma bodies.[27] In other organs, they are found more commonly in sarcoidosis than in infectious granulomatous inflammation; however, they are certainly not specific.[26-29]

Asteroid bodies are visually striking stellate-shaped inclusion bodies usually found within a cytoplasmic clearing. They are composed of noncollagenous filaments and myelinoid membranes and can be stained with antiubiquitin antibodies.[27]

In 1993, Devaney and colleagues,[30] at the Armed Forces Institute of Pathology in Washington, DC, reported on the histomorphology of 100 sarcoid biopsies with granulomas. Findings present in association with granulomas included parenchymal necroinflammatory foci in 40% of biopsies and portal inflammation in 31%, with 12% displaying interface hepatitis. The necroinflammation may closely resemble that of chronic hepatitis, and serologic exclusion of infection by hepatitis B virus (HBV) or HCV may be warranted in some cases.Loss of bile ducts was reported in 37% of patients, and 31% had features of acute or chronic cholangitis.

Sarcoid granulomas only rarely exhibit extensive true necrosis[31] that should not be confused microscopically with the common dense hyaline fibrosis associated with sarcoidosis (**Fig. 2**).

Other Noninfectious Causes

Crohn disease commonly causes granulomatous inflammation in the luminal gastrointestinal tract but only exceptionally in the liver.[25]

Vasculitis such as Wegener granulomatosis can involve the liver, and an association between hepatic granulomas and Sjögren syndrome has been described.[32]

Granulomas in liver allografts after liver transplant are relatively rare occurrences. In one study of posttransplant biopsies, granulomas were found in 42 of 563 patients and were thought to be acute rejection–related in 2 patients.[33] These granulomas originated in portal tracts and extended outward. Hypothetically, the release of antigenic material from bile ducts or vascular endothelium damaged by the rejection infiltrate could promote the granulomatous response. Rather than being a component of the acute-rejection response, posttransplant granulomas may also be attributable to other causes, and drug hepatotoxicity and infection must be considered.[34]

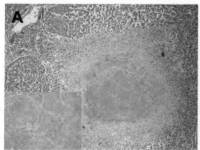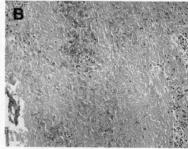

Fig. 2. (*A*) A large hyalinized granuloma in a well-established case of sarcoidosis (hematoxylin-eosin, original magnification ×4). Note the lack of cellular debris in the areas of hyalinization (inset; hematoxylin-eosin, original magnification ×40). This lack of cellular debris is one of the useful features in differentiating hyalinization (pseudonecrosis) from true necrosis. (*B*) A truly necrotic granuloma in a patient who had positive acid-fast bacilli (AFB) staining (hematoxylin-eosin, original magnification ×10). Note the ample cellular debris in the necrotic region.

The authors reviewed their departmental database of posttransplant allograft biopsies for a 6-year period and found 10 of 762 biopsies with acute rejection and granulomas without other obvious causes beyond acute rejection. Cases in which the native liver disease was known to prominently feature granulomas (eg, sarcoid, PBC) were excluded. In 8 of 10 cases, acid-fast bacilli (AFB) and Gomori methenamine silver (GMS) staining techniques had been performed and the results were negative.

In the 10 cases in which the granulomas were attributed to acute rejection, their location was intraportal, periportal, and rarely, pericentral (adjacent to a central vein with endotheliitis). In portal or periportal regions, the granulomas were noted to be contiguous with, or in close proximity to, the typical lesions of acute rejection. The presence of eosinophils within both the acute-rejection response and the granulomas further supported the granuloma being a part of the rejection process. The absence of granulomas with eosinophils elsewhere within the lobules in such cases was evidence against the possible alternative diagnosis of drug hepatotoxicity. The occasional granulomas that appeared to lie outside, but near the portal tracts, on deeper levels were shown to be contiguous with the typical portal immune infiltrates of acute rejection. Multinucleated giant cells were rare (1 case). In the cases studied by the authors, the granulomas were absent in subsequent biopsies in all patients (usually associated with significant improvement or resolution of the acute rejection).

Recurrent HCV infection in the allograft is an alternative cause of granulomas, although the HCV-related granuloma is usually small, histiocytic, and can be found deep within the lobular parenchyma away from portal tracts and may be present in subsequent allograft biopsies.[35]

Based on the authors' experience, the factors that favor acute rejection as the cause of posttransplant granulomas include (1) proximity to portal tracts demonstrating acute rejection, (2) presence of eosinophils, (3) negative AFB staining and GMS staining, (4) absence of granulomatous disease in the native liver, and (5) disappearance of granulomas on improvement of the rejection.

INFECTIOUS DISEASES AND HEPATIC GRANULOMAS

Infectious disease is the most common cause of hepatic granulomas in the developing world. Most infectious granulomas are epithelioid and some have necrosis (**Fig. 3**). Fibrin-ring granulomas are an unusual variant characterized by the presence of an epithelioid granuloma with a central lipid vacuole and a surrounding ring of fibrin. These granulomas are more common in infection and were classically associated with Q fever (*Coxiella burnetii*) but also can be seen in toxoplasmosis; salmonella, cytomegalovirus, and Epstein-Barr virus infections; drug reactions (allopurinol); and systemic lupus erythematous.[36]

In 1993, HCV was first reported as a cause of hepatic granulomas by Emile and colleagues,[37] who found granulomas in approximately 10% of cirrhotic livers explanted for HCV. By biopsy, the finding is rare, with one large series reporting an incidence of 1.3%.[38] Another large study reported a similar incidence of 1.24%.[39] Granulomas can also be found after a transplant for HCV. One study found granulomas in 8% of patients who underwent a transplant for HCV.[35] A large study of granulomas in biopsies of patients who received a transplant for HCV found an incidence of 0.24%.[40]

Histologically, HCV granulomas are typically epithelioid, nonnecrotizing, and located within the lobules. Additional features can include the presence of giant cells and a rim of lypmphocytes.[37]

HBV can rarely cause hepatic granulomas.[41] The incidence has not been studied extensively, but one study found granulomas in 3 of 151 (approximately 2%) biopsies

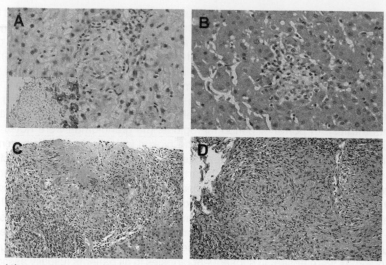

Fig. 3. (*A*) A nonnecrotizing periportal epithelioid granuloma in a patient with chronic hepatitis B (hematoxylin-eosin, original magnification ×20). The inset shows the immunoperoxidase staining for hepatitis B core antigen (immunoperoxidase, original magnification ×20). (*B*) A small, nonnecrotizing, epithelioid lobular granuloma in a patient with chronic HCV (hematoxylin-eosin, original magnification ×20). (*C*) A large necrotizing granuloma in a patient with Lyme disease (hematoxylin-eosin, original magnification ×10). (*D*) An area containing nonnecrotizing granulomas in a patient with positive AFB staining (hematoxylin-eosin, original magnification ×10) (the same biopsy specimen as **Fig. 2**B).

of patients with HBV.[42] A larger study put the number at about 1.5%, suggesting that the rates of granulomas in HBV are fairly similar to those of HCV.[43] As with HCV-related granulomas, they are described as epithelioid and nonnecrotizing.[43]

Mycobacterium tuberculosis often causes hepatic granulomas in infected patients (particularly those with the miliary form) and can have an associated reactive hepatitis. The granulomas tend to be caseating with giant cells and can coalesce to form nodules referred to as tubercles. Resolution often displays fibrosis and calcification.[36] Tuberculosis can present as an isolated finding in the liver, although this is exceptional.[44] The workup of any hepatic granuloma should start with a stain for AFB and a silver stain for fungi (such as GMS), and this is doubly true for caseating granulomas.

Mycobacterium avium-intracellulare complex (classically found in patients with immunosuppression) causes hepatic granulomas in more than half of patients with the disease.[36] There are striking differences between the histologic findings of patients with immunocompetence and immunosuppression. Immunocompetent patients have more classic epithelioid granulomas with an associated mixed inflammatory infiltrate (lymphocytes and granulocytes) without many organisms on AFB staining. Patients lacking an intact immune system show aggregates of foamy macrophages without much inflammation and with numerous organisms on AFB staining,[36] as was exemplified at the height of the AIDS epidemic.

Lyme disease is the most common tick-borne illness in the United States. Humans become infected through the bite of the *Ixodes* ticks that transfers the causative pathogen, *Borrelia burgdorferi*.[45] Abnormal liver function tests occur rarely in this condition, and necrotizing hepatic granulomas have recently been reported (see **Fig. 3**C).[46]

Other known causes of hepatic granulomas include *Mycobacterium leprae, Bartonella henselae, Rickettsia,* tularemia, *Listeria,* Whipple disease, *Salmonella* (including as part of typhoid fever), syphilis, *Chlamydia, Rhodococcus, Yersinia,* and bacille Calmette-Guérin disease.[36,47,48]

Hepatic involvement by *Candida* spp frequently causes suppurative granulomatous inflammation. Other fungi such as *Histoplasma, Aspergillus,* and *Mucor;* the protozoan *Toxoplasma;* and diseases such as nocardiosis, actinomycosis, and coccidiomycosis can also cause granulomas.[36,47] Staining with GMS, periodic acid–Schiff, and mucicarmine is often helpful in identification of fungi.

Parasitic infections can also cause hepatic granulomas. Schistosomal granulomas often contain abundant eosinophils and develop several weeks after infection in response to eggs laid by the infective worms. Clinically, this can lead to cirrhosis and portal hypertension.[49] The granulomatous response is usually of the T_H2 variety, and it has recently been demonstrated that IL-13 blockade may aid in preventing fibrosis, which is responsible for much of the morbidity and mortality.[50]

FOREIGN BODIES AND HEPATIC GRANULOMAS

Foreign body–type granulomas require few T-lymphocyte interactions and are composed almost entirely of macrophages forming giant cells as part of innate immunity.[4] The clinical history may disclose the source (eg, talc in intravenous drug users or suture material after surgery). Morphologically, demonstration of polarizable material in the granulomas helps to make the diagnosis.

DRUGS AND HEPATIC GRANULOMAS

Granulomas caused by drugs often have nonspecific features (**Fig. 4**) and may be located anywhere in the liver. They may have variable sizes, and eosinophils are often helpful in assigning drug causation. Drug hepatotoxicity may also induce accompanying changes of an acute hepatitis, cholestasis, or steatosis. A lengthy list of medications may result in hepatic granulomas (**Table 2**).[51] Newer agents, such as etanercept, continue to be identified as causes.[52]

NEOPLASIA AND HEPATIC GRANULOMAS

Benign and malignant neoplasms, including primary and metastatic tumors, have been reported in association with hepatic granulomas. Hodgkin disease may be the

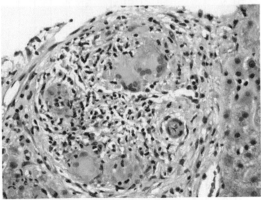

Fig. 4. A large epithelioid portal granuloma with many eosinophils is noted (hematoxylin-eosin, original magnification ×40). This granuloma was attributed to drug reaction.

Table 2
Drugs associated with hepatic granulomas

Miscellaneous	Neurologic	Antimicrobial	Cardiovascular	Biologic	Hypoglycemic	Herbal/ Alternative	Antiinflammatory	Antineoplastic
Allopurinol	Carbamazepine	Cephalexin	Chinidine (antiarrythmic)	Etanercept[52]	Glyburide	Seatone	Aspirin	Procarbazine
BCG	Chlorpromazine	Dapsone	Diltiazem[54]	Peginterferon[40]	Tolbutamide	Green juice[55]	Dimethicone	
Feprazone	Methyldopa	Isoniazid	Disopyramide		Rosiglitazone[56]		Gold	
Contraceptives	Diazepam	Nitrofurantoin	Hydralazine				Phenazone	
Halothane	Phenytoin	Oxacillin	Metolazone				Sulfasalazine	
Mineral oil		Penicillin	Phenprocoumon				Mesalamine[57]	
Papaverine		Sulfa antibiotics	Prajmalium					
Ranitidine			Procainamide					
Quinine			Quinidine					
Propylthiouracil[58]			Tocainide					
Saridon (Excedrin)[59]			Trichlormethiazide					
			Hydrochlorothiazide[60]					
			Clofibrate[61]					

Data from Ishak KG, Zimmerman HJ. Drug-induced and toxic granulomatous hepatitis. Baillieres Clin Gastroenterol 1986;2:463–80.

cause of hepatic granulomas in 8% to 17% of cases.[10] Other neoplasms including leukemias, gastrointestinal adenocarcinomas, and hepatocellular carcinomas have also been reported.[10–14]

SUMMARY

Identification of granulomas in liver biopsy and postmortem specimens requires consideration of systemic immunologic disorders, infectious diseases, drug hepatotoxicity and, occasionally, reaction to an intra- or extrahepatic neoplasm. Based on studies from Western countries, the current incidence of granulomas in liver biopsies is approximately 4%, a statistic that should replace older data that suggest an incidence as high as 15%. Staining procedures (AFB and GMS), the presence or absence of necrosis within the granuloma, the clinical setting, and laboratory data all come to bear on establishing the cause whenever possible. The lobular distribution of granulomas and their cellular constituents provides important diagnostic clues. Despite careful evaluation of histologic features, clinical data, and laboratory test results, the cause of hepatic granulomas may remain uncertain in up to 5 to 10% of cases.

REFERENCES

1. Zaba LC, Smith GP, Sanchez M, et al. Dendritic cells in the pathogenesis of sarcoidosis. Am J Respir Cell Mol Biol 2010;42(1):32–9.
2. Ma J, Chen T, Mandelin J, et al. Regulation of macrophage activation. Cell Mol Life Sci 2003;60(11):2334–46.
3. Robbins SL, Kumar V, Cotran RS. Robbins and Cotran pathologic basis of disease. 8th edition. Philadelphia: Saunders/Elsevier; 2010. p. 1450, xiv.
4. Co DO, Hogan LH, Il-Kim S, et al. T cell contributions to the different phases of granuloma formation. Immunol Lett 2004;92(1–2):135–42.
5. Wallis RS, Ehlers S. Tumor necrosis factor and granuloma biology: explaining the differential infection risk of etanercept and infliximab. Semin Arthritis Rheum 2005;34(5 Suppl 1):34–8.
6. Schoppet M, Pankuweit S, Maisch B. Cardiac sarcoidosis: cytokine patterns in the course of the disease. Arch Pathol Lab Med 2003;127(9):1207–10.
7. Lefkowitch JH. Hepatic granulomas. J Hepatol 1999;30(Suppl 1):40–5.
8. Satti MB, al-Freihi H, Ibrahim EM, et al. Hepatic granuloma in Saudi Arabia: a clinicopathological study of 59 cases. Am J Gastroenterol 1990;85(6):669–74.
9. Sanai FM, Ashraf S, Abdo AA, et al. Hepatic granuloma: decreasing trend in a high-incidence area. Liver Int 2008;28(10):1402–7.
10. Gaya DR, Thorburn D, Oien KA, et al. Hepatic granulomas: a 10 year single centre experience. J Clin Pathol 2003;56(11):850–3.
11. McCluggage WG, Sloan JM. Hepatic granulomas in Northern Ireland: a thirteen year review. Histopathology 1994;25(3):219–28.
12. Drebber U, Kasper HU, Ratering J, et al. Hepatic granulomas: histological and molecular pathological approach to differential diagnosis–a study of 442 cases. Liver Int 2008;28(6):828–34.
13. Dourakis SP, Saramadou R, Alexopoulou A, et al. Hepatic granulomas: a 6-year experience in a single center in Greece. Eur J Gastroenterol Hepatol 2007; 19(2):101–4.
14. Martin-Blondel G, Camara B, Selves J, et al. [Etiology and outcome of liver granulomatosis: a retrospective study of 21 cases]. Rev Med Interne 2010;31(2): 97–106 [in French].

15. Gershwin ME, Mackay IR. The causes of primary biliary cirrhosis: convenient and inconvenient truths. Hepatology 2008;47(2):737–45.
16. Myers RP, Shaheen AA, Fong A, et al. Epidemiology and natural history of primary biliary cirrhosis in a Canadian health region: a population-based study. Hepatology 2009;50(10):1–9.
17. Lleo A, Invernizzi P, Mackay IR, et al. Etiopathogenesis of primary biliary cirrhosis. World J Gastroenterol 2008;14(21):3328–37.
18. Drebber U, Mueller JJ, Klein E, et al. Liver biopsy in primary biliary cirrhosis: clinicopathological data and stage. Pathol Int 2009;59(8):546–54.
19. Rybicki BA, Iannuzzi MC. Epidemiology of sarcoidosis: recent advances and future prospects. Semin Respir Crit Care Med 2007;28(1):22–35.
20. Doughan AR, Williams BR. Cardiac sarcoidosis. Heart 2006;92:282–8.
21. Ayyala US, Padilla ML. Diagnosis and treatment of hepatic sarcoidosis. Curr Treat Options Gastroenterol 2006;9(6):475–83.
22. Ebert EC, Kierson M, Hagspiel KD. Gastrointestinal and hepatic manifestations of sarcoidosis. Am J Gastroenterol 2008;103(12):3184–92 [quiz 3193].
23. Roberts WC, McAllister HA Jr, Ferrans VJ. Sarcoidosis of the heart. A clinicopathologic study of 35 necropsy patients (group 1) and review of 78 previously described necropsy patients (group 11). Am J Med 1977;63(1):86–108.
24. Moreno-Merlo F, Wanless IR, Shimamatsu K, et al. The role of granulomatous phlebitis and thrombosis in the pathogenesis of cirrhosis and portal hypertension in sarcoidosis. Hepatology 1997;26(3):554–60.
25. Mueller S, Boehme MW, Hofmann WJ, et al. Extrapulmonary sarcoidosis primarily diagnosed in the liver. Scand J Gastroenterol 2000;35(9):1003–8.
26. Rosen Y. Pathology of sarcoidosis. Semin Respir Crit Care Med 2007;28(1): 36–52.
27. Ishak KG. Sarcoidosis of the liver and bile ducts. Mayo Clin Proc 1998;73(5): 467–72.
28. Hsu RM, Connors AF Jr, Tomashefski JF Jr. Histologic, microbiologic, and clinical correlates of the diagnosis of sarcoidosis by transbronchial biopsy. Arch Pathol Lab Med 1996;120(4):364–8.
29. Jones Williams W. The nature and origin of Schaumann bodies. J Pathol Bacteriol 1960;79:193–201.
30. Devaney K, Goodman ZD, Epstein MS, et al. Hepatic sarcoidosis. Clinicopathologic features in 100 patients. Am J Surg Pathol 1993;17(12):1272–80.
31. Scheuer PJ. Hepatic granulomas. Br Med J (Clin Res Ed) 1982;285(6345):833–4.
32. Miller EB, Shichmanter R, Friedman JA, et al. Granulomatous hepatitis and Sjogren's syndrome: an association. Semin Arthritis Rheum 2006;36(3):153–8.
33. Ferrell LD, Lee R, Brixko C, et al. Hepatic granulomas following liver transplantation. Clinicopathologic features in 42 patients. Transplantation 1995;60(9):926–33.
34. Odze RD, Goldblum JR, Crawford JM. Surgical pathology of the GI tract, liver, biliary tract, and pancreas. Philadelphia: Saunders; 2004. p. 1067.
35. Vakiani E, Hunt KK, Mazziotta RM, et al. Hepatitis C-associated granulomas after liver transplantation: morphologic spectrum and clinical implications. Am J Clin Pathol 2007;127(1):128–34.
36. Lamps LW. Hepatic granulomas, with an emphasis on infectious causes. Adv Anat Pathol 2008;15(6):309–18.
37. Emile JF, Sebagh M, Féray C, et al. The presence of epithelioid granulomas in hepatitis C virus-related cirrhosis. Hum Pathol 1993;24(10):1095–7.
38. Ozaras R, Tahan V, Mert A, et al. The prevalence of hepatic granulomas in chronic hepatitis C. J Clin Gastroenterol 2004;38(5):449–52.

39. Snyder N, Martinez JG, Xiao SY. Chronic hepatitis C is a common associated with hepatic granulomas. World J Gastroenterol 2008;14(41):6366–9.
40. Fiel MI, Shukla D, Saraf N, et al. Development of hepatic granulomas in patients receiving pegylated interferon therapy for recurrent hepatitis C virus post liver transplantation. Transpl Infect Dis 2008;10(3):184–9.
41. Kanno A, Murakami K. A transient emergence of hepatic granulomas in a patient with chronic hepatitis B. Tohoku J Exp Med 1998;185(4):281–5.
42. Goldin RD, Levine TS, Foster GR, et al. Granulomas and hepatitis C. Histopathology 1996;28(3):265–7.
43. Tahan V, Ozaras R, Lacevic N, et al. Prevalence of hepatic granulomas in chronic hepatitis B. Dig Dis Sci 2004;49(10):1575–7.
44. Hayashi M, Yamawaki I, Okajima K, et al. Tuberculous liver abscess not associated with lung involvement. Intern Med 2004;43(6):521–3.
45. Bratton RL, Whiteside JW, Hovan MJ, et al. Diagnosis and treatment of Lyme disease. Mayo Clin Proc 2008;83(5):566–71.
46. Zanchi AC, Gingold AR, Theise ND, et al. Necrotizing granulomatous hepatitis as an unusual manifestation of Lyme disease. Dig Dis Sci 2007;52(10):2629–32.
47. Wong P, Houston S, Power B, et al. A case of *Histoplasma capsulatum* causing granulomatous liver disease and Addisonian crisis. Can J Gastroenterol 2001; 15(10):687–91.
48. Mert A, Tabak F, Ozaras R, et al. Typhoid fever as a rare cause of hepatic, splenic, and bone marrow granulomas. Intern Med 2004;43(5):436–9.
49. Mentink-Kane MM, Cheever AW, Thompson RW, et al. IL-13 receptor alpha 2 down-modulates granulomatous inflammation and prolongs host survival in schistosomiasis. Proc Natl Acad Sci U S A 2004;101(2):586–90.
50. Chiaramonte MG, Donaldson DD, Cheever AW, et al. An IL-13 inhibitor blocks the development of hepatic fibrosis during a T-helper type 2-dominated inflammatory response. J Clin Invest 1999;104(6):777–85.
51. Ishak KG, Zimmerman HJ. Drug-induced and toxic granulomatous hepatitis. Baillieres Clin Gastroenterol 1986;2:463–80.
52. Farah M, Al Rashidi A, Owen DA, et al. Granulomatous hepatitis associated with etanercept therapy. J Rheumatol 2008;35(2):349–51.
53. Sartin JS, Walker RC. Granulomatous hepatitis: a retrospective review of 88 cases at the Mayo clinic. Mayo Clin Proc 1991;66(9):914–8.
54. Sarachek NS, London RL, Matulewicz TJ. Diltiazem and granulomatous hepatitis. Gastroenterology 1985;88(5 Pt 1):1260–2.
55. Mifuji R, Iwasa M, Tanaka Y, et al. "Green juice"-associated granulomatous hepatitis. Am J Gastroenterol 2003;98(10):2334–5.
56. Dhawan M, Agrawal R, Ravi J, et al. Rosiglitazone-induced granulomatous hepatitis. J Clin Gastroenterol 2002;34(5):582–4.
57. Braun M, Fraser GM, Kunin M, et al. Mesalamine-induced granulomatous hepatitis. Am J Gastroenterol 1999;94(7):1973–4.
58. Liaw YF, Huang MJ, Fan KD, et al. Hepatic injury during propylthiouracil therapy in patients with hyperthyroidism. A cohort study. Ann Intern Med 1993;118(6): 424–8.
59. Abe M, Kumagi T, Nakanishi S, et al. Drug-induced hepatitis with hepatic granuloma due to saridon. J Gastroenterol 2002;37(12):1068–72.
60. Hussain H, Black M. Granulomatous liver disease. Curr Treat Options Gastroenterol 2000;3(6):473–80.
61. Harrington PT, Guiterrez JJ, Ramirez-Ronda CH, et al. Granulomatous hepatitis. Rev Infect Dis 1982;4(3):638–55.

Trafficking and Transporter Disorders in Pediatric Cholestasis

A.S. Knisely, MD[a],*, Paul Gissen, MBChB, PhD[b,c]

KEYWORDS

- Pediatric cholestasis • Bile salt export pump
- Multidrug resistance protein • Genetic diagnosis • Cell polarity

Many sorts of insult to the liver and biliary tract can lead to cholestasis, with and without jaundice. Distinguishing among the causes of cholestasis is important for assigning prognosis and recommending therapy. Such distinctions can be drawn in part with findings in liver-biopsy specimens. Considerable overlap exists, however, in sets of liver-biopsy findings associated with individual causes of cholestasis.

Certain instances of cholestasis in infancy and childhood have been traced to defects in genes that encode proteins expressed at the bile canaliculus or in genes that subserve mechanisms by which the bile-canaliculus wall is populated with its constituent proteins. Correlation of genetic findings with liver-biopsy findings in children with such disorders has facilitated biopsy diagnosis in pediatric materials, raised hopes for extending the utility of biopsy diagnosis in cholestasis of adult onset, and uncovered questions of interest in hepatobiliary physiology.

THE INACCESSIBILITY OF BILE FORMATION

Bile is the product of active secretion and postsecretory modification, from centrilobular hepatocyte to septal-duct cholangiocyte. It unfortunately is not a fluid easily available to physiological investigation. In the kidney, an ultrafiltrate of plasma within the lumen of the nephron can be sampled at various levels. Shifts in its composition after its initial passive generation then can be studied and inferences on the functions of cells lining different portions of the nephron can be drawn. In the liver, such stop-flow studies are practicable only in the extrahepatic biliary tract, which contains

[a] Institute of Liver Studies, King's College Hospital, Denmark Hill, London SE5 9RS, UK
[b] School of Clinical and Experimental Medicine, University of Birmingham, Wolfson Drive, Edgbaston, Birmingham, B15 2TT, UK
[c] The Metabolic Unit, Birmingham Children's Hospital, Steelhouse Lane, Birmingham, B4 6NH, UK
* Corresponding author.
E-mail address: alex.knisely@kcl.ac.uk

Clin Liver Dis 14 (2010) 619–633
doi:10.1016/j.cld.2010.08.001
1089-3261/10/$ – see front matter © 2010 Elsevier Inc. All rights reserved.

posthepatic bile that is effectively mature. Understanding of the processes by which bile is formed and modified, and of the disruptions in these processes that lead to cholestasis, has thus been gained relatively slowly. Studies in cohorts of infants with cholestasis, however, have recently led to better appreciation of the physiology of bile formation.

These studies largely have relied on extrapolation from mouse or rat models of hepatobiliary disease, with demonstration that lesions in orthologous genes underlie similar phenotypes; on identification of shared chromosomal segments (autozygosity) in distantly related probands with the same phenotype; and on identification of shared regions of homozygosity in nonrelated probands with the same phenotype. (In the latter two settings, genes within the shared regions are evaluated for sequence variants that are specific to probands and are predicted to be likely to impair expression or function of encoded proteins. These genes, or their expression, are then disrupted in animal or cellular models, and the consequences of the disruption are observed to see if they match features of the human disorder). Gene identification permits not only studies of function, and dysfunction, of encoded proteins. It also permits correlative attempts to determine what aspects of clinical disease, and what aspects of liver-biopsy findings, typify mutations in particular genes—and thereby to develop for diagnosis tools other than gene sequencing.

A SKETCH OF BILE SALT HANDLING, WITH STEPS IMPLICATED IN FORMS OF INTRAHEPATIC CHOLESTASIS

Different forms of intrahepatic cholestasis have been associated with mutations in genes encoding various proteins involved in bile production and in bile-acid circulation from liver to gut and back again. Not all of these, but most, are denoted below with an asterisk.

Hepatocytes synthesize primary bile acids (cholic acid [CA] and chenodeoxycholic acid [CDCA]) from cholesterol by modifying a sterol nucleus in many steps.[1] CA and CDCA are amidated, that is, conjugated with glycine or taurine, by *bile acid-CoA : amino acid N-acyltransferase (BAAT). The resulting bile salts are more hydrophilic, and thus less likely to traverse membranes spontaneously, than are the precursor bile acids.[2] These salts are the substrate of the canalicular transporter *bile salt export pump (BSEP), which transfers them into the canalicular lumen against a concentration gradient.[3] The microdomain environment optimal for function of BSEP and other transporters is in part maintained by the flippase *familial intrahepatic cholestasis 1 (FIC1). In association with CDC50A, a protein of undetermined function, FIC1 enriches the cytoplasmic leaflet of the canalicular membrane in phosphoserine transferred from the exoplasmic leaflet.[3,4] Cholangiocytes take up some bile salts via the apical sodium-dependent bile acid transporter (ASBT) and export them via the heterodimeric basolateral organic solute transporter alpha/beta (OSTαβ) into the cholangioportal circulation, returning them to the liver lobule.[5,6] However, most bile salts are conveyed into the duodenum as micelles in combination with cholesterol and phospholipid. Cholesterol and phospholipid reach the bile through elution from the canalicular membrane by bile salts. Cholesterol is made available for elution by the heterodimeric transporter ABCG5/G8 and phospholipid by the floppase *multidrug resistance protein 3 (MDR3), both of which enrich the exoplasmic leaflet of the canalicular membrane in their substrate.[7,8] Micellar chaperonage reduces detergent effects of bile salts on canalicular and cholangiocyte-apex membranes. These micelles break down upon dilution in the more acidic environment of the small bowel lumen, where emulsification by amphipathic bile salts facilitates absorption of lipids and fat-soluble vitamins. Most bile salts are taken up from chyme in the distal ileum and forwarded into the portal venous circulation via ASBT on enterocyte brush borders, intestinal bile salt binding protein (IBABP) within enterocytes, and OSTαβ on enterocyte basolateral aspects.[6] Some bile salts enter the large bowel, where bacteria separate the bile-acid and amino-acid moieties. Bacteria also remove a hydroxyl group at position C7 of the sterol nucleus of CA and CDCA to yield secondary bile acids (respectively deoxycholic acid [DCA] and lithocholic acid [LCA]). These also traverse the bowel wall into the portal venous circulation. From there bile salts and bile acids reach the space of Disse, where *microsomal epoxide hydroxylase (EPHX1), natrium taurocholate cotransporting polypeptide (NTCP), and organic anion-transporting polypeptide (OATP) 1A2 and OATP1B2 forward them into the hepatocyte.[4,9] BAAT there conjugates DCA and LCA with glycine or taurine. LCA also undergoes hydroxylation via cytochrome P450 3A (CYP3A4) and sulfation via sulfotransferase (SULT2A1).[10] Sulfated LCA is a substrate for *multidrug resistance-associated protein 2 (MRP2), a canalicular transport protein homologous to BSEP. MRP2 also transports conjugated bilirubin into the canalicular lumen.[11] (Failure to conjugate bilirubin, a process mediated by uridine diphosphate glycosyl transferase 1, underlies the hyperbilirubinemia of both Gilbert syndrome and Crigler-Najjar syndrome, not further addressed here.) The expression of many of these species is regulated by bile salt levels. When bile salts bind to the *farnesoid X receptor (FXR) in enterocytes, the bile salt—FXR complex induces the expression of IBABP and OSTαβ (tending to lower intracellular bile salt concentrations). In hepatocytes, the complex activates transcription of BAAT, BSEP, and MDR3 (favoring secretion of bile salts and supplying phospholipid as their chaperone) as well as of short heterodimer partner (SHP). In turn, SHP in the hepatocyte inhibits transcription of genes involved in bile salt uptake (NTCP, OATP1A2, OATP1B2) and bile acid synthesis, whereas in the enterocyte it inhibits transcription of ASBT and thereby again of bile salt uptake.[12]

Also implicated in forms of intrahepatic cholestasis are mutations in genes encoding proteins that subserve sorting and distribution of various cell constituents. Such mutations lead, it appears, to multisystem disorders; cholestasis is only one of several manifestations. These disorders include arthrogryposis—renal dysfunction—cholestasis syndrome (ARC)[13,14] and microvillus inclusion disease (MVID).[15] These might better be considered not as primary forms of intrahepatic cholestasis but as inhabiting the borderlands of secondary intrahepatic cholestasis (see later discussion).

CLASSES OF CHOLESTASIS

Short of genetic analysis, cholestatic hepatobiliary disease can be sorted clinicopathologically between the two principal categories of obstructive, often extrahepatic, cholestasis, and nonobstructive, or intrahepatic, cholestasis. In the former, cholestasis results when bile flow is mechanically blocked, as by gallstones or tumor, or as in extrahepatic biliary atresia. (The origins of the inflammation that leads to biliary atresia are interesting, but they likely do not touch on the physiology of bile formation itself.)

Persons in the latter group, who have nonobstructive intrahepatic cholestasis, in turn fall into two principal subgroups. In the first subgroup, cholestasis results when processes of bile secretion and modification, or of synthesis of constituents of bile, are caught up secondarily in hepatocellular injury so severe that nonspecific impairment of many functions can be expected, including those subserving bile formation. In the second subgroup, no presumed cause of hepatocellular injury can be identified. Cholestasis in such patients appears to result when one of the steps in bile secretion or modification, or of synthesis of constituents of bile, is constitutively damaged. Such cholestasis is considered primary.

VARIABILITY IN, AND PREDISPOSITION TO, SECONDARY INTRAHEPATIC CHOLESTASIS

In the borderlands between these groups are instances of intrahepatic cholestasis without particularly severe liver injury. Examples in infancy include some, but not all, patients with alpha-1-antitrypsin storage disorder, recipients of parenteral alimentation, and patients with septo-optic dysplasia. In these settings cholestasis is not accorded the status of a cholestatic disorder per se; it is instead regarded as a concomitant, almost as an optional feature, of an underlying illness. Concern is generally not strong for how it is that one patient receiving parenteral alimentation, or with hypopituitarism, becomes jaundiced while another does not. The factors that conduce to icterus await definition. They may include mutation in genes implicated in primary cholestasis.

With cholestasis in later childhood and adulthood, the perspective shifts. When a bout of cholestasis occurs, an antecedent or associated event is generally sought. If found, it is invoked to classify the type of cholestasis present. Such classes of cholestatic disorder include paraneoplastic cholestasis (Stauffer syndrome); intrahepatic cholestasis of pregnancy; contraceptive-associated cholestasis; drug-associated cholestasis; and infection-associated cholestasis, as with *Leptospira* sp or hepatitis A virus. However, in clinical practice no particular weight is generally laid on what links the infection, the perturbation in hormonal milieu, or the malignancy to the development of jaundice, and again, the factors that conduce to icterus await definition.

PRIMARY INTRAHEPATIC CHOLESTASIS

Infants whose intrahepatic cholestasis can not be subsumed into a coexistent definable disorder often have disease in which jaundice fails to remit and liver scarring develops. These features, together with recurrence of such disease within sibships, have defined a syndrome, long considered idiopathic, that is known as progressive familial intrahepatic cholestasis (PFIC). In later life, if no presumed precipitant in the list above can be found for a bout of cholestasis, the clinical diagnosis of benign and recurrent intrahepatic cholestasis (BRIC) may be assigned. (Bouts of cholestasis in BRIC have been noted to follow intercurrent minor illness. Perhaps shifts in enteric bacterial populations alter aspects of enterohepatic bile acid handling and disturb a precarious equilibrium.) BRIC differs from PFIC clinically in that jaundice remits in BRIC and, by histopathologic criteria, in that liver scarring does not develop. With respect to fibrosis, however, intergrades between BRIC and PFIC are acknowledged; and early in the course of PFIC, cholestasis may transiently wane.[3,16]

SERUM GAMMA-GLUTAMYL TRANSPEPTIDASE VALUES, PFIC, AND LOW- GAMMA-GLUTAMYL TRANSPEPTIDASE CHOLESTASIS

The first form of PFIC identified was "Byler disease," given the surname of the couple identified as progenitors of the extended Amish kindred to which the first recognized cases belonged. Jaundice in Byler disease appears in early infancy, persists, and leads to liver scarring. As jaundice in some instances of familial intrahepatic cholestasis (FIC) is mild or intermittent, and liver architecture may remain normal on repeated sampling over years, cholestasis with clinicopathologic features like those in Byler disease came to be called "progressive" or PFIC. With the recognition of an association in intrahepatic cholestasis between poor prognosis and failure of serum gamma-glutamyl transpeptidase (GGT) values to rise more than slightly, remaining in or near the range expected in health, low-GGT and high-GGT intrahepatic cholestasis were discriminated. In low-GGT PFIC, concentrations of bile salts in bile were very low. Byler disease itself was low-GGT, as was BRIC.[3,16]

A particular subset of low-GGT PFIC was rapidly differentiated: the broad category of bile acid synthesis disorders. Synthesis of primary bile acids is a multistep process with well-understood pathways. When one step along a pathway is blocked, intermediate or precursor bile-acid species may accumulate behind that step. These bile-acid species are not normally found in plasma or urine, and to identify them as present in a child with intrahepatic cholestasis can direct specific investigation, with eventual diagnosis on the basis of both clinical-chemistry and genetic findings.[17] Although cholestasis that can be traced to mutation in genes encoding enzymes in this pathway is intrahepatic and familial, and although without proper treatment it leads to liver scarring, such cholestasis was definitionally excluded from "idiopathic" PFIC. Also distinct from idiopathic PFIC were the low-GGT disorders ARC and MVID. These were considered distinct not because a cause could be assigned, but because clinical and histopathologic features set them apart.

FROM BRIC TO PFIC AND BACK AGAIN

Soon after shared-segment mapping in Dutch persons with BRIC defined a locus for the undefined gene presumed to be mutated in their disorder,[18] the hypothesis that PFIC and BRIC represented points on a continuum of low-GGT intrahepatic cholestasis was supported when similar studies in the eponymous Byler kindred found homozygosity for markers at the same locus in children with PFIC.[19] Children of consanguine parentage who had PFIC and were not demonstrably homozygous at that locus thus could be defined as suffering from something other than Byler disease—termed "Byler syndrome" or "non-Byler low-GGT PFIC." In Amish children with Byler disease, hepatocytes were small and orderly, with bile pigment principally in canalicular lumina. On ultrastructural study, the canalicular contents were loose and coarsely granular (Byler and bile). In Byler syndrome, giant-cell change of hepatocytes, with cytoplasmic bile staining, was prominent, and on transmission electron microscopy the bile was amorphous or finely filamentous.[20] A gene (ATP8B1, encoding FIC1) at the implicated locus was found to be mutated in persons with BRIC, in Amish children with Byler disease, and in non-Amish children with PFIC whose liver-biopsy findings recapitulated those in Amish children with Byler disease.[21] Identification of FIC1 as a phosphoserine flippase,[22] like its association with CDC50A,[23] drew largely on work with the gene's orthologue in yeast. Deficiency of FIC1 seems to lead to deficiency of membrane integrity, with accelerated breakdown of inner-ear cilia[24] and, in the liver, loss of microvillus components into the canalicular lumen (underlying the vesicular appearance of Byler bile).[25] Whether impairment of function of BSEP, demonstrated in FIC1 deficiency, results only from disordered membrane composition[26,27] or also from the loss of an activating effect of FIC1 on synthesis of FXR, and thereby of BSEP,[28–30] is an open question. BSEP is, at any rate, expressed at the canalicular membrane in FIC1 deficiency.[31] GGT and other canalicular ectoenzymes, however, are not.[25] Immunostaining for these species, like an ultrastructural search for Byler bile, can be of diagnostic value in PFIC (**Fig. 1**). A disorder like FIC1 deficiency, although without ATP8B1 mutation, theoretically might result from lesions in the gene encoding CDC50A. No patient with PFIC or BRIC attributable to such a cause has yet been described.

Homozygosity mapping (distinct from shared-segment mapping in that the probands studied were not known to be distant relatives) in patients with non-Byler PFIC soon identified a locus likely to harbor a gene mutated in a second form of low-GGT PFIC.[32] The gene itself (ABCB11, encoding BSEP) and the function of its product had been known for some time,[33] but their role in human disease was

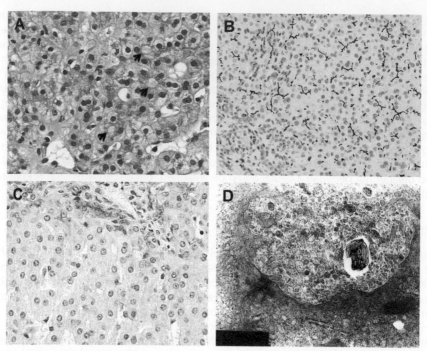

Fig. 1. *ATP8B1* mutation, FIC1 deficiency: PFIC-1. Liver at presentation, term infant, 12 weeks. (*A*) Slight hepatocellular disarray with large pale canalicular bile plugs (*arrowheads*) (hematoxylin and eosin (H&E), original magnification 400×). (*B*) Canalicular expression of BSEP (anti-BSEP antibody/diaminobenzidine chromogen (DAB), hematoxylin counterstain, (original magnification 200×). (*C*) Lack of canalicular expression of GGT; marking persists at cholangiocytes and portal-tract margins (anti-GGT antibody/DAB, hematoxylin counterstain, (original magnification 400×). (*D*) Canaliculus lacking microvilli distended by loose, coarsely granular contents (Byler bile) (osmium tetroxide/uranyl acetate/lead citrate, (original magnification 32,500×).

appreciated only when mutations in *ABCB11* were associated with PFIC.[34] PFIC caused by *ATP8B1* mutation quickly was termed PFIC, type 1 (PFIC-1) whereas PFIC caused by *ABCB11* mutation was termed PFIC-2.[16] (Some patients with low-GGT PFIC can not be shown to have coding-region mutations in either gene or, although of consanguine parentage, are not homozygous for markers at either the *ATP8B1* or the *ABCB11* locus.[31,35] Perhaps other forms of PFIC remain to be defined.) Some patients with BRIC, when studied after this second gene had been implicated in PFIC, also proved to have mutations in *ABCB11*. Their disorder then was termed BRIC-2, with BRIC owing to *ATP8B1* mutations termed BRIC-1.[36] As mentioned above, non-Byler PFIC—including PFIC-2—is characterized histopathologically by substantial lobular disarray, with anisocytosis, giant-cell change and rosetting of hepatocytes, and bile pigment in both hepatocyte cytoplasm and canalicular lumina. Necrosis of individual hepatocytes also is seen.[20,31] Byler bile is not a feature ultrastructurally.[20] In PFIC-2, although exceptions exist, BSEP can not be detected on immunostaining or is only focally and weakly expressed.[31,37] GGT and other ectoenzymes are present along remnants of a distorted, interrupted canalicular network (**Fig. 2**). These points can be of diagnostic use to the histopathologist. Their

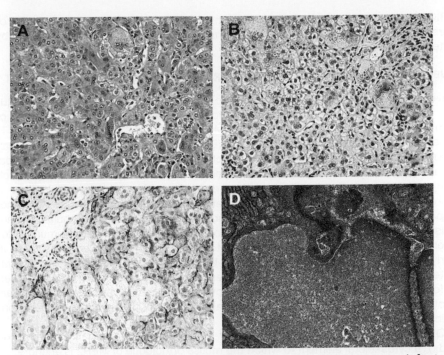

Fig. 2. *ABCB11* mutation, BSEP deficiency: PFIC-2. Liver at presentation, term infant, 8 weeks. (*A*) Giant-cell hepatitis with bile-stained hepatocytes (H&E). (*B*) Lack of canalicular expression of BSEP (anti-BSEP antibody/DAB, hematoxylin counterstain). (*C*) Canalicular expression of GGT (anti-GGT antibody/DAB, hematoxylin counterstain). (*A–C*, original magnification 200×). (*D*) Canaliculus lacking microvilli and distended by electron-dense, amorphous contents (osmium tetroxide/uranyl acetate/lead citrate, original magnification 35,000×).

clinical-biochemistry correlate manifests as a tendency for transaminase-activity values in BSEP deficiency to be higher than in FIC1 deficiency.[31,38]

Distinction between FIC1 deficiency and BSEP deficiency is worth attempting as part of assigning prognosis. While BSEP is expressed only in the liver,[34] FIC1 is expressed at many sites,[21] with deficiency predisposing to deafness, malabsorption, and other disorders that may declare themselves only well after liver transplantation (LTX) has abrogated cholestasis.[5] In addition, BSEP deficiency predisposes to hepatobiliary malignancy in even the first few years of life,[39,40] whereas FIC1 deficiency has not yet been described in association with such malignancy. This difference may affect monitoring before LTX as well as assessment of need for LTX. Finally, anti-BSEP antibodies that impede BSEP function may develop after LTX, leading to recurrence of PFIC.[41,42] No parallel complication after LTX for FIC1 deficiency has been described.

With respect to both BRIC-1 and BRIC-2, patterns of canalicular-antigen expression are not yet defined, and distinctions have not yet been drawn. Correlations between clinical state resulting from *ATP8B1* or *ABCB11* mutation and types of demonstrable mutations suggest that mutations predicted to terminate protein transcription result in PFIC, with abrogation of protein expression.[37,43] Mutations predicted to substitute one amino-acid residue for another, however, vary in their effects. Sometimes an altered protein is trafficked abnormally and is expressed poorly, and sometimes it is trafficked normally but functions poorly.[44] The consequences may be either PFIC or

BRIC, so that, as an example, expression of BSEP may conceivably either fail or persist in BRIC-2. This likely will impede immunohistochemical diagnosis in BRIC by criteria developed in PFIC.

DUBIN-JOHNSON SYNDROME (WITH ROTOR SYNDROME): OF MICE AND MEN. PART 1

Several years before PFIC lost its idiopathic status, the TR- rat, a strain with constitutive jaundice, was shown to harbor a deletion in the gene encoding the orthologue of MRP2.[45] Mutations in *ABCC2*, encoding MRP2, shortly thereafter were identified in persons with Dubin-Johnson syndrome (DJS).[46] Although MRP2 deficiency may lead to inadvertent overdosage of some chemotherapeutic agents,[10,47] the clinical significance of DJS lies principally in the need to recognize it as a condition in which conjugated hyperbilirubinemia requires only clinical-biochemistry evaluation. If increased urinary coproporphyrin I excretion is documented, concern for other hepatobiliary disease can be allayed.[48] In adults with DJS, coarsely granular pigment clustered about canaliculi turns the liver brown-black. To demonstrate immunohistochemically that MRP2 is not expressed is of interest rather than of diagnostic value. In early infancy, however, when extrahepatic biliary atresia, a potential cause of conjugated hyperbilirubinemia, must be excluded timely, liver biopsy may be conducted before urinary coproporphyrin fractionation results are in hand. To immunostain sections for MRP2 then can be diagnostically useful, as DJS pigment may be inconspicuous in early life (**Fig. 3**).

Of interest is that a partial phenocopy of DJS develops in mice deficient in radixin (Rdx), a cytoskeletal element to which the mouse orthologue of MPR2 is anchored.[49] Although humans with a parallel disorder have not been described, one must bear in mind that various forms of intrahepatic cholestasis in which a particular step in bile formation or bile-acid handling appears deficient may result secondarily, as a sequela of a lesion affecting the environment of a protein rather than the protein itself.

Rotor syndrome, an autosomal-recessive form of constitutive conjugated hyperbilirubinaemia, differs from DJS in handling of coproporphyrin and in lacking hepatocyte pigment accumulation. It is not caused by *ABCC2* lesions or MRP2 deficiency.[50] At present it must be considered idiopathic.

MDR3 DEFICIENCY (PFIC-3): OF MICE AND MEN. PART 2

Mice in which the homologue of human *ABCB4*, encoding MDR3, was disturbed had, as expected from work in yeast,[51] bile lacking in phospholipid. They also developed a cholangiopathy, ascribed to corrosion of biliary-tract membranes by nonmicellar bile salts.[52] Instances of a similar cholangiopathy in infants were soon traced to deficiency of MDR3 with lesions in *ABCB4*.[53] This disorder is marked by high serum GGT values; nonetheless, it has come to be regarded as a form of PFIC and, as it was identified after PFIC-1 and PFIC-2, it is known as PFIC-3.[8]

Forms of MDR3 deficiency less severe than PFIC-3 are known. No description of "BRIC-3" has yet appeared; however, haploinsufficiency for MDR3 (as in mothers of infants with PFIC-3) predisposes to intrahepatic cholestasis of pregnancy.[8,53,54] Injury in MDR3 deficiency, including PFIC-3, seems more severe histopathologically in portal tracts than in the lobule, with fibrosis, mixed inflammation, and a spectrum of disease that ranges from ductular reaction to bile-duct loss.[8,55,56] Perhaps this lack of lobular involvement helps to explain why intermittent, relatively mild MDR3 dysfunction does not generally cause icterus. Immunostaining for MDR3 expression is variably informative. In severe disease manifest in infancy MDR3 generally is not demonstrable, but in material from older patients with documented *ABCB4* lesions, if marking for MDR3 is

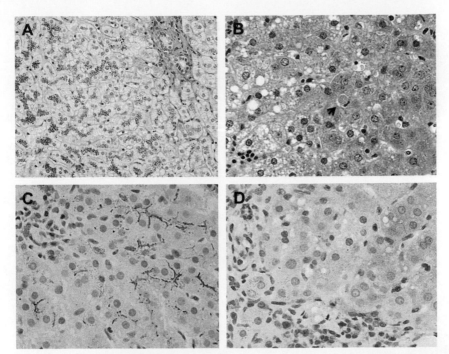

Fig. 3. *ABCC2* mutation, MRP2 deficiency: Dubin-Johnson syndrome. (*A*) Adult liver: coarsely granular brown-black pigment at canalicular poles of hepatocytes (diastase and periodic acid—Schiff reaction, original magnification 200×). (*B–D*) Infant liver (original magnification 400×). (*B*) Moderate lobular disarray with necrotic individual hepatocyte (*arrowhead*), steatosis, and scant pigmentation (H&E). (*C*) Canalicular expression of MRP2 homologue BSEP (anti-BSEP antibody/DAB, hematoxylin counterstain). (*D*) Lack of canalicular expression of MRP2 (anti-MRP2 antibody/DAB, hematoxylin counterstain).

patchy or weak, whether this is to be ascribed to technical issues or to faulty MDR3 expression is hard to decide. A feature of MDR3 deficiency occasionally helpful in histopathologic diagnosis results from decreased solubility of cholesterol in phospholipid-deficient bile: to see cholesterol clefts distorting the epithelium of small bile-duct radicles (**Fig. 4**) should prompt consideration of *ABCB4* disease.[55] Cholesterol sludging and cholesterol cholelithiasis are recognized aspects of MDR3 deficiency.[57]

DEFECTS IN THE MASTER SWITCH: CHOLESTASIS AND FXR SEQUENCE VARIATION

Intrahepatic cholestasis of pregnancy has been associated with FXR polymorphisms. Some of these, studied in vitro, altered FXR activity or translation efficiency.[58] Decreased FXR activity might be expected to conduce to cholestasis. Histopathologic features of such cholestasis are not described.

FAMILIAL HYPERCHOLANEMIA: ONLY THREE TYPES?

As noted for milder MDR3 deficiency, cholestasis can be anicteric, with the principal clinical features those of malabsorption and pruritus. One patient was described in whom high circulating concentrations of bile salts were associated with mutations in the gene encoding EPHXI.[59] Such mutations might reasonably be expected to impede hepatocyte uptake of bile salts without necessarily impeding bilirubin secretion.

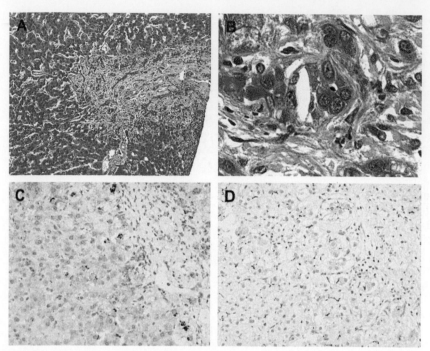

Fig. 4. *ABCB4* mutation, MDR3 deficiency: PFIC-3. Liver of 4-year-old child. (*A*) Portal tract expanded by fibrosis, with increased numbers of bile-duct profiles (H&E, original magnification 100×). (*B*) Cholesterol cleft within bile duct, distorting cholangiocytes (H&E, original magnification 1,000×). (*C*) Lack of canalicular expression of MDR3 (anti-MDR3 antibody/DAB, hematoxylin counterstain). (*D*) Canalicular expression of MRP2 (anti-MRP2 antibody/DAB, hematoxylin counterstain). (*C* and *D*, original magnification 200×).

Patients with lesions in genes that encode other basolateral bile salt uptake proteins, such as NTCP, OATP1A2, and OATP1B2, have not been described. Whether some instances of hypercholanemia will be associated with such lesions is an open question. Amish children are known who have mutations in the genes encoding BAAT and the hepatocyte tight-junction protein TJP2. They suffer principally from pruritus and malabsorption, although a bland canalicular cholestasis may be encountered. With defects in TJP2, "leaky" tight junctions are thought to permit reflux of intracanalicular bile salts between hepatocytes into plasma. With defects in BAAT, nonamidated bile acids, poorer substrates for BSEP activity, as well as less amphophilic than bile salts, are thought to accumulate within hepatocytes and to re-enter plasma from hepatocyte and canalicular lumen alike.[2] GGT values are not elevated in these forms of hypercholanemia,[2] and GGT is unremarkably expressed along the canaliculus (A.S. Knisely, personal observations). Of interest is that bile acids are readied for BAAT-mediated amidation by choloyl : CoA synthetase (SLC27A5); defects in the gene encoding this enzyme also can be expected to lead to hypercholanemia, although patients with hypercholanemia on this basis have yet to be described.

LOW-GGT INTRAHEPATIC CHOLESTASIS AND TRAFFICKING OR POLARITY DEFECTS

Instances of MVID are associated with mutation in the gene encoding myosin 5b (MYO5B), a protein involved in establishing polarity within epithelial cells.[15]

Intrahepatic cholestasis may develop in MVID, particularly after small-bowel transplantation, even when the hepatopathy of parenteral alimentation is not a contributing factor. Cholestasis in this setting is bland, with little lobular disarray and predominantly intracanalicular accumulations of bile pigment. GGT expression at canalicular membranes is deficient, and serum GGT values do not rise despite hyperbilirubinemia.[60] Whether a failure in the trafficking of GGT itself, or of a component of the canalicular membrane necessary for normal GGT expression, to the apical aspect of the hepatocyte underlies lack of GGT expression in MVID is unknown. Better elucidated are the mechanisms that underlie ARC, in which either mutation in *VPS33B* or *VIPAR* can produce a phenotype that includes loss of polarity in hepatocytes.[13,14] *VPS33B* encodes a protein important in coordinating membrane fusion between vesicle and destination site.[13] Some ARC patients lacking *VPS33B* mutations were found to harbor mutations in *VIPAR*, which encodes a protein that interacts with the product of *VPS33B*.[14] Both proteins thus, like MYO5B, act to establish cell polarity through directed sorting to basolateral or apical aspects of epithelium. Hepatocytes express GGT and other canalicular ectoenzymes diffusely in both forms of ARC, rather than restricting their expression to canalicular domains. As in MVID, GGT values in ARC are not elevated, despite conjugated hyperbilirubinemia.[13] As in BRIC-1 and PFIC-1, then, the failure of GGT values to rise can be ascribed to unavailability of GGT for elution into bile, with reflux into plasma. Of interest is that hepatocytes in ARC may accumulate DJS-like pigment,[13,61] suggesting dysfunction of MRP2. The genes involved in MVID and ARC, like those in PFIC-1 and PFIC-2, were identified by homozygosity mapping rather than as orthologues of genes implicated in hepatobiliary disease of animals.

IMMUNOHISTOCHEMICAL STUDIES IN INTRAHEPATIC CHOLESTASIS: A SUMMARY

To immunostain for BSEP and MDR3 in severe hepatobiliary disease manifest early in life can rapidly identify, under best conditions, whether or not sequencing of *ABCB11* or *ABCB4*, respectively, is likely to yield a genetic diagnosis. In low-GGT intrahepatic cholestasis, to demonstrate BSEP expression can direct attention to bile acid synthesis disorders, if lobular disarray is pronounced. If, instead, bland canalicular cholestasis is seen, FIC1 deficiency can be suspected. To immunostain for ectoenzymes, in particular GGT, also can be useful in FIC1 deficiency, as antibodies that mark FIC1 in formalin-fixed, paraffin-embedded material are not available. Immunostaining for MRP2 may identify DJS in early life. Otherwise, to immunostain for MRP2 serves principally as a control for adequacy of processing. To demonstrate MRP2 expression but not BSEP expression, for example, permits the inference that absence of BSEP expression may not be nonspecific. Uses in diagnosis for immunostaining of other species implicated in cholestasis await definition.

REFERENCES

1. Chiang JY. Regulation of bile acid synthesis: pathways, nuclear receptors, and mechanisms. J Hepatol 2004;40:539–51.
2. Carlton VE, Harris BZ, Puffenberger EG, et al. Complex inheritance of familial hypercholanemia with associated mutations in TJP2 and BAAT. Nat Genet 2003;34:91–6.
3. Lam P, Soroka CJ, Boyer JL. The bile salt export pump: clinical and experimental aspects of genetic and acquired cholestatic liver disease. Semin Liver Dis 2010; 30:125–33.
4. Dawson PA, Lan T, Rao A. Bile acid transporters. J Lipid Res 2009;50:2340–57.

5. Paulusma CC, Elferink RP, Jansen PL. Progressive familial intrahepatic cholestasis type 1. Semin Liver Dis 2010;30:117–24.
6. Xia X, Francis H, Glaser S, et al. Bile acid interactions with cholangiocytes. World J Gastroenterol 2006;12:3553–63.
7. Soroka CJ, Ballatori N, Boyer JL. Organic solute transporter, OSTalpha-OSTbeta: its role in bile acid transport and cholestasis. Semin Liver Dis 2010;30:178–85.
8. Davit-Spraul A, Gonzales E, Baussan C, et al. The spectrum of liver diseases related to ABCB4 gene mutations: pathophysiology and clinical aspects. Semin Liver Dis 2010;30:134–46.
9. von Dippe P, Amoui M, Stellwagen RH, et al. The functional expression of sodium-dependent bile acid transport in Madin-Darby canine kidney cells transfected with the cDNA for microsomal epoxide hydrolase. J Biol Chem 1996;271: 18176–80.
10. Elias E, Mills CO. Coordinated defence and the liver. Clin Med 2007;7:180–4.
11. Jedlitschky G, Hoffmann U, Kroemer HK. Structure and function of the MRP2 (ABCC2) protein and its role in drug disposition. Expert Opin Drug Metab Toxicol 2006;2:351–66.
12. Wagner M, Zollner G, Trauner M. Nuclear receptor regulation of the adaptive response of bile acid transporters in cholestasis. Semin Liver Dis 2010;30: 160–77.
13. Gissen P, Johnson CA, Morgan NV, et al. Mutations in VPS33B, encoding a regulator of SNARE-dependent membrane fusion, cause arthrogryposis-renal dysfunction-cholestasis (ARC) syndrome. Nat Genet 2004;36:400–4.
14. Cullinane AR, Straatman-Iwanowska A, Zaucker A, et al. Mutations in VIPAR cause an arthrogryposis, renal dysfunction and cholestasis syndrome phenotype with defects in epithelial polarization. Nat Genet 2010;42:303–12.
15. Müller T, Hess MW, Schiefermeier N, et al. MYO5B mutations cause microvillus inclusion disease and disrupt epithelial cell polarity. Nat Genet 2008;40: 1163–5.
16. Knisely AS. Progressive familial intrahepatic cholestasis: a personal perspective. Pediatr Dev Pathol 2000;3:113–25.
17. Heubi JE, Setchell KD, Bove KE. Inborn errors of bile acid metabolism. Semin Liver Dis 2007;27:282–94.
18. Houwen RH, Baharloo S, Blankenship K, et al. Genome screening by searching for shared segments: mapping a gene for benign recurrent intrahepatic cholestasis. Nat Genet 1994;8:380–6.
19. Carlton VE, Knisely AS, Freimer NB. Mapping of a locus for progressive familial intrahepatic cholestasis (Byler disease) to 18q21-q22, the benign recurrent intrahepatic cholestasis region. Hum Mol Genet 1995;4:1049–53.
20. Bull LN, Carlton VE, Stricker NL, et al. Genetic and morphological findings in progressive familial intrahepatic cholestasis (Byler disease [PFIC-1] and Byler syndrome): evidence for heterogeneity. Hepatology 1997;26:155–64.
21. Bull LN, van Eijk MJ, Pawlikowska L, et al. A gene encoding a P-type ATPase mutated in two forms of hereditary cholestasis. Nat Genet 1998;18:219–24.
22. Ujhazy P, Ortiz D, Misra S, et al. Familial intrahepatic cholestasis 1: studies of localization and function. Hepatology 2001;34:768–75, Hepatology 2002;35:246.
23. Paulusma CC, Folmer DE, Ho-Mok KS, et al. ATP8B1 requires an accessory protein for endoplasmic reticulum exit and plasma membrane lipid flippase activity. Hepatology 2008;47:268–78.
24. Stapelbroek JM, Peters TA, van Beurden DH, et al. ATP8B1 is essential for maintaining normal hearing. Proc Natl Acad Sci U S A 2009;106:9709–14.

25. Paulusma CC, Groen A, Kunne C, et al. Atp8b1 deficiency in mice reduces resistance of the canalicular membrane to hydrophobic bile salts and impairs bile salt transport. Hepatology 2006;44:195–204.
26. Paulusma CC, de Waart DR, Kunne C, et al. Activity of the bile salt export pump (ABCB11) is critically dependent on canalicular membrane cholesterol content. J Biol Chem 2009;284:9947–54.
27. Cai SY, Gautam S, Nguyen T, et al. ATP8B1 deficiency disrupts the bile canalicular membrane bilayer structure in hepatocytes, but FXR expression and activity are maintained. Gastroenterology 2009;136:1060–9.
28. Martínez-Fernández P, Hierro L, Jara P, et al. Knockdown of ATP8B1 expression leads to specific downregulation of the bile acid sensor FXR in HepG2 cells: effect of the FXR agonist GW4064. Am J Physiol Gastrointest Liver Physiol 2009;296:G1119–29.
29. Koh S, Takada T, Kukuu I, et al. FIC1-mediated stimulation of FXR activity is decreased with PFIC1 mutations in HepG2 cells. J Gastroenterol 2009;44: 592–600.
30. Chen F, Ellis E, Strom SC, et al. ATPase class I type 8B member 1 and protein kinase C zeta induce the expression of the canalicular bile salt export pump in human hepatocytes. Pediatr Res 2010;67:183–7.
31. Davit-Spraul A, Fabre M, Branchereau S, et al. ATP8B1 and ABCB11 analysis in 62 children with normal gamma-glutamyl transferase progressive familial intrahepatic cholestasis (PFIC): phenotypic differences between PFIC1 and PFIC2 and natural history. Hepatology 2010;51:1645–55.
32. Strautnieks SS, Kagalwalla AF, Tanner MS, et al. Identification of a locus for progressive familial intrahepatic cholestasis PFIC2 on chromosome 2q24. Am J Hum Genet 1997;61:630–3.
33. Gerloff T, Stieger B, Hagenbuch B, et al. The sister of P-glycoprotein represents the canalicular bile salt export pump of mammalian liver. J Biol Chem 1998;273: 10046–50.
34. Strautnieks SS, Bull LN, Knisely AS, et al. A gene encoding a liver-specific ABC transporter is mutated in progressive familial intrahepatic cholestasis. Nat Genet 1998;20:233–8.
35. Strautnicks S, Byrne J, Knisely A, et al. There must be a third locus for low GGT PFIC [abstract]. Hepatology 2001;34:240A.
36. van Mil SW, van der Woerd WL, van der Brugge G, et al. Benign recurrent intrahepatic cholestasis type 2 is caused by mutations in ABCB11. Gastroenterology 2004;127:379–84.
37. Strautnieks SS, Byrne JA, Pawlikowska L, et al. Severe bile salt export pump deficiency: 82 different ABCB11 mutations in 109 families. Gastroenterology 2008; 134:1203–14.
38. Pawlikowska L, Strautnieks S, Jankowska I, et al. Differences in presentation and progression between severe FIC1 and BSEP deficiencies. J Hepatol 2010;53:170–8.
39. Knisely AS, Strautnieks SS, Meier Y, et al. Hepatocellular carcinoma in ten children under five years old with bile salt export pump deficiency. Hepatology 2006;44:478–86.
40. Scheimann AO, Strautnieks SS, Knisely AS, et al. Mutations in bile salt export pump (ABCB11) in two children with progressive familial intrahepatic cholestasis and cholangiocarcinoma. J Pediatr 2007;150:556–9.
41. Keitel V, Burdelski M, Vojnisek Z, et al. De novo bile salt transporter antibodies as a possible cause of recurrent graft failure after liver transplantation: a novel mechanism of cholestasis. Hepatology 2009;50:510–7.

42. Jara P, Hierro L, Martínez-Fernández P, et al. Recurrence of bile salt export pump deficiency after liver transplantation. N Engl J Med 2009;361:1359–67.
43. Klomp LW, Vargas JC, van Mil SW, et al. Characterization of mutations in ATP8B1 associated with hereditary cholestasis. Hepatology 2004;40:27–38.
44. Byrne JA, Strautnieks SS, Ihrke G, et al. Missense mutations and single nucleotide polymorphisms in ABCB11 impair bile salt export pump processing and function or disrupt pre-messenger RNA splicing. Hepatology 2009; 49:553–67.
45. Paulusma CC, Bosma PJ, Zaman GJ, et al. Congenital jaundice in rats with a mutation in a multidrug resistance-associated protein gene. Science 1996; 271:1126–8.
46. Paulusma CC, Kool M, Bosma PJ, et al. A mutation in the human canalicular multispecific organic anion transporter gene causes the Dubin-Johnson syndrome. Hepatology 1997;25:1539–42.
47. Hulot JS, Villard E, Maguy A, et al. A mutation in the drug transporter gene ABCC2 associated with impaired methotrexate elimination. Pharmacogenet Genomics 2005;15:277–85.
48. Wolkoff AW. Inheritable disorders manifested by conjugated hyperbilirubinemia. Semin Liver Dis 1983;3:65–72.
49. Kikuchi S, Hata M, Fukumoto K, et al. Radixin deficiency causes conjugated hyperbilirubinemia with loss of Mrp2 from bile canalicular membranes. Nat Genet 2002;31:320–5.
50. Hrebícek M, Jirásek T, Hartmannová H, et al. Rotor-type hyperbilirubinaemia has no defect in the canalicular bilirubin export pump. Liver Int 2007;27: 485–91.
51. Ruetz S, Gros P. Phosphatidylcholine translocase: a physiological role for the mdr2 gene. Cell 1994;77:1071–81.
52. Smit JJ, Schinkel AH, Oude Elferink RP, et al. Homozygous disruption of the murine mdr2 P-glycoprotein gene leads to a complete absence of phospholipid from bile and to liver disease. Cell 1993;75:451–62.
53. de Vree JM, Jacquemin E, Sturm E, et al. Mutations in the MDR3 gene cause progressive familial intrahepatic cholestasis. Proc Natl Acad Sci U S A 1998; 95:282–7.
54. Pauli-Magnus C, Meier PJ, Stieger B. Genetic determinants of drug-induced cholestasis and intrahepatic cholestasis of pregnancy. Semin Liver Dis 2010; 30:147–59.
55. Ziol M, Barbu V, Rosmorduc O, et al. ABCB4 heterozygous gene mutations associated with fibrosing cholestatic liver disease in adults. Gastroenterology 2008; 135:131–41, 2008;135:1429.
56. Gotthardt D, Runz H, Keitel V, et al. A mutation in the canalicular phospholipid transporter gene, ABCB4, is associated with cholestasis, ductopenia, and cirrhosis in adults. Hepatology 2008;48:1157–66.
57. Poupon R, Barbu V, Chamouard P, et al. Combined features of low phospholipid-associated cholelithiasis and progressive familial intrahepatic cholestasis 3. Liver Int 2010;30:327–31.
58. van Mil SW, Milona A, Dixon PH, et al. Functional variants of the central bile acid sensor FXR identified in intrahepatic cholestasis of pregnancy. Gastroenterology 2007;133:507–16.
59. Zhu QS, Xing W, Qian B, et al. Inhibition of human m-epoxide hydrolase gene expression in a case of hypercholanemia. Biochim Biophys Acta 2003;1638: 208–16.

60. Peters J, Lacaille F, Horslen S, et al. Microvillus inclusion disease treated by small bowel transplantation: development of progressive intrahepatic cholestasis with low serum concentrations of γ-glutamyl transpeptidase activity [abstract]. Hepatology 2001;34:213A.
61. Nezelof C, Dupart MC, Jaubert F, et al. A lethal familial syndrome associating arthrogryposis multiplex congenita, renal dysfunction, and a cholestatic and pigmentary liver disease. J Pediatr 1979;94:258–60.

Vascular Disorders of the Liver

James M. Crawford, MD, PhD*

KEYWORDS

• Vascular disorder • Liver • Blood flow • Hepatic compromise

The normal adult liver weighs 1400 to 1600 g, constituting approximately 2.5% of body weight. The liver has a dual blood supply: the portal vein provides 60% to 70% of hepatic blood flow, and the hepatic artery supplies 30% to 40%. Given the enormous flow of blood through the liver, it is not surprising that systemic circulatory disturbances may have a considerable effect on hepatic vascular physiology. In most instances, clinically significant abnormalities of liver function do not develop, but hepatic morphology may be strikingly affected. Conversely, primary vascular disorders of the liver can have profound effects on hepatic function, and potentially the survival of the individual so affected. In the midst of otherwise common causes of hepatic dysfunction such as hepatitis, lack of clinical suspicion for a vascular disorder can have detrimental consequences for patient management. Collectively, vascular disorders of the liver can be grouped according to whether blood flow into, through, or from the liver is impaired (**Box 1**).

ANATOMY

The hepatic vascular anatomy merits review, because dramatic clinical events may occur with compromise of the larger segments of the hepatic vasculature. The branching pattern of the hepatic arterial and portal vein trees within the liver are key determinants of hepatic anatomy, because they define both the physiologic patterns of microcirculatory blood flow, and also the planes along which the liver may be subdivided during surgery. Entering the hilum through the porta hepatis, the branches of the portal veins, hepatic arteries (and bile ducts) travel in parallel in portal tracts. The first branch, which is extrahepatic, is into the right and left systems. Within the liver corpus, the vascular watershed between the right and left portal vein and hepatic artery systems (and hence the right and left hepatic lobes) is not midline, but is 2 to 3 cm to the right of midline.

Hofstra North Shore-LIJ School of Medicine and North Shore-Long Island Jewish Health System, Manhasset, NY, USA
* Corresponding author. North Shore-LIJ Core Laboratories, 10 Nevada Drive, Lake Success, NY 11042–1114.
E-mail address: jcrawford1@nshs.edu

Clin Liver Dis 14 (2010) 635–650
doi:10.1016/j.cld.2010.08.002
1089-3261/10/$ – see front matter © 2010 Elsevier Inc. All rights reserved.

Box 1
Classification of vascular disorders of the liver

Obstruction to hepatic vascular inflow
   Portal vein thrombosis
      Surgical complications
      Trauma
      Phlebitis
         Intraabdominal sepsis
         Umbilical vein catheterization
      Thrombogenic disorders
         Inherited coagulative disorders
         Pancreatitis
         Cirrhosis.
      Hepatocellular carcinoma
      Intraabdominal malignancy
   Hepatic artery occlusion
      Polyarteritis nodosa
      Rheumatologic disorders with vasculitis
      Systemic amyloidosis
      Hyaline arteriosclerosis
Presinusoidal obstruction (noncirrhotic portal hypertension)
   Hepatoportal sclerosis
   Nodular hyperplasias
      Focal nodular hyperplasia
      Nodular regenerative hyperplasia
Obstruction to sinusoidal blood flow
   Cirrhosis
   Sickle cell disease
   Eclampsia (intravascular coagulation)
   Infiltrative malignancy (breast, lung, leukemia, melanoma)
   Infection: congenital syphilis
   Peliosis hepatis (not obstructive, but involves sinusoidal blood lakes)
Venous outflow obstruction
   Centrilobular congestion
      Centrilobular hemorrhagic necrosis
      Cardiac sclerosis
   Hepatic venous thrombosis (Budd-Chiari syndrome)
   Obliterative hepatocavopathy (inferior vena cava thrombosis)
   Venoocclusive disease (sinusoidal obstruction syndrome)

Once within the liver, the next 2 primary vascular branches divide vertically and horizontally. Allowing for the dorsal bulge of the liver between the groove of the inferior vena cava and midline (the caudate lobe), there are 9 designated segments in the liver: (1) caudate lobe; (2) left lobe, mediosuperior; (3) left lobe, medioinferior; (4a) left lobe, laterosuperior; (4b) left lobe, lateroinferior; (5) right lobe, medioinferior; (6) right lobe, lateroinferior; (7) right lobe, laterosuperior; (8) right lobe, mediosuperior. Because segment 4b lies between the falciform ligament and the gallbladder fossa and groove for the inferior vena cava laterally, this region is also designated the quadrate lobe.[1]

The intrahepatic branches of the portal vein, hepatic artery, and bile duct run together within the portal tract system, ramifying through approximately 17 to 20 orders of branches to supply the entire corpus of the liver.[2] However, the subdivisions are not strictly dichotomous, in that one branch may have fewer subbranches than another. Hence, the liver ultimately has an irregular lobular organization at the microscopic level.

The hepatic venous anatomy does not strictly parallel the distribution of the portal system, because hepatic veins traverse between portal system–defined lobules as the venous system exits the liver. This is understandable, because ultimately the hepatic veins have to exit through the dorsum of the liver, whereas the portal system enters the liver ventrally. The hepatic venous system also does not ramify as extensively as the portal system, so there is a slight preponderance of terminal portal tracts to terminal hepatic veins throughout the liver.[3] The 3 major hepatic veins, the right, intermediate, and left (the intermediate and left often forming a common trunk), enter the inferior vena cava in the superior portion of its retrohepatic segment. Several smaller accessory hepatic veins open into the lower part of the hepatic segment of the inferior vena cava.[4] The caudate lobe drains directly into the inferior vena cava.

MICROANATOMY

A detailed examination of the hepatic microvasculature is beyond the scope of this article, and the reader is referred to a definitive source.[5] However, some key facts have direct relevance to hepatic vascular disorders. First is the vascular supply of the intrahepatic biliary tree. As stated earlier, the hepatic arterial system travels in parallel to the portal vein system, sending branches throughout the portal tract system. In the largest interlobar portal tracts, there are typically 4 hepatic arteries accompanying the interlobar bile ducts.[6] The hepatic artery/bile duct ratio lessens until, in the most distal portal tracts, hepatic arteries are paired in close proximity with interlobular bile ducts in a 1:1 ratio.[7] Even at this level, there are typically 2 hepatic artery/bile duct pairs per portal vein in traditional portal triads. Eventually, in the most terminal portions of the portal tract system, only hepatic artery/terminal bile duct dyads may remain, leaving behind the terminal branches of portal veins. These terminal branches also diminish and come to an end.

Blood exits hepatic arteries by 3 routes: into a plexus around portal veins, into a plexus around bile ducts, and into terminal hepatic arterioles.[8] These plexuses drain into hepatic sinusoids. Occasional arterioportal anastomoses between periportal arterioles and terminal portal venules have been observed but the frequency of these in normal human livers is uncertain.[9] For the portal venous system, the arteriolar plexus disappears by the level of terminal portal veins. In contrast, a peribiliary arterial-fed plexus supplies all the intrahepatic bile ducts. Around the larger ducts, the peribiliary plexus is 2-layered, with a rich inner, subepithelial layer of fine capillaries and an outer, periductular venous network that receives blood from the inner layer. The smallest, terminal bile ducts have only a single layer of fine capillaries. Terminal hepatic arterioles are believed to empty directly into hepatic sinusoids, although the veracity of this possibility in humans has been debated for decades.[10,11] To the extent that such terminal arterioles do contribute blood directly to sinusoids, independently contractile smooth muscle sphincters in the walls of hepatic arterioles and their arteriolosinusoidal branches control blood flow.

Blood exits portal veins via terminal (penetrating) portal venules, from which a series of sinusoids originates. The inlets to the portal venules are controlled by sphincters composed of sinusoidal endothelial cells. Sinusoidal architecture itself is heterogeneous: upstream sinusoids form an interconnecting polygonal network, whereas downstream the sinusoids become organized as convergent parallel channels that drain into the terminal hepatic venule, a convergent architecture that is evident histologically at medium power. Short intersinusoidal channels connect adjacent parallel sinusoids in the downstream region.[12]

Portal vein blood flow is not directly controlled, except indirectly by regulation of splanchnic blood supply.[13] Hence, the only direct control of blood flow within the liver is via the hepatic artery and its tributaries.[14]

Impaired Blood Flow into the Liver

Hepatic artery compromise

Liver infarcts are rare, thanks to the double blood supply to the liver. Nonetheless, thrombosis or compression of an intrahepatic branch of the hepatic artery by neoplasia, or occlusion by embolism or polyarteritis nodosa, may result in a localized infarct that is usually anemic and pale tan, sometimes with a hemorrhagic suffusion from portal blood. Although transient increases in serum markers of liver injury, particularly transaminases, may occur, compromise to overall hepatic function is not usually a concern.

Interruption of blood flow in the main hepatic artery is a different consideration. If the liver is native and otherwise normal, ischemic necrosis of the organ may be avoided. Retrograde arterial flow through accessory vessels, when coupled with the portal venous supply, is usually sufficient to sustain the liver parenchyma, including the intrahepatic biliary tree. The only exception is hepatic artery thrombosis in a transplanted liver, which is a feared complication and can lead to infarction of the major ducts of the biliary tree and loss of the organ (**Fig. 1**).[15] Hepatic artery thrombosis is the most common vascular complication after liver transplantation, occurring in 2% to 5% of liver transplant recipients. There are numerous interdependent risk factors for this complication, including older age of the donor, younger age of the recipient, ABO incompatibility, and hepatic artery anatomy (particularly the size of the anastomosis).[16]

Portal vein obstruction and thrombosis

Blockage of the extrahepatic portal vein may be insidious and well tolerated or may be a catastrophic and potentially lethal event; most cases are somewhere in between.[17] Occlusive disease of the portal vein or its major radicals typically produces abdominal pain and, in most instances, ascites and other manifestations of portal hypertension, principally esophageal varices that are prone to rupture. The ascites, when present, is often massive and intractable. Acute impairment of visceral blood flow leads to profound congestion and bowel infarction.

Extrahepatic portal vein obstruction may arise from the following conditions, but in about 50% of cases, no cause can be implicated:

- Banti syndrome, in which subclinical occlusion of the portal vein (as from neonatal umbilical sepsis or umbilical vein catheterization) presents as variceal

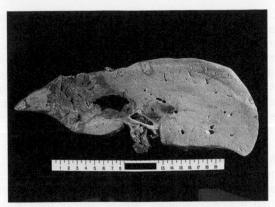

Fig. 1. Explanted liver graft, following initial orthotopic liver transplantation that was complicated by hepatic artery thrombosis. Hilar infarction involves the major bile ducts, and extends into the corpus of the liver.

> bleeding and ascites years later (Banti syndrome is distinct from Bantu syndrome, involving accumulation of excess iron in the liver)
>
> - Intraabdominal sepsis; for example, acute diverticulitis or appendicitis leading to pylephlebitis in the splanchnic circulation, with anterograde thrombosis extending into the portal vein itself
> - Ulcerative colitis, without or with celiac disease
> - Thrombogenic disorders, including the presence of anticardiolipin antibody, postsurgical thromboses, and perinatal umbilical vein catheterization (**Fig. 2**)
> - Trauma
> - Pancreatitis that initiates splenic vein thrombosis, which propagates into the portal vein
> - Retrograde portal vein invasion by hepatocellular carcinoma, which may further incite upstream portal vein thrombosis.

The portal hypertension arising from portal vein thrombosis generally has a benign prognosis. Transplant-free survival from the time of first presentation is 94%, 84%,

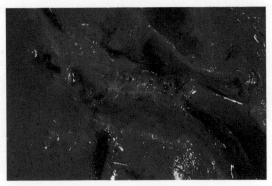

Fig. 2. Long-term outcome of portal vein thrombosis at birth following umbilical vein catheterization for exchange transfusion. Postmortem examination at 18 years of age revealed remote thrombotic occlusion of the portal vein (opened longitudinally), with fibrosis and recanalization by multiple small channels.

and 69% at 1, 5, and 10 years, respectively, although progression to clinical liver failure still eventually occurs in 53% of these patients.[18]

Intrahepatic portal vein radicles may also be obstructed by acute thrombosis. However, the thrombosis does not cause ischemic infarction, but instead results in a sharply demarcated area of red-blue discoloration called infarct of Zahn. There is no necrosis, only severe hepatocellular atrophy and marked hemostasis in distended sinusoids. Invasion of the portal vein system by primary or secondary cancer in the liver can progressively occlude portal inflow to the liver; tongues of hepatocellular carcinoma can even occlude the extrahepatic portal vein.

Idiopathic portal hypertension

Idiopathic portal hypertension is a clinical designation for impaired portal vein inflow and portal hypertension in the absence of cirrhosis. Esophageal varices and splenomegaly are common accompaniments, with or without hypersplenism. Ascites is uncommon, but decompensation of liver function with development of massive ascites may occur.[19] If a cause can be identified, it may be associated with hypercoagulability of the blood, myeloproliferative disorders, peritonitis, chronic exposure to arsenicals, or autoimmune disorders. Idiopathic portal hypertension has an unusually high incidence in some parts of the world; up to 25% of esophageal variceal bleeding in India is attributed to the presence of idiopathic portal hypertension.

The histologic manifestation of idiopathic portal hypertension is termed hepatoportal sclerosis, owing to dense fibrosis of intrahepatic portal tracts with obliteration of portal vein channels.[20] At low power, the liver histopathology is striking for expansion of the portal tract by fibrous tissue, and difficulty in identifying portal veins (**Fig. 3**A). At higher power, sclerotic obliteration of portal veins may be evident (see **Fig. 3**B). The sclerotic tissue is confined to portal tracts; there are no fibrous septa, and no nodular transformation of the hepatic parenchyma.

Whether this striking histology represents a primary progressive disorder or partially healed, more-severe hepatic fibrotic injury is unclear. In the first instance, toxic injury to the hepatic vasculature, as from arsenical exposure, provides ample causation for sclerotic obliteration. In the second instance, regression of cirrhosis with resorption of most of the fibrotic scar tissue has now been well documented in the literature, for conditions ranging from treated hepatitis C viral infection to long-term therapy for genetic hemochromatosis.[21] However, regression of the vascular injury induced by cirrhosis may remain for many years after regression of cirrhosis. Hepatoportal sclerosis may constitute one such manifestation of partially reversed cirrhosis. Resolution

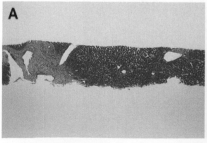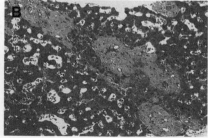

Fig. 3. Hepatoportal sclerosis. (*A*) At low power, prominent fibrotic portal tracts are evident, without evidence of the nodular transformation of cirrhosis. (*B*) At higher power, portal tract sclerosis is present, without evident portal veins. (*A* and *B*, Masson trichrome stain, original magnifications 40× and 100×, respectively.)

of this conundrum is difficult, owing to the observational nature of the retrospective studies of individuals with this malady.[22,23]

Impaired Blood Flow Through the Liver

The hepatic sinusoids comprise one of the largest-caliber vascular beds in the body. Impairment of blood flow through this vascular bed constitutes a major loss of physiologic function, with profound influence on homeostasis for the entire human organism. The most common cause of sinusoidal blood flow obstruction is cirrhosis. As has been documented by Wanless and colleagues[26] among others,[24,25] a central pathophysiologic mechanism in cirrhosis is obliteration of the small vascular channels within the liver, centering on the sinusoids.

Pathophysiology of obstruction to intrahepatic blood flow in cirrhosis

Arterialization of the liver in cirrhosis has been known for more than a century, whereby resistance to blood flow in the hepatic artery is decreased, whereas there is sluggish or even reversed flow in the portal vein.[21] Fundamental structural reasons include

- Capillarization of sinusoids, whereby the number and size of sinusoidal endothelial fenestrations decrease, subendothelial basement membrane is deposited, and the normally permeable sinusoids become impermeable vascular channels that shunt blood from portal tracts to the terminal hepatic veins[12]
- Acquisition of myofibers by perisinusoidal stellate cells, converting them into activated myofibroblasts. Tonic contraction constricts the sinusoidal vascular channels, increasing sinusoidal vascular resistance
- Fibrosis in the perivenular region of the lobule may partially obstruct vascular outflow, creating postsinusoidal vascular resistance
- In the midst of the increased resistance of the sinusoidal channels, rapid blood flow caused by the increased source arterial pressure creates an effective arteriovenous shunt, further decreasing solute exchange
- Arterialization also occurs at the level of portal tracts, where an increased number (and size) of arterial profiles correlates with formation of arterio(portal) venous connections. The portal venous system is thus partially exposed to hepatic arterial blood pressure.

Sclerosis of the portal tracts, and their vascular branches, increases presinusoidal vascular resistance for blood inflow via the splanchnic system. Hence, resistance to hepatic arterial blood flow decreases owing to an increased arterial capacity, whereas resistance to portal vein blood inflow increases. Hepatic arterial blood pressure is sufficient to supply blood to the liver, but the low pressure of the splanchnic system is not able to overcome the pressure impedance, leading to portal hypertension and its ensuing features, such as splenomegaly and esophageal varices.

To add insult to this injury, parenchymal extinction occurs as a result of frank occlusion of hepatic vascular channels. Parenchymal extinction is defined as a focal loss of contiguous hepatocytes.[27] The contiguous cell loss is the result of focal ischemia resulting from thrombotic obstruction of veins or sinusoids. The size of extinction lesions depends on the size of the obstructed vessels, and whether upstream arteries or veins, or downstream veins, or both, are occluded. In angiographic and ultrasonographic studies, portal vein thrombosis has been detected in 0.6% to 16.6% of patients with cirrhosis,[28,29] and grossly visible portal vein fibrosis, or thrombosis, has been found in 39% of cirrhotic livers at autopsy.[26,30] Venoocclusive lesions of hepatic veins less than 0.2 mm in diameter have been found in up to 74% of cirrhotic livers examined at autopsy.[23,24,30] Obliterative lesions are found in 36% of portal veins and 70% of hepatic veins in livers removed at liver transplantation.[26] The distribution of portal vein obliterative lesions is more uniform than those in hepatic veins, each consistent with the concept of propagation of multifocal thrombi downstream from their site of origin. Portal vein lesions are associated with prominent regional variation in the size of cirrhotic nodules. Hepatic vein lesions are associated with regions of confluent fibrosis and parenchymal extinction. The compelling conclusion is that thrombosis of medium- and large-sized portal veins and hepatic veins is a common occurrence in cirrhosis, and may represent a final common pathway for the propagation of parenchymal extinction to full-blown cirrhosis.

The concept of parenchymal extinction is important because it indicates that

- Parenchymal extinction is not directly caused by the initial hepatocellular injury but is an epiphenomenon caused by innocent bystander injury of the local vessels
- Each parenchymal extinction lesion has its own natural history and may be in an early or late stage of healing
- Cirrhosis develops simultaneously with the accumulation of numerous independent and discrete parenchymal extinction lesions throughout the liver
- The form of cirrhosis is largely determined by the distribution of the vascular injury.

When a region of parenchyma becomes extinct, it collapses so that a portal tract becomes closely associated with an adjacent terminal hepatic vein. This close approximation offers an opportunity for the artery in the portal tract to drain directly into the collapsed perivenous tissue, creating a stable high-flow and high-pressure conduit connecting a small artery to a small hepatic vein. Short of parenchymal extinction, the formation of bona fide bridging fibrous septa between portal tracts and terminal hepatic veins in cirrhosis enables portovenous and arteriovenous shunting through de novo vascular channels, effectively bypassing the parenchymal nodules. Shunted blood flow through the fast vascular channels leaves the remainder of the hepatic parenchyma almost bereft of meaningful blood flow.[31,32] This would also help explain the increased blood flow observed in sinusoids of the cirrhotic liver, in the midst of relative underperfusion of the liver parenchyma as a whole. A remarkable fraction of nutritive blood flow may therefore pass through these intrahepatic functional shunts, contributing to ongoing hepatocellular necrosis and, hence, further parenchymal extinction. This vicious cycle contributes to transformation of the liver into a scarred, misshapen organ through which blood can barely pass, with the ensuing complications of portal hypertension and functional failure.

Physical occlusion of the sinusoids
Physical occlusion of the sinusoids occurs in a small but important group of diseases.

- In sickle cell disease, the hepatic sinusoids may become packed with sickled erythrocytes, free in the sinusoids, or phagocytosed by Kupffer cells (**Fig. 4**), leading to panlobular parenchymal necrosis.
- Disseminated intravascular coagulation may occlude sinusoids. This condition is usually inconsequential except for the periportal sinusoidal occlusion and parenchymal necrosis that may arise in pregnancy as part of eclampsia (**Fig. 5**).
- Metastatic tumor cells (eg, breast carcinoma, lymphoma, malignant melanoma) may fill the hepatic sinusoids in the absence of a mass lesion (**Fig. 6**). The attendant obstruction to blood flow and massive necrosis of hepatocytes can lead to fulminant hepatic failure.

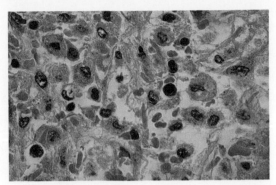

Fig. 4. Sickle cell disease, in which sinusoids are filled with sickled erythrocytes. This field was immediately adjacent to a macroscopic area of hepatic infarction (hematoxylin and eosin stain, original magnification 400×.)

- Amyloidosis may lead to massive deposition of proteinaceous material in the space of Disse. The sinusoidal lumen is narrowed or obliterated, and hepatocytes also atrophy (**Fig. 7**). Even severe hepatic amyloidosis may be clinically silent, until vague manifestations of hepatic dysfunction become evident.

Passive congestion and centrilobular necrosis
These hepatic manifestations of systemic circulatory compromise are considered together because they represent a morphologic continuum. Both changes are commonly seen at autopsy because there is an element of preterminal circulatory failure with virtually every death.

Right-sided cardiac decompensation leads to passive congestion of the liver. The liver is slightly enlarged, tense, and cyanotic, with rounded edges. Microscopically, there is congestion of centrilobular sinusoids. With time, centrilobular hepatocytes become atrophic, resulting in markedly attenuated liver cell plates. Left-sided cardiac failure or shock may lead to hepatic hypoperfusion and hypoxia, causing ischemic coagulative necrosis of hepatocytes in the central region of the lobule (centrilobular necrosis). In most instances, the only clinical evidence of centrilobular necrosis or

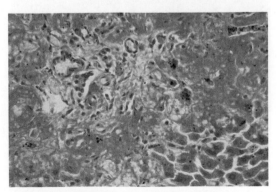

Fig. 5. Eclampsia, in which disseminated intravascular coagulation led to occlusion of periportal sinusoids, with ensuing periportal necrosis. The portal tract is in the center of the image (hematoxylin and eosin stain, original magnification 100×.)

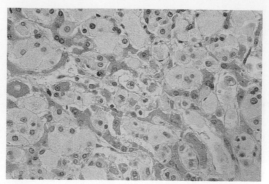

Fig. 6. Sinusoidal infiltration by malignant melanoma (hematoxylin and eosin stain, original magnification 400×.)

its variants is mild to moderate transient increase of serum aminotransferases, but the parenchymal damage may be sufficient to induce mild to moderate jaundice.

The combination of hypoperfusion and retrograde congestion acts synergistically to generate centrilobular hemorrhagic necrosis. The liver takes on a variegated mottled appearance, reflecting hemorrhage and necrosis in the centrilobular regions, known as the nutmeg liver (**Fig. 8**). By microscopy, there is a sharp demarcation of viable periportal and necrotic pericentral hepatocytes, with suffusion of blood through the centrilobular region. An uncommon complication of sustained chronic severe congestive heart failure is so-called cardiac sclerosis. The pattern of liver fibrosis is distinctive, in that it is mostly centrilobular.[33,34] The damage rarely fulfills the criteria for the diagnosis of cirrhosis, but the historically sanctified term cardiac cirrhosis cannot easily be replaced.

Peliosis hepatis

Sinusoidal dilation occurs in any condition in which efflux of hepatic blood is impeded. Peliosis hepatitis is a rare condition in which the dilation is primary.[35] The liver contains blood-filled cystic spaces, either nonlined or lined with sinusoidal endothelial cells.[36]

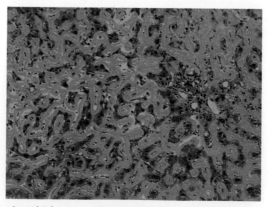

Fig. 7. Amyloidosis, in which sinusoids are obliterated by subendothelial deposition of amyloid protein within the space of Disse (hematoxylin and eosin stain, original magnification 400×.)

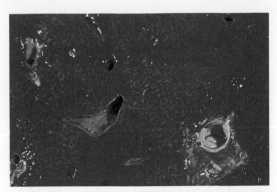

Fig. 8. Centrilobular hemorrhagic necrosis, showing variegated appearance of cut liver surface at autopsy.

The pathogenesis of peliosis hepatis is unknown. Focal apoptosis of hepatocytes or sinusoidal endothelial cells, and disruption of liver extracellular matrix, seems to play a role in the pathogenesis. *Bartonella* species have been seen in the sinusoidal endothelial cells in AIDS-associated peliosis.[37] Clinically, it is associated with many diseases, including cancer, tuberculosis, AIDS, or posttransplantation immunodeficiency. It is also associated with exposure to anabolic steroids and, rarely, oral contraceptives and danazol. Clinical signs are generally absent even in advanced peliosis, but potentially fatal intraabdominal hemorrhage or hepatic failure may occur. Peliotic lesions usually disappear after correction of underlying causes.

Hepatic Venous Outflow Obstruction

Hepatic vein thrombosis and inferior vena cava thrombosis
Obstruction of a single main hepatic vein by thrombosis is clinically silent. The obstruction of 2 or more major hepatic veins produces liver enlargement, pain, and ascites, a condition known as Budd-Chiari syndrome. It is the consequence of increased intrahepatic blood pressure, and an inability of the massive hepatic blood flow to shunt around the blocked outflow tract. Hepatic vein thrombosis is associated with primary myeloproliferative disorders (including polycythemia vera), inherited disorders of coagulation (eg, deficiencies in antithrombin, protein S, or protein C, or mutations of factor V), antiphospholipid syndrome, paroxysmal nocturnal hemoglobinuria, and intraabdominal cancers, particularly hepatocellular carcinoma. The occurrence of hepatic vein thrombosis in the setting of pregnancy or oral contraceptive use is usually through interaction with an underlying thrombogenic disorder. About 10% of cases are idiopathic in origin, presumably unrecognized thrombogenic disorders.

A separate distinction is made for inferior vena cava obstruction at its hepatic portion (obliterative hepatocavopathy). This disorder is caused by inferior vena cava thrombosis or membranous obstruction of the inferior vena cava. It is endemic in Nepal, with a suspected association with infections.[38]

With acutely developing thrombosis of the major hepatic veins or the hepatic portion of the inferior vena cava, the liver is swollen and red-purple and has a tense capsule. Microscopically, the affected hepatic parenchyma reveals severe centrilobular congestion and necrosis (**Fig. 9**). Centrilobular fibrosis develops in instances in which the thrombosis is more slowly developing. The major veins may contain totally

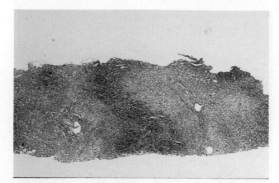

Fig. 9. Budd-Chiari syndrome. Low power microscopic image showing hemorrhage into cen-trilobular region, located midway between unaffected portal tracts (Masson trichrome stain, original magnification 40×).

occlusive fresh thrombi, subtotal occlusion, or, in chronic cases, organized adherent thrombi.

The mortality of untreated acute hepatic vein thrombosis is high. Prompt surgical creation of a portosystemic venous shunt permits reverse flow through the portal vein and considerably improves the prognosis. In vena caval thrombosis, direct dila-tion of caval obstruction may be possible during angiography. The chronic forms of these thrombotic syndromes are less lethal, and more than two-thirds of patients are alive after 5 years.

Sinusoidal obstruction syndrome (venoocclusive disease)

Originally described in Jamaican drinkers of pyrrolizidine alkaloid–containing bush tea and named venoocclusive disease, the disease is now called sinusoidal obstructive syndrome, and occurs primarily in the immediate weeks following bone marrow trans-plantation.[39] The incidence approaches 25% in recipients of allogeneic marrow trans-plants, usually within the first 3 weeks. Sinusoidal obstructive syndrome can occur in patients who have cancer and are receiving chemotherapy, especially with agents such as gemtuzumab ozogamicin (used in the treatment of acute myeloid leukemia),

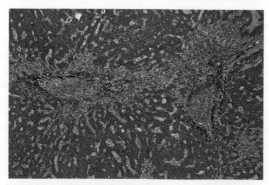

Fig. 10. Venoocclusive disease. Medium power image showing occlusion of terminal hepatic veins by cellular debris and retained erythrocytes, with partial fibrotic organization. The perivenular (centrilobular) parenchyma shows hepatocyte loss and hemorrhage (Masson tri-chrome stain, original magnification 100×).

actinomycin D (in the treatment of Wilms tumors), dacarbazine (a drug that is activated by sinusoidal endothelial cells), and in patients who receive cytotoxic agents such as cyclophosphamide before bone marrow transplantation. Mortality can be more than 30%. Although histology is the gold standard for the diagnosis, a diagnosis of sinusoidal obstruction syndrome is frequently made solely on clinical grounds (tender hepatomegaly, ascites, weight gain, and jaundice), owing to the high risk of liver biopsy in these patients.

Sinusoidal obstructive syndrome is characterized by obliteration of hepatic vein radicles by varying amounts of subendothelial swelling and fine reticulated collagen.[40] In acute disease, there is striking centrilobular congestion with hepatocellular necrosis and accumulation of hemosiderin-laden macrophages. As the disease progresses, obliteration of the lumen of the venule is easily identified by using special stains for connective tissue (**Fig. 10**). In chronic or healed sinusoidal obstruction syndrome, dense perivenular fibrosis radiating out into the parenchyma may be present, frequently with total obliteration of the venule; hemosiderin deposition is evident in the scar tissue, and congestion is minimal.

Sinusoidal obstructive syndrome arises from toxic injury to the sinusoidal endothelium,[40,41] which presumably starts with the depolymerization of actin in sinusoidal endothelial cells and increased production of metalloproteinases. Endothelial lining cells round up and slough off the sinusoidal wall, embolizing downstream and obstructing sinusoidal blood flow. This process is accompanied by entry of erythrocytes into the space of Disse, necrosis of perivenular hepatocytes, and downstream accumulation of cellular debris in the terminal hepatic vein. Proliferation of perisinusoidal stellate cells and subendothelial fibroblasts in the terminal hepatic vein follows, with fibrosis and deposition of extracellular matrix in the sinusoids.

Nodular Hyperplasias

Liver tumors would not readily be classified as vascular disorders. However, 2 nodular conditions merit discussion because their underlying pathophysiology is vascular: focal nodular hyperplasia, and nodular regenerative hyperplasia. The common factor in both types of nodules seems to be alterations in hepatic blood supply arising from focal obliteration of portal vein radicles with compensatory augmentation of arterial blood supply. In focal nodular hyperplasia, the obliteration is localized, whereas in nodular regenerative hyperplasia the lesions are present throughout the liver.[27,42]

Focal nodular hyperplasia appears as a well-demarcated but poorly encapsulated nodule, ranging up to many centimeters in diameter. The lesion is generally lighter than the surrounding liver and is sometimes yellow. Typically, there is a central gray-white, depressed stellate scar from which fibrous septa radiate to the periphery. The central scar contains large vessels, usually arterial, that typically exhibit fibromuscular hyperplasia with eccentric or concentric narrowing of the lumen. The radiating septa exhibit foci of intense lymphocytic infiltrates and exuberant bile duct proliferation along septal margins. The parenchyma between the septa exhibits essentially normal hepatocytes but with a thickened plate architecture characteristic of regeneration. Focal nodular hyperplasia presents as a spontaneous mass lesion, most frequently in young to middle-aged adults, either women or men. Although the pathogenesis is unknown, long-term use of anabolic hormones or of contraceptives have been implicated in the development of focal nodular hyperplasia. These nodules are usually found incidentally, although symptoms from a mass lesion may bring this lesion to clinical attention.

Nodular regenerative hyperplasia affects the entire liver with roughly spherical nodules, in the absence of fibrosis. Microscopically, plump hepatocytes are surrounded by rims of atrophic cells. The variation in parenchymal architecture may be missed on a hematoxylin and eosin stain, and reticulin staining is required to appreciate the changes in hepatocellular architecture. Nodular regenerative hyperplasia is associated with the development of portal hypertension with its attendant clinical manifestations. The latter lesion occurs in association with conditions affecting intrahepatic blood flow, including solid organ (particularly renal) transplantation, bone marrow transplantation, and vasculitic conditions. Nodular regenerative hyperplasia may also occur in patients infected with human immunodeficiency virus. A common theme is smoldering vascular injury, affecting the hepatic vascular circulation over a period of many years.

REFERENCES

1. Couinaud C. Le foie; études anatomiques et chirurgicales. Paris: Masson et Cie; 1957 [in French].
2. Crawford JM. Development of the intrahepatic biliary tree. Semin Liver Dis 2002; 22:213–26.
3. Teutsch HF. The modular microarchitecture of human liver. Hepatology 2005;42: 317–25.
4. Chang RW, Quan S-S, Yen WW. An applied anatomic study of the ostia venae hepaticae and the retrohepatic segment of the inferior vena cava. J Anat 1989;164:41–8.
5. Roskams T, Desmet VJ, Verslype C. Development, structure and function of the liver. In: Burt AD, Portmann BC, Ferrell LD, editors. MacSween's pathology of the liver. Philadelphia (PA): Churchill Livingstone/Elsevier; 2007. p. 1–76.
6. Washington K, Clavien PA, Killenberg P. Peribiliary vascular plexus in primary sclerosing cholangitis and primary biliary cirrhosis. Hum Pathol 1997;28:791–5.
7. Crawford AR, Lin XZ, Crawford JM. The normal adult human liver biopsy: a quantitative reference standard. Hepatology 1998;28:323–31.
8. Takasaki S, Hano H. Three dimensional observation of the human hepatic artery (arterial system in the liver). J Hepatol 2001;34:455–66.
9. McCuskey RS. Morphological mechanisms for regulating blood flow through hepatic sinusoids. Liver 2000;20:3–7.
10. Ekataksin W, Kaneda K. Liver microvascular architecture: an insight into the pathophysiology of portal hypertension. Semin Liver Dis 1999;19:359–82.
11. Ekataksin W. The isolated artery: an intrahepatic arterial pathway that can bypass the lobular parenchyma in mammalian livers. Hepatology 2000;31:269–79.
12. Le Beil B, Bioulac-Sage P, Senuita R, et al. Fine structure of hepatic sinusoids and sinusoidal cells in disease. J Electron Microsc Tech 1990;14:257–82.
13. More N, Lobosotomayor G, Basse-Cathalinat B, et al. Splanchnic arterial blood flow in rats with portacaval shunts. Am J Physiol 1984;246:G331–4.
14. Oda M, Yokomori H, Han JY. Regulatory mechanisms of hepatic microcirculatory hemodynamics: hepatic arterial system. Clin Hemorheol Microcirc 2006;34:11–26.
15. Khalaf H. Vascular complications after deceased and living donor liver transplantation: a single-center experience. Transplant Proc 2010;42:865–70.
16. Proposito D, Loinaz Segurola C, Garcia Garcia I, et al. Assessment of risk factors in the incidence of hepatic artery thrombosis in a consecutive series of 687 liver transplantation. Ann Ital Chir 2001;72:187–205.
17. Spaander MC, van Buuren HR, Hansen BE, et al. Ascites in patients with noncirrhotic non-malignant extrahepatic portal vein thrombosis. Aliment Pharmacol Ther 2010;32(4):529–30.

18. Eapen CE, Nightingale P, Hubscher SG, et al. Non-cirrhotic intrahepatic portal hypertension: associated gut diseases and prognostic factors. Dig Dis Sci 2010. [Epub ahead of print, PMID: 20499175].
19. Inokuma T, Eguchi S, Tomonaga T, et al. Acute deterioration of idiopathic portal hypertension requiring living donor liver transplantation: a case report. Dig Dis Sci 2009;54:1597–601.
20. Bioulac-Sage P, Le Bail B, Bernard PH, et al. Hepatoportal sclerosis. Semin Liver Dis 1995;15:329–39.
21. Wanless I, Crawford JM. Cirrhosis. In: Odze RD, Goldblum JR, editors. Pathology of the gastrointestinal tract, pancreas, liver and biliary tree. 2nd edition. Philadelphia: WB Saunders; 2008. p. 1147–68.
22. Nakashima E, Kage M, Wanless IR. Idiopathic portal hypertension: histologic evidence that some cases may be regressed cirrhosis with portal vein thrombosis. Hepatology 1999;30:218A.
23. Wanless IR, Nakashima E, Sherman M. Regression of human cirrhosis: morphologic features and the genesis of incomplete septal cirrhosis. Arch Pathol Lab Med 2000;124:1599–607.
24. Goodman ZD, Ishak KG. Occlusive venous lesions in alcoholic liver disease: a study of 200 cases. Gastroenterology 1982;83:786–96.
25. Nakanuma Y, Ohta G, Doishita K. Quantitation and serial section observations of focal veno-occlusive lesions of hepatic veins in liver cirrhosis. Virchows Arch A Pathol Anat Histopathol 1985;405:429–38.
26. Wanless IR, Wong F, Blendis LM, et al. Hepatic and portal vein thrombosis in cirrhosis: possible role in development of parenchymal extinction and portal hypertension. Hepatology 1995;21:1238–47.
27. Shimamatsu K, Wanless IR. Role of ischemia in causing apoptosis, atrophy, and nodular hyperplasia in human liver. Hepatology 1997;26:343–50.
28. Okuda K, Ohnishi K, Kimura K, et al. Incidence of portal vein thrombosis in liver cirrhosis. An angiographic study in 708 patients. Gastroenterology 1985;89: 279–86.
29. Hou PC, McFadzean AJ. Thrombosis and intimal thickening in the portal system of cirrhosis of the liver. J Pathol Bacteriol 1965;89:473–80.
30. Burt AD, MacSween RNM. Hepatic vein lesions in alcoholic liver disease: retrospective biopsy and necropsy study. J Clin Pathol 1986;39:63–7.
31. Sherman IA, Pappas SC, Fisher MM. Hepatic microvascular changes associated with development of liver fibrosis and cirrhosis. Am J Physiol 1990;258: H460–5.
32. Wanless IR, Shimamatsu K. Phlebitis in viral and autoimmune chronic hepatitis and primary biliary cirrhosis. Possible role in the histogenesis of cirrhosis. Mod Pathol 1997;10:147A.
33. Tanaka M, Wanless IR. Pathology of the liver in Budd-Chiari syndrome: portal vein thrombosis and the histogenesis of veno-centric cirrhosis, veno-portal cirrhosis, and large regenerative nodules. Hepatology 1998;27:488–96.
34. Wanless IR, Liu JJ, Butany J. Role of thrombosis in the pathogenesis of congestive hepatic fibrosis (cardiac cirrhosis). Hepatology 1995;21:1232–7.
35. DeLeve LD. Hepatic microvasculature in liver injury. Semin Liver Dis 2007;27: 390–400.
36. Tsokos M, Erbersdobler A. Pathology of peliosis. Forensic Sci Int 2005;20: 25–33.
37. Koehler JE, Tappero JW. Bacillary angiomatosis and bacillary peliosis in patients infected with human immunodeficiency virus. Clin Infect Dis 1993;17:612–24.

38. Kew MC, Hodkinson HJ. Membranous obstruction of the inferior vena cava and its causal relation to hepatocellular carcinoma. Liver Int 2006;26:1–7.
39. Bayraktar UD, Seren S, Bayraktar Y. Hepatic venous outflow obstruction: three similar syndromes. World J Gastroenterol 2007;13:1912–27.
40. Helmy A. Review article: updates in the pathogenesis and therapy of hepatic sinusoidal obstruction syndrome. Aliment Pharmacol Ther 2006;23:11–25.
41. Chojkier M. Hepatic sinusoidal-obstruction syndrome: toxicity of pyrrolizidine alkaloids. J Hepatol 2003;39:437–46.
42. Bioulac-Sage P, Balabaud C, Wanless IR. Diagnosis of focal nodular hyperplasia: not so easy. Am J Surg Pathol 2001;25:1322–5.

Sinusoidal Obstruction Syndrome

Laura Rubbia-Brandt, MD, PhD*

KEYWORDS

- Oxaliplatin • Colorectal liver metastases • Hepatotoxicity
- Drugs • Chemotherapy • Hepatic vascular lesions

Hepatic sinusoidal obstruction syndrome (SOS) is caused by toxic injury to sinusoidal endothelial cells (SECs). It is characterized by the loss of sinusoidal wall integrity with consequent sinusoidal congestive obstruction and is occasionally associated with perisinusoidal fibrosis, centrilobular hepatic vein fibrotic obstruction, nodular regenerative hyperplasia (NRH), or peliosis. Initial reports of this condition date from 100 years ago with causative agents being senecio poisoning in South Africa,[1] consumption of pyrrolizidine alkaloid–rich herbal bush tea in Jamaica,[2] and inadequately winnowed wheat or herbal traditional remedies in countries such as India or Egypt.[3] More recently, it has become a well-established complication of myeloablative high-dose chemoirradiation treatment in the context of hematopoietic stem cell transplantation.[4] Today, SOS has been associated with more than 20 drugs including conventional doses of some immunosuppressive and chemotherapeutic agents (**Box 1**).

The disease was originally known as hepatic venoocclusive disease (VOD), in reference to histologically evident centrilobular vein occlusion. At that time, these hepatic venous lesions were necessary for the diagnosis. However, recent experimental studies have clarified the pathogenesis of SOS, and shown that centrilobular vein involvement is not essential to the development of SOS and that the main injury occurs at the level of the hepatic sinusoids.[5,6] In pathologic studies, occlusion of the centrilobular veins occurs only in 50% to 75% of patients who develop SOS after hematopoietic stem cell transplantation[7] and approximately 50% of patient with SOS after oxaliplatin (OX)-based chemotherapy.[8–10] This has led to a general acceptance of the term SOS in preference to VOD. The diagnosis is currently based on sinusoidal lesions, independently of hepatic venous lesions.

The current increase in the diagnosis of SOS has resulted from its recognition as a complication in a range of situations such as solid organ transplantation, inflammatory bowel diseases requiring the use of immunosuppression, and colorectal liver metastases (CRLM) treated by preoperative chemotherapy. Recommendations for

Division of Clinical Pathology of University Hospital, Geneva, Switzerland
* Service de Pathologie Clinique, Hôpitaux Universitaires de Genève, 1 rue Michel Servet, 1211 Geneva, Switzerland
E-mail address: laura.rubbia-brandt@hcuge.ch

Clin Liver Dis 14 (2010) 651–668
doi:10.1016/j.cld.2010.07.009
1089-3261/10/$ – see front matter © 2010 Elsevier Inc. All rights reserved.

liver.theclinics.com

Box 1
Major causes of SOS in humans

Actinomycin D

Azathioprine

Busulfan

Carmustine

Cytosine arabinoside

Cyclophosphamide

Dacarbazine

Gemtuzumab ozogamicin

Melphalan

Mercaptopurine

Mitomycin

Oxaliplatin

Pyrrozolidine alkaloids

Urethane

Terbinafine

Traditional herbal remedies

6-Mercaptopurine

6-Thioguanine

Bone marrow transplantation

Total-body irradiation

Hepatic irradiation (high doses)

Platelet transfusion containing ABO-incompatible plasma

---

dealing with hepatotoxicity from CRLM have been proposed.[11] Although some preventive strategies are being studied, surgeons, oncologists, hepatologists, radiologists, and pathologists dealing with patients with colorectal cancer should be aware that this distinctive vascular lesion is common, that its management strategy and surgical risks can alter, and that it can engender significant morbidity and mortality.

SOS PATHOLOGIC LESIONS IN HUMANS

Regardless of its cause, SOS has similar morphologic features. A liver with severe SOS has a typical bluish red, marbled appearance (**Figs. 1** and **2**). The lesion may occasionally predominate in the subcapsular region or be associated with hemorrhagic lakes resembling peliosis hepatitis. This appearance, commonly known as blue liver, can result in surgical anxiety and frequent requests for frozen section examination.

The microscopic lesions are randomly distributed with affected lobules intermingled with intact parenchyma. SOS is characterized by distinct areas of dilated sinusoids filled with plugs of erythrocytes. These are predominately observed in centrilobular zones

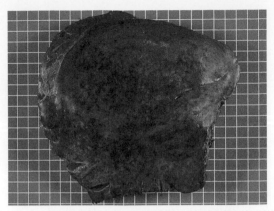

Fig. 1. Macroscopically, the liver appears bluish red and marbled.

and form bridging congestive bands (**Fig. 3**). This sinusoidal congestion is associated with perisinusoidal hemorrhage characterized by extravasation of erythrocytes into the perisinusoidal space (**Figs. 4** and **5**) consistent with sinusoidal wall rupture. The extravasation of erythrocytes may be focal or diffuse along the dilated sinusoids. Occasionally, centrilobular veins show focal endothelial cell rounding and/or intimal hemorrhage, and the venular inlets are dilated and easily visible where they join the centrilobular veins. These sinusoidal areas may be associated with atrophy of hepatocellular plates, dissociation of hepatocytes, or focal hepatocellular necrosis. At the ultrastructural level, endothelial cells are rounded up and protrude into the lumen of the sinusoid.[8] The perisinusoidal space may be completely denuded of endothelial cells. The sinusoidal lumen is filled with cytoplasmic blebs and erythrocytes (see **Fig. 5**).

Morphologic studies have shown that drug-related SOS may be associated with 1 or more other lesions such as centrilobular perisinusoidal and venular fibrosis, peliosis, and NRH.[9,10,12] These lesions are morphologically distinct from sinusoidal changes, although they are related to its severity.[9]

When present, perisinusoidal fibrosis often affects only a segment of the centrilobular zone (see **Fig. 4**) and may be accompanied by variable degrees of centrilobular vein occlusion (see **Fig. 4**) that is only rarely complete. Centrilobular vein occlusion and perisinusoidal fibrosis are related to SOS severity.

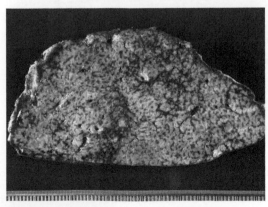

Fig. 2. Macroscopically, the cut surface of the liver is congested.

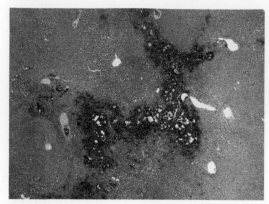

Fig. 3. At low-power examination, the liver revealed areas of sinusoidal congestion involving centrilobular and mediolobular areas, forming bridging congestive bands.

SOS may be associated with nodular transformation of the liver (or NRH in its diffuse form), which is characterized by small, bulging nodules composed of enlarged hepatocytic cells. These cells may be centered on portal tracts and delineated at their periphery by atrophic hepatocytes or dilated sinusoids (**Figs. 6** and **7**).

A detailed pathologic grading system of human SOS and associated lesions has recently been published.[9] This should serve as a common language in the multidisciplinary team managing patients with CRLM.

PATHOGENESIS

Most drugs that induce SOS have been shown in vitro to be more toxic to SEC than to hepatocytes.[13,14] Glutathione depletion in SEC exacerbates SEC injury, whereas depletion in hepatocytes does not increase hepatocyte injury.

Normal Sinusoids and SECs

The complex functions of the liver are tightly dependent on an adequate microcirculation, with sinusoids playing a crucial role.

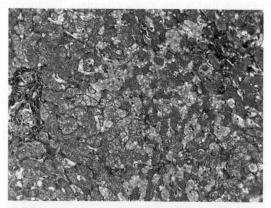

Fig. 4. On Masson trichrome stain at higher-power examination, sinusoidal congestion is severe in centrilobular and mediolobular zones, outlined by atrophic hepatocyte trabeculae. The small hepatic vein is partially occluded by fibrous tissue. Fibrosis is present focally along centrilobular sinusoids.

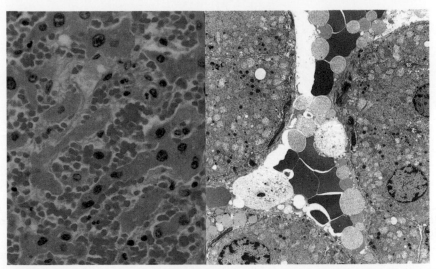

Fig. 5. At high-power field, the perisinusoidal space of Disse is extensively dilated and contains several erythrocytes in close contact with hepatocytes. At ultrastructure, erythrocytes are intermingled with cytoplasmic blebs.

The sinusoid is a unique vessel lined by fenestrated endothelium and lacking a basement membrane.[13,14] It is surrounded by the perisinusoidal space of Disse, which contains a minimal collagen network. The sinusoid is the principal hepatic vessel involved in transvascular exchange between the blood and the parenchymal cells. It supplies parenchymal tissue with oxygen and nutriments and serves as a gate controlling leukocyte egress in hepatic inflammation.[15] In addition, it is responsible for clearing toxins and foreign bodies from the bloodstream. Intact microvascular function requires distinct sinusoidal cell populations (ie, Kupffer cells [KCs], SECs, and hepatic stellate cells [HSCs]) (**Fig. 8**).

Several SEC functions are related to their morphologic characteristics. SECs are flattened, with processes perforated by pores known as fenestrae that occupy 6% to 8% of the endothelial surface.[16] The fenestrae are organized in clusters of 10 to 50 pores, 150 nm in diameter and unevenly distributed along the sinusoid. The highest

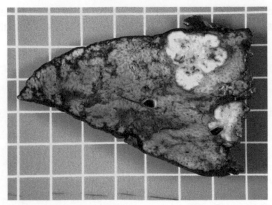

Fig. 6. Macroscopically, on the cut surface, the liver is diffusely nodular. Nodules are outlined by congested areas.

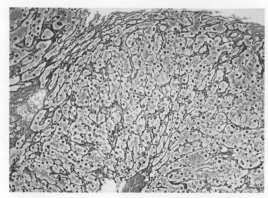

Fig. 7. High-power examination on reticulin stain shows a regenerative nodule made of enlarged hepatocytic cells centered by portal tracts and delineated at the periphery by atrophic hepatocytes.

concentration of these pores is localized in the centilobular zone. Fenestrae are dynamic structures that contract and dilate, functioning as a selective sieving barrier to control the exchange. The absence of basement membrane around SECs also contributes to direct contact of soluble and insoluble blood constituents with hepatocytes, resulting in the enhancement of hepatic metabolic activity.[13,14] SECs have a scavenger function, eliminating a variety of macromolecules from the blood by receptor-mediated endocytosis, and an antigen-presenting function similar to dendritic cells. In cooperation with KCs and hepatic dendritic cells, they may thus participate in the immunoregulatory functions of the liver.[15]

HSCs are fat- and vitamin A–storing perisinusoidal cells that have a major role in retinol metabolism and the regulation of sinusoidal blood flow.[13] When activated, they acquire a more myofibroblastic phenotype and are essential actors in hepatic fibrosis.[17]

KCs are anchored to the luminal face of the sinusoids, they are attached to endothelium, and are exposed to bloodstream.[13] They have a heterogeneous distribution along the sinusoids, resulting in zonal distribution of phagocytosis. Their cell bodies protrude into the lumen, induce flow hindrance, and contribute to blood flow regulation.

Sinusoids play a major role in regulating hepatic blood flow, in part through autoregulation of sinusoidal blood flow. This autoregulation occurs through a critical

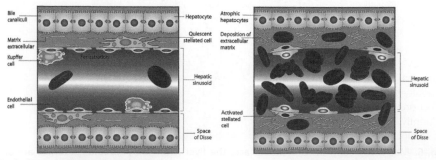

Fig. 8. Normal sinusoid and SOS.

balance between vasoconstrictive and vasodilative agents. In normal liver, nitric oxide (NO) is predominantly synthesized by the constitutive NO synthetase of endothelial cells in large vessels and sinusoids. NO regulates the vascular tone of the hepatic circulation. It acts as a potent vasodilator of arterial circulation, but exerts only a minor effect on the portal venous bed. NO also regulates hepatic sinusoid flow by acting on HSCs. In addition to its role in blood flow regulation, NO influences extracellular matrix remodeling by inhibiting matrix metalloproteinase (MMP) expression.

The hepatic microenvironment is responsible for the unique features of SECs.[13,14,18] Both vascular endothelial growth factor (VEGF) produced by hepatocytes and HSCs and NO released by SECs themselves in response to VEGF have a major role in maintaining SEC differentiation, notably SEC fenestration. SECs themselves play a major role in maintenance of normal sinusoid structure. SECs express matrix metalloprotein-9 (MMP-9) and matrix metalloprotein-2 (MMP-2), enzymes responsible for extracellular remodeling. SECs maintain HSCs in a quiescent state through VEGF-stimulated NO production, and promote reversion of activated collagen–producing HSC to a quiescent state.[19] Activation of SEC exerts proinflammatory and proadhesive, as well as procoagulant, properties.

SECs are a major cellular target for several toxins.[14] One explanation for this is their location, which results in their direct exposure to drugs absorbed by the intestinal tract and transported to the liver by portal circulation. Hepatocytes and SECs are rich in cytochrome P450 and thus activate drugs and export their toxic metabolites into the perisinusoidal space.

Animal Model

The development of a rat model based on monocrotaline gavage by Deleve and colleagues[20] has led to a better understanding of SOS pathogenesis, both at the morphologic and biochemical levels. These mechanisms are summarized in **Fig. 9**.

Monocotaline is a pyrrolizidine alkaloid metabolized into the toxic compound monocrotaline pyrrole by cytochrome P450 enzymes present in hepatic SECs and subsequently detoxified by glutathione. Pathologic changes are seen in centrilobular zones of hepatic lobules within 48 hours after monocrotaline administration.[21] The initial target of injury is the SEC. Monocrotaline binds to actin filaments in the cytoplasm of SECs and causes their depolymerization.[22] This alteration in the cytoskeleton results in morphologic changes of SECs, which round up, swell, and lose their fenestration. This rupture of the sinusoidal endothelial barrier allows erythrocytes to penetrate the perisinusoidal space and dissect the sinusoidal lining. Additional events aggravate SEC injury and detachment. An increase in expression of MMP-9 (and to a lesser extent MMP-2) from SECs and KCs coincides with sinusoidal lining denudation in the first 48 hours and continues for several days.[22] Perisinusoidal extracellular matrix degradation may occur and further contributes to SEC detachment and dehiscence. Two mechanisms cause this upregulation in MMPs activity: actin depolymerization and the loss of SECs, which results in a decline in NO synthesis and thus the removal NO-related inhibition of MMPs synthesis.[22,23] Oxidative stress also contributes to SEC injury through monocrotaline-induced in vitro and in vivo depletion of cellular glutathione and augmentation of reactive oxygen species (ROS) production.[23] Sloughed SECs, cytoplasmic blebs, and KCs intermingle with erythrocytes subsequently embolize downstream within the sinusoid lumen toward venular inlets and centrilobular veins.[24] This increase in microvascular plugging causes a reduction of blood flow in the sinusoids. SOS therefore corresponds to the rupture of perisinusoidal space integrity and sinusoidal obstruction.

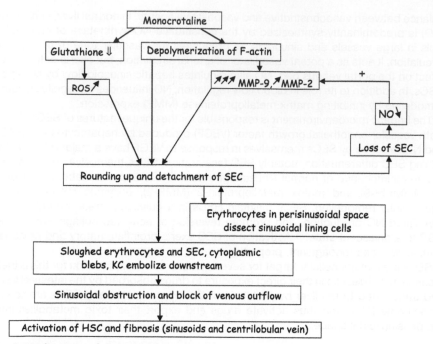

Fig. 9. Mechanisms of sinusoidal injury.

Between 3 and 5 days after monocrotaline exposure, heptocyte necrosis begins.[20] This can lead to widespread zonal liver disruption and centrilobular hemorrhagic necrosis. Lobular microvascular dysfunction occurs along with parenchymal injury, leading to a self-sustaining functional perfusion deficient–injury relationship.[13] Microcirculation disturbances lead to insufficient energy supply, alteration of mitochondrial redox state, subsequent decline of hepatic tissue oxygenation, and impairment of adenosine triphosphate regeneration. There is a tight relationship between intact microcirculation and the viability of parenchymal cells. Progressively mononuclear cells adhere to denuded sinusoids and to endothelium of centrilobular veins; this new cellular accumulation contributes to sinusoidal obstruction.[20] In parallel to this sinusoidal damage, hepatic VEGF mRNA expression is significantly increased.[21] VEGF plays an important role in maintaining the fenestrated endothelial barrier and preventing the capillarization of sinusoids.[13] High VEGF mRNA expression could be a response to endothelial barrier disruption or to cellular hypoxia following sinusoidal obstruction.[13]

Finally, at days 6 to 7, deposition of collagen in the sinusoids occurs with fibrosis of centrilobular venular lumens, leading to centrilobular venular occlusion and inlet vein occlusion (see **Fig. 8**).[20] Monocrotaline-related SOS according to the Deleve protocol is not associated with NRH development.

Injury to SEC possibly creates a procoagulant condition in the sinusoid. Overexpression of MMP-2 and MMP-9 is associated with increased platelet adhesion to sinusoidal cells after cold preservation of liver or sinusoidal cells.[21] Nevertheless, the role of clotting abnormalities in the experimental SOS model is the subject of debate.

It results in hepatomegaly, hyperbilirubinemia, and ascites.[20] It increases portal pressure and delays liver regeneration after major hepatectomy in an experimental animal model.[25]

Human SOS

The mechanisms involved human SOS have not been conclusively established. Morphologically, the lesions observed in chemotherapy-related SOS are similar to the monocrotaline rat model and the molecular causes might be similar. For instance, several drugs, such as OX and some platinum compounds, lead to generation of ROS and glutathione depletion in SEC, resulting in SEC injury.[26] Cisplatin may cause actin depolymerization and upregulation of MMP-9 activity.[27,28] Patients with SOS show increased serum VEGF that is synchronized with the development of SOS.[29] HSC activation has been reported in patients with SOS.[8]

As in rat, the role of clotting factors in the pathogenesis of human SOS is unclear. Ultrastructural studies of liver obtained from individuals with bush tea disease revealed no evidence of clotting abnormalities.[30] In addition, immunohistochemical studies of autopsy livers did not detect platelets, although fibrinogen and factor VIII were detected in the hepatic veins.[31] However, thrombocytopenia has recently been associated with severe OX-related SOS.[32] Because of the role of platelets in liver regeneration through a serotonin-mediated mechanism,[33] alteration in platelet function could play a role in postoperative liver insufficiency following severe SOS lesions.

SEC toxic injury in humans may manifest as NRH,[5,6] a lesion that is morphologically distinct from SOS, although its development is related to SOS severity.[9] The pathogenesis of NRH is poorly understood.[34–41] It is thought to be related to changes in intrahepatic blood flow that lead to atrophic hypoperfused areas interspersed with hyperperfused regenerative areas. Circulatory impairment can start either as obstructive portal vein injury[37,38] or at the level of the sinusoids, as in drug-associated NRH.[36] The role of inactivation of Notch1 as been shown in a mouse model but has yet to be evaluated in humans.[42] Platelet dysfunction has been associated with NRH in patients with human immunodeficiency virus.[43]

EFFECT OF CHEMOTHERAPY-ASSOCIATED SOS IN TREATMENT OF HEPATIC COLORECTAL METASTASES

Liver metastases develop either synchronously or metachronously in approximately 60% of patients with colorectal cancer, and are the most common complication of colorectal cancer. In about 30% of patients, the liver is the only site of metastatic involvement, heralding a 5-year survival rate of less than 10%. Thus, CRLM play a major role in colorectal cancer mortality.[44] Hepatic resection currently offers the best chance of long-term survival to these patients, with 5-year survival following complete resection reaching 60%.[45] However, less than 20% of CRLM are surgically resectable at diagnosis. Several factors have significantly increased the number of patients with CRLM who benefit from surgery: progress of surgical techniques, better knowledge of the functional anatomy of the liver, detection of metastases at an earlier stage, introduction of new therapeutic approaches (eg, cryosurgery, radiofrequency), and use of preoperative chemotherapy. The aim of preoperative chemotherapy is to reduce the size of metastases, thus allowing the resection of a significant number of metastases previously considered unresectable. Initially, only palliative treatment of metastatic colorectal cancer with 5-fluorouracil and leucovorin were available, yielding response rates of only 10% to 20%. Tumor size reduction to the point that would permit surgical resection was rare. Chemotherapy for CRLM has dramatically improved in the last decade, with tumoral response rates increasing to 80% using different combinations of new chemotherapeutic agents such as irinotecan, a topoisomerase I inhibitor, or OX, the only platinum derivative with significant activity in colorectal cancer, possibly combined with biologic agents such as bevacizumab, a monoclonal antibody against VEGF and cetuximab, a monoclonal antibody against epidermal growth factor receptor.[44–52] Such effective chemotherapies are thus increasingly used before hepatic surgery as neoadjuvant treatment to render unresectable CRLM resectable, to identify selective good responders before surgery, and because response to chemotherapy may be a good predictor of a tumors' biologic aggressiveness because those who progress less than chemotherapy may not benefit from resection. This management approach has resulted in an increased number of patients qualifying for curative surgical procedures, and a significant improvement in response rate, disease-free, and even overall survival in metastatic disease. This modern multidisciplinary management has become standard of care in most specialized European and North American centers.

One side effect of this approach has been an increased hepatotoxicity in the nontumoral liver, notably in association with OX. Since the initial report of OX-related SOS,[8] several reports have confirmed the presence of hepatic adverse effects of OX, and their relevance to preoperative management and postoperative outcomes.[10,12,53–57] Although a more cautious approach in the use of preoperative chemotherapy has been recommended,[11] and new surgical strategies are implemented considering OX-related liver damage,[58] investigations of SOS prevalence, OX spectrum of hepatic lesions, and the potential protective effect of bevacizumab are ongoing. Today, the clinical significance of OX-related SOS is widely recognized.[59–61]

Some differences in the prevalence of OX-related SOS exist in the literature.[8–10,32,50,53–56] These differences may be explained by heterogeneous populations amongst studies; differences in administration and number of cycles of chemotherapy; underrecognition, because lesions may be overlooked in centers that do not systematically perform special staining, such as reticulin, or that do not focus on sampling of the nontumoral parenchyma; some studies reporting only the prevalence of moderate to severe grades of SOS lesion, whereas others also report the prevalence of mild SOS; and the absence of a full consensus between pathologists on the definition of sinusoidal lesions related to chemotherapy.

SOS in the context of hematopoietic stem cell transplantation presents with a wide spectrum of clinical severity.[4–6] It is characterized by weight gain caused by fluid retention, with or without ascites, right upper quadrant pain of liver origin, hepatomegaly, and jaundice and can be divided into mild, moderate, and severe disease with clinical severity correlating closely with the severity of microvascular lesions. Mild SOS does not require treatment and has a self-limiting course. Moderate SOS requires treatment but resolves completely. Severe SOS may lead to death or does not resolve. Clinically severe SOS is not uniquely caused by occlusion of centrilobular veins but correlates with the other centrilobular changes.[7] The incidence of SOS after high-dose myeloablative conditioning regimens varies from 0% to 50% and mortality is currently in the range of 15% to 20%.[4] These variations are largely caused by the type of conditioning regimen, by the size of the patient cohort in different published series, and by diverse criteria or diagnoses. At autopsy, 50% of patients with liver dysfunction who did not meet clinical diagnostic criteria of SOS had evidence of SOS lesion on histology.[4] It is likely that some degree of sinusoidal injury occurs in most patients who receive liver toxic conditioning regimens, even in the absence of the characteristic symptoms.

Clinical consequences of SOS after OX treatment of CRLM have been a matter of debate. Today, its importance is clearly recognized. In the operative or postoperative period, patients treated with OX have a higher incidence of complications than patients who had surgery alone.[10–12,32,53–55,62] Postoperative morbidity is observed in 25% to 36% of patients, with typical clinical manifestations of OX-related liver injury being a longer duration of surgery, increase risk of preoperative hemorrhage, longer hospital stay, postoperative liver failure because of delayed regeneration, portal hypertension including ascites, splenomegaly, persistent thrombocytopenia, bleeding from esophageal and hemorrhoidal varices, and rare cases of unexplained mortality. Several investigators have reported that clinical complications were related to the duration of preoperative chemotherapy, with higher morbidity among patients who received at least 6 cycles or more compared with those who received fewer than 6 cycles or who were treated by surgery alone. Splenomegaly and thrombocytopenia have been shown to correlate with the number of cycles administered, but no direct relationship has been established between the dose of administered chemotherapy before liver resection and severity of SOS.[32] Based on several case reports, clinical manifestations can arise over a long period of time.[62] For instance, in patients with stage III cancer treated by systemic adjuvant chemotherapy, portal hypertension may develop within 2 to 3 weeks after hepatectomy, but also several months after the end of treatment.

Clinical complications such as portal hypertension following OX-based chemotherapy and more complicated surgery may also be related to the presence of NRH. NRH may have a prolonged silent clinical course but, when symptomatic, patients develop cholestasis with increased alkaline phosphatases and/or signs of portal hypertension that may dominate the clinical presentation. Large autopsy series have established the prevalence of NRH at 2.5% and revealed associations with various conditions, including chemotherapeutic agents.[37]

DIAGNOSIS OF SOS RELATED TO OX-BASED CHEMOTHERAPY FOR CRLM

Reliable preoperative diagnosis of SOS is essential to allow selection of patients before liver surgery, especially in complicated cases (eg, a major resection, a patient with CRLM, a potentially altered liver function reservoir because of OX pretreatment). However, the absence of a specific diagnostic tool makes recognizing SOS a challenge. Some risk factors of SOS have been identified, such as abnormal preoperative γ-glutamyltransferase, age, female gender, indocyanine green retention rate at 15 minutes, number of cycles of chemotherapy, and a short interval between the end of chemotherapy and liver resection.[54,63]

A recent study suggests that preoperative platelet count (to a value less than 167,000), aspartate aminotransferase (AST) platelet ratio index (APRI) value (a ratio index of aspartate aminotransferase to platelet count), or FIB-4 scoring system (calculated with a formula based on AST, platelet count, and age) may represent predictive noninvasive blood tests for high-grade lesions of SOS.[32] APRI scores have been evaluated as predictors of liver fibrosis in patients with hepatitis C virus–related liver disease. In multivariate analysis, a high APRI score was associated with severe histologic SOS. Although promising, the routine use of these scoring systems needs to be further assessed.

Although imaging is not independently diagnostic, it can play a role in supporting the diagnosis by demonstrating the presence of hepatomegaly and ascites. The best-studied modality seems to be magnetic resonance imaging for diagnosis of severe SOS, whereas computed tomography (CT) is unable to identify SOS accurately.[64,65]

In hematopoietic stem cell transplantation, the current standard for confirming the diagnosis of clinically apparent SOS is measurement of the wedged hepatic venous pressure gradient and liver histology.[66] Hepatic venous pressure gradient greater than 10 mm Hg has specificity greater than 90% and positive predictive value greater than 85% for the diagnosis of SOS. By analogy, this approach could raise the question of preoperative liver biopsy to confirm the severity of SOS lesions in patients with CRLM who are candidates for a major liver resection. The reliability of a liver biopsy suffers because SOS lesions can be heterogeneously distributed and thus liver biopsy can be falsely negative. Combining liver biopsy with hemodynamic evaluation could help the overall sensitivity. The benefit of a preoperative needle biopsy of the liver to evaluate the severity of SOS lesions in patients receiving preoperative OX-based chemotherapy has not been evaluated. Despite sensitive modern imaging modalities, histology is the only way to diagnose NRH with confidence. For pathologists, the diagnosis of NRH can be challenging, and reticulin staining is mandatory.

PREVENTION OF POSTOPERATIVE COMPLICATIONS

Knowledge of chemotherapy-associated hepatotoxicity has led to investigation of preventive strategies for the management of SOS in patients treated with OX. The multidisciplinary approach to the treatment of patients with CRLM has allowed more patients to undergo potentially curative hepatic resection. When resection with curative intent is planned, oncologists should avoid extended preoperative chemotherapy and address patients for surgery early. A tumor response can already be observed after 2 to 3 cycles of chemotherapy, and additional cycles of chemotherapy provide only a minor therapeutic benefit.[45] The objectives of chemotherapy are to control disease before surgery (not necessarily a radiologic remission) and to avoid adverse outcomes from chemotherapy-associated liver injury.[45,59–61] Radiologists should be aware of the limited accuracy of CT in CRLM detection after chemotherapy and that radiological tumor response is often not predictive of histologic tumor response.[64,65] Surgeons should be increasingly alert to chemotherapy-associated hepatotoxicity and pay attention not only to the liver that has to be removed but also to what will remain following resection. Pathologists should be aware that their role in this context is changing. Pathology reports for surgical CRLM resection should mention not only the resection margin status but also the degree of tumor response to preoperative chemotherapy (tumor regression grade)[52] and the type and degree of lesions in the surrounding nontumoral liver. Samplings of nontumoral liver and special stains are highly advisable. Pathologists can be solicited for frozen section or preoperative liver biopsy.

Evaluation of residual functional liver volume after hepatectomy has become a key component in the selection of patients for hepatic resection. The ratio of future liver remnant to total estimated liver volume is a surrogate parameter that indicates the potential function of the remnant liver and is a predictor of surgical outcome. In patients with normal liver function, a minimum of 20% is needed to prevent complications after a major hepatectomy. In patients with substantial chemotherapy-induced liver damage, a liver remnant of 30% has been proposed as the minimum volume needed for a safe hepatic resection.[59–61] Another method that predicts the function of the expected remnant liver is hepatic clearance of indocyanine green.[54]

Patients who have chemotherapy-associated liver injury and a hepatic residual volume that is expected to be insufficient after surgery may benefit from preoperative embolization of the portal vein branches supplying the liver tissue to be resected.[67–70] This procedure results in atrophy of the resected liver and induces hypertrophy of the future liver remnant. Inadequate liver hypertrophy following portal vein embolization is an important indicator of the inability of the liver to adequately recover and may be associated with increased postoperative morbidity. Two-stage hepatectomy is an interesting alternative that can minimize chemotherapy-associated liver complications but enable complete resection of metastases.[71]

The optimal interval between end of preoperative chemotherapy and liver surgery remains an open question. Some studies show that a longer interval between chemotherapy and hepatic resection reduces surgical complications for patients with CRLM but not postoperative morbidity.[72] However, this interval should be balanced with the risk of tumor progression during the treatment-free interval. Tumoral regrowth occurs rapidly, notably at the periphery of the tumor mass (dangerous halo) and major regrowth can already be seen only 4 to 7 weeks after chemotherapy.[71]

The potential for regression of chemotherapy-associated liver injury, notably SOS and NRH, remains unknown, as does the time frame for this regression and whether delayed hepatic complications can arise. Short-term studies have revealed the persistence of SOS and NRH in 2-stage hepatectomies in which the liver of a patient was available with an interval of 4 to 7 weeks, suggesting that there is no advantage in delaying an operation that is otherwise optimally scheduled for tumor response to chemotherapy.[71] In the long-term, the issue remains open: analogies with the toxic oil syndrome, in which NRH and portal hypertension were noted 2.5 years after consuming the oil, azathioprine, and 6-thioguanine, suggest that the changes may persist and become symptomatic in time.[73] In cases that underwent iterative hepatic surgery for recurrence, several cases of a persistence of sinusoidal dilatation or fibrosis were observed.[8] The level of portal hypertension, evaluated by spleen size, seems to improve only between 1 and 3 years after the end of OX treatment.[62] Thus, if cases of regression have been observed, the risks of persistence or progression of the disease exist, particularly for patients who receive multiple cycles of adjuvant or maintenance chemotherapy. Despite an apparently indolent course, delayed complications may develop.

Better comprehension of the molecular events underlying chemotherapy-associated hepatic injury might also be a source of potential medical prevention. Several options are beginning to emerge from studies in animal models. In the rat, administration of MMP-2/-9 inhibitors or infusion of glutathione prevented the development of SOS by reducing SEC damage.[22,23,74] In hematopoietic stem cell transplantation, preserved hepatic function was seen in patients treated with glutamine, a possible inducer of glutathione synthesis.[75] These approaches could be therapeutically viable strategies for prevention of OX-associated liver injury. Aspirin intake has been associated with reduced risk for sinusoidal lesions.[76]

Targeted biologic molecules are increasingly being used for the systemic treatment of CRLM. Bevacizumab has been shown to increase response rates in patients with stage IV colorectal cancer and to improved progression-free survival.[50] It also has a protective effect against OX-induced sinusoidal injury.[9,50,77] The mechanism by which this protective effect might occur is suggested by experimental studies in animal models and offers a rationale for the pathologic findings. Notably, VEGF induces MMP-9 expression by SEC.[13,17] Thus, VEGF blockade by bevacizumab may lead to downregulation of MMP-9 production and release, and thus may attenuate sinusoidal lesions. The preventive action of MMP-9 inactivation on SOS development is consistent with experiments in which other inhibitors of MMP-9 prevented the histologic changes, thus implicitly confirming a major causative role of MMPs in the pathogenesis of SOS.[5,6] The current study showing the decrease of both SOS and NRH in patients treated by OX and bevacizumab suggests a common pathogenic mechanism or link between them. However, if anti-VEGF therapy acts on sinusoidal dilatation, it may not act on endothelial injury itself. With bevacizumab, the effect of

VEGF on SEC differentiation and HSC quiescence can potentially be avoided.[19] This area is in need of further detailed studies.

Anticoagulants such as heparin and defibrotide, prostaglandin E1, plasminogen activator, ursodeoxycholic acid, and pentoxifylline have been examined for their ability to prevent hematopoietic stem cell transplantation–related SOS.[5,6] They modulate endothelial cell injury and protect the sinusoidal endothelium from SOS. They have yet to be evaluated in OX-related hepatotoxicity. New perspective will possibly emerge from the use of bone marrow–derived SEC progenitors.[78]

SUMMARY

Current management of several cancers is based on the use of effective systemic chemotherapy. One major drawback is hepatotoxicity. A target of drug toxicity is SECs, resulting in hepatic microcirculation. Based on recent clinicopathologic and experimental studies, there is now a general acceptance of the term SOS in preference to VOD. Injury to SECs is the key initiating event in SOS. Several open questions are the object of intense study, including its pathogenesis, diagnosis, and prevention.

REFERENCES

1. Willmot F. Senecio disease, or cirrhosis of the liver due to senecio poisoning. Lancet 1920;196:848.
2. Bras G, Jeliffe DB, Stuart KL. Veno-occlusive disease of the liver with non-portal type of cirrhosis occurring in Jamaica. Arch Pathol 1954;57:285–300.
3. Stuart KL, Bras G. Veno-occlusive diseases of the liver. Q J Med 1957;26:291.
4. Levitsky J, Sorrell MF. Hepatic complications of hematopoietic cell transplantation. Curr Gastroenterol Rep 2007;9:60–5.
5. Deleve LD. Hepatic microvasculature in liver injury. Semin Liver Dis 2007;27:390–400.
6. DeLeve LD, Valla D, Garcia-Tsao G. Vascular disorders of the liver. Hepatology 2009;49:1729–64.
7. Shulman HM, Fisher LB, Schoch HG, et al. Venoocclusive disease of the liver after marrow transplantation: histological correlates of clinical signs and symptoms. Hepatology 1994;19:1171–80.
8. Rubbia-Brandt L, Audard V, Sartoretti P, et al. Severe hepatic sinusoidal obstruction associated with oxaliplatin-based chemotherapy in patients with metastatic colorectal cancer. Ann Oncol 2004;15:460–6.
9. Rubbia-Brandt L, Lauwers GY, Wuang H, et al. Sinusoidal obstruction syndrome and nodular regenerative hyperplasia are frequent oxaliplatin associated liver lesions and partially prevented by bevacizumab in patients with hepatic colorectal metastasis. Histopathology 2010;56:430–9.
10. Aloia T, Sebagh M, Plasse M, et al. Liver histology and surgical outcomes after preoperative chemotherapy with fluorouracil plus oxaliplatin in colorectal cancer liver metastases. J Clin Oncol 2006;24:4983–90.
11. Bilchik AJ, Poston G, Curley SA, et al. Neoadjuvant chemotherapy for metastatic colon cancer: a cautionary note. J Clin Oncol 2005;23:9073–8.
12. Hubert C, Sempoux C, Horsmans Y, et al. Nodular regenerative hyperplasia: a deleterious consequence of chemotherapy for colorectal liver metastases? Liver Int 2007;1478:938–42.
13. Vollmar B, Menger MD. The hepatic microcirculation: mechanistic contributions and therapeutic targets in liver injury and repair. Physiol Rev 2009;89:1269–339.

14. McCuskey RS. Sinusoidal endothelial cells as an early target for hepatic toxicants. Clin Hemorheol Microcirc 2006;34(1–2):5–10.
15. Crispe IN. The liver as a lymphoid organ. Annu Rev Immunol 2009;27:147–63.
16. Yokomori H. New insights into the dynamics of sinusoidal endothelial fenestrae in liver sinusoidal endothelial cells. Med Mol Morphol 2008;41(1):1–4.
17. Jiao J, Friedman SL, Aloman C. Hepatic fibrosis. Curr Opin Gastroenterol 2009; 25(3):223–9.
18. DeLeve LD, Wang X, Hu L, et al. Rat liver sinusoidal endothelial cell phenotype is maintained by paracrine and autocrine regulation. Am J Physiol Gastrointest Liver Physiol 2004;287(4):G757–63.
19. Deleve LD, Wang X, Guo Y, et al. Sinusoidal endothelial cells prevent rat stellate cell activation and promote reversion to quiescence. Hepatology 2008;48: 920–30.
20. Deleve LD, McCuskey RS, Wang X, et al. Characterization of a reproducible rat model of hepatic veno-occlusive disease. Hepatology 1999;29:1779–91.
21. Murata S, Ohkohchi N, Matsuo R, et al. Platelets promote liver regeneration in early period after hepatectomy in mice. World J Surg 2007;31:808–16.
22. Deleve LD, Wang X, Tsai J, et al. Sinusoidal obstruction syndrome (veno-occlusive disease) in the rat is prevented by matrix metalloproteinase inhibition. Gastroenterology 2003;125:882–90.
23. DeLeve LD, Wang X, Kanel GC, et al. Decreased hepatic nitric oxide production contributes to the development of rat sinusoidal obstruction syndrome. Hepatology 2003;38:900–8.
24. DeLeve LD, Ito I, Bethea NW, et al. Embolization by sinusoidal lining cells obstructs the microcirculation in rat sinusoidal obstruction syndrome. Am J Physiol Gastrointest Liver Physiol 2003;284:G1045–52.
25. Schiffer E, Frossard JL, Rubbia-Brandt L, et al. Hepatic regeneration is decreased in a rat model of sinusoidal obstruction syndrome. J Surg Oncol 2009;99(7):439–46.
26. Laurent A, Nicco C, Chereau C, et al. Controlling tumour growth by modulating endogenous production of reactive oxygen species. Cancer Res 2005;65: 948–56.
27. Alexandre J, Nicco C, Chereau C, et al. Improvement of the therapeutic index of anticancer drugs by the superoxide dismutase mimic mangafodipir. J Natl Cancer Inst 2006;98:236–44.
28. Zeng HH, Lu JF, Wang K. The effect of cisplatin and transplatin on the conformation and association of F-actin. Cell Biol Int 1995;19:491–7.
29. Iguchi A, Kobayashi R, Yoshida M, et al. Vascular endothelial growth factor (VEGF) is one of the cytokines causative and predictive of hepatic veno-occlusive disease (VOD) in stem cell transplantation. Bone Marrow Transplant 2001;27(11):1173–80.
30. Brooks SEH, Miller CG, McKenzie K. Acute veno-occlusive diseases of the liver. Arch pathol 1970;89:507–20.
31. Shulman HM, Gown AM, Nugent DJ. Hepatic veno-occlusive disease after bone marrow transplantation. Immunohistochemical identification of the material within occluded central venules. Am J Pathol 1987;127(3):549–58.
32. Soubrane O, Brouquet A, Zalinski S, et al. Predicting high grade lesions of sinusoidal obstruction syndrome related to oxaliplatin-based chemotherapy for colorectal liver metastases correlation with post-hepatectomy outcome. Ann Surg 2010;251:454–60.
33. Lesurtel M, Graf R, Aleil B, et al. Platelet-derived serotonin mediates liver regeneration. Science 2006;312:104–7.

34. Reshamwala P, Kleiner DE, Heller T. Nodular regenerative hyperplasia: not all nodules are created equal. Hepatology 2006;44:1407–44.
35. Al-Mukhaizeem K, Rosenberg A, Sherker AH. Nodular regenerative hyperplasia of the liver: an under-recognized cause of portal hypertension in hematological disorders. Am J Hematol 2004;75:225–30.
36. Roskams T, Baptista A, Bianchi L, et al. Histopathology of portal hypertension: a practical guideline. Histopathology 2003;42:2–13.
37. Wanless IR. Micronodular transformation (nodular regenerative hyperplasia) of the liver: a report of 64 cases among 2,500 autopsies and a new classification of benign hepatocellular nodules. Hepatology 1990;11:787–97.
38. Wanless IR, Godwin TA, Allen F, et al. Nodular regenerative hyperplasia of the liver in hematologic disorders: a possible response to obliterative portal venopathy. A morphometric study of nine cases with an hypothesis on the pathogenesis. Medicine 1980;59:367–79.
39. Bayraktar UD, Bayraktar UD, Bayraktar Y. Hepatic venous outflow obstruction: three similar syndromes. World J Gastroenterol 2007;13:1912–27.
40. Ueno S, Tanabe G, Sueyoshi K, et al. Hepatic hemodynamics in a patient with nodular regenerative hyperplasia. Am J Gastroenterol 1996;91:1012–5.
41. Naber AH, Van Haelst U, Yap SH. Nodular regenerative hyperplasia of the liver: an important cause of portal hypertension in non-cirrhotic patients. J Hepatol 1991;12:94–9.
42. Croquelois A, Blindenbacher A, Terracciano L, et al. Inducible inactivation of Notch1 causes nodular regenerative hyperplasia in mice. Hepatology 2005;41:487–96.
43. Mendizabal M, Craviotto S, Chen T, et al. Noncirrhotic portal hypertension: another cause of liver disease in HIV patients. Ann Hepatol 2009;8(4):390–5.
44. Adam R. Colorectal cancer with synchronous liver metastases. Br J Surg 2007;94:129–31.
45. Mentha G, Majno PE, Terraz S, et al. Treatment strategies for the management of advanced colorectal liver metastases detected synchronously with the primary tumour. Eur J Surg Oncol 2007;33:S76–83.
46. Andres A, Majno P, Morel P, et al. Improved long-term outcome of surgery for advanced colorectal liver metastases: reasons and implications for management on the basis of a severity score. Ann Surg Oncol 2008;15:134–43.
47. Andre T, Boni C, Mounedji-Boudiaf L, et al. Oxaliplatin, fluorouracil, and leucovorin as adjuvant treatment for colon cancer. N Engl J Med 2004;350:2343–51.
48. Nordlinger B, Van Cutsem E, Rougier P, et al. Does chemotherapy prior to liver resection increase the potential for cure in patients with metastatic colorectal cancer? A report from the European Colorectal Metastases Treatment Group. Eur J Cancer 2007;43:2037–45.
49. Mentha G, Majno PE, Andres A, et al. Neoadjuvant chemotherapy and resection of advanced synchronous liver metastases before treatment of the colorectal primary. Br J Surg 2006;93:872–8.
50. Ribero D, Wuang H, Matteo D, et al. Bevacizumab improves pathologic response and protects against hepatic injury in patients treated with oxaliplatin-based chemotherapy for colorectal liver metastases. Cancer 2007;110:2761–7.
51. Seium Y, Stupp R, Ruhstaller T, et al. Oxaliplatin combined with irinotecan and 5-fluorouracil/leucovorin (OCFL) in metastatic colorectal cancer: a phase I-II study. Ann Oncol 2005;16:762–6.
52. Rubbia-Brandt L, Giostra E, Brezault C, et al. Importance of histological tumor response assessment in predicting the outcome in patients with colorectal liver

metastases treated with neo-adjuvant chemotherapy followed by liver surgery. Ann Oncol 2007;18:299–304.

53. Arotcarena R, Calès V, Berthelemy PH, et al. Severe sinusoidal lesions: a serious and overlooked complication of oxaliplatin-containing chemotherapy? Gastroenlerol Clin Biol 2006;30:1313–6.

54. Nakano H, Oussoultzoglou E, Rosso E, et al. Sinusoidal injury increases morbidity after major hepatectomy in patients with colorectal liver metastases receiving preoperative chemotherapy. Ann Surg 2008;247:118–24.

55. Vauthey JN, Pawlik TM, Ribero D, et al. Chemotherapy regimen predicts steatohepatitis and an increase in 90-day mortality after surgery for hepatic colorectal metastases. J Clin Oncol 2006;24:2065–72.

56. Kandutsch S, Klinger M, Hacker S, et al. Patterns of hepatotoxicity after chemotherapy for colorectal cancer liver metastases. Eur J Surg Oncol 2008;34(11): 1231–6.

57. Tisman G, MacDonald D, Shindell N, et al. Oxaliplatin toxicity masquerading as recurrent colon cancer. J Clin Oncol 2004;22:3202–4.

58. Mentha G, Roth AD, Terraz S, et al. Liver first approach in the treatment of colorectal cancer with synchronous liver metastases. Dig Surg 2008;25:430–5.

59. Zorzi D, Laurent A, Pawlik TM, et al. Chemotherapy-associated hepatotoxicity and surgery for colorectal liver metastases. Br J Surg 2007;94:274–86.

60. Chun YS, Laurent A, Maru D, et al. Management of chemotherapy-associated hepatotoxicity in colorectal liver metastases. Lancet Oncol 2009;10(3):278–86.

61. Floyd J, Sachs B, Perry MC. Hepatotoxicity of chemotherapy. Semin Oncol 2006; 33:50–67.

62. Slade JH, Alattar ML, Fogelman DR, et al. Portal hypertension associated with oxaliplatin administration: clinical manifestations of hepatic sinusoidal injury. Clin Colorectal Cancer 2009;8(4):225–30.

63. Karoui M, Penna C, Amin-Hashem M, et al. Influence of preoperative chemotherapy on the risk of major hepatectomy for colorectal liver metastases. Ann Surg 2006;243(1):1–7.

64. Ward J, Guthrie JA, Boyes S, et al. Sinusoidal obstructive syndrome diagnosed with superparamagnetic iron oxide-enhanced magnetic resonance imaging in patients with chemotherapy-treated colorectal liver metastases. J Clin Oncol 2008;26:4304–10.

65. O'Rourke TR, Welsh FK, Tekkis PP, et al. Accuracy of liver-specific magnetic resonance imaging as a predictor of chemotherapy-associated hepatic cellular injury prior to liver resection. Eur J Surg Oncol 2009;35(10):1085–91.

66. Shulman HM, Gooley T, Dudley MD, et al. Utility of transvenous liver biopsies and wedged hepatic venous pressure measurements in sixty marrow transplant recipients. Transplantation 1995;59(7):1015–22.

67. Abdalla EK, Hicks ME, Vauthey JN. Portal vein embolization: rationale, technique and future prospects. Br J Surg 2001;88:165–75.

68. Abdalla EK, Barnett CC, Doherty D, et al. Extended hepatectomy in patients with hepatobiliary malignancies with and without preoperative portal vein embolization. Arch Surg 2002;137:675–80.

69. Azoulay D, Castaing D, Krissat J, et al. Percutaneous portal vein embolization increases the feasibility and safety of major resection for hepatocellular carcinoma in injured liver. Ann Surg 2000;232:665–72.

70. Di Stefano DR, de Baere T, Denys A, et al. Preoperative percutaneous portal vein embolization: evaluation of adverse events in 188 patients. Radiology 2005;234: 625–30.

71. Mentha G, Terraz S, Morel P, et al. Dangerous halo after neoadjuvant chemotherapy and two-step hepatectomy for colorectal liver metastases. Br J Surg 2009;96(1):95–103.

72. Welsh FK, Tilney HS, Tekkis PP, et al. Safe liver resection following chemotherapy for colorectal metastases is a matter of timing. Br J Cancer 2007;96(7):1037–42.

73. Solis-Herruzo JA, Vidal JV, Colina F, et al. Nodular regenerative hyperplasia of the liver associated with the toxic oil syndrome: report of five cases. Hepatology 1986;6:687–93.

74. DeLeve LD, Wang X, Kuhlenkamp JF, et al. Toxicity of azathioprine and monocrotaline in murine sinusoidal endothelial cells and hepatocytes: the role of glutathione and relevance to hepatic venoocclusive disease. Hepatology 1996;23: 589–99.

75. Goringe AP, Brown S, O'Callaghan U, et al. Glutamine and vitamin E in the treatment of hepatic veno-occlusive disease following high-dose chemotherapy. Bone Marrow Transplant 1998;21(8):829–32.

76. Brouquet A, Benoist S, Julie C, et al. Risk factors for chemotherapy-associated liver injuries: a multivariate analysis of a group of 146 patients with colorectal metastases. Surgery 2009;145(4):362–71.

77. Klinger M, Eipeldauer S, Hacker S, et al. Bevacizumab protects against sinusoidal obstruction syndrome and does not increase response rate in neoadjuvant XELOX/FOLFOX therapy of colorectal cancer liver metastases. Eur J Surg Oncol 2009;35(5):515–20.

78. Harb R, Xie G, Lutzko C, et al. Bone marrow progenitor cells repair rat hepatic sinusoidal endothelial cells after liver injury. Gastroenterology 2009;137(2): 704–12.

Adding Value to Liver (and Allograft) Biopsy Evaluation Using a Combination of Multiplex Quantum Dot Immunostaining, High-Resolution Whole-Slide Digital Imaging, and Automated Image Analysis

Kumiko Isse, MD, PhD[a], Kedar Grama, MS[b],
Isaac Morse Abbott, MS[b], Andrew Lesniak[a], John G. Lunz, PhD[a],
William M.F. Lee, MD, PhD[c], Susan Specht, MS[a],
Natasha Corbitt, BS[a], Yoshiaki Mizuguchi, MD, PhD[a],
Badrinath Roysam, PhD[b], A.J. Demetris, MD[a],*

KEYWORDS

• Multiplex immunostaining • Digital pathology
• Liver allograft pathology • Automated image analysis
• Liver biopsy

Supported by: P01 A1081678, N01-AI-15416, U01 A1077867, and PO1A1064343 (A.J.D.); R01 EB005157 (B.R.); and RO1 CA135509 (W.M.L. and B.R.).
Disclosures: Dr Demetris is a member of the clinical development team for Omnyx (www.omnyx.com), a corporation developing a complete digital pathology solution. He also serves as a consultant for Bristol-Myers Squibb and DCL/Novartis.
[a] Department of Pathology, Division of Transplantation, University of Pittsburgh Medical Center, E741 Montefiore, 200 Lothrop Street, Pittsburgh, PA 15231, USA
[b] Electrical & Computer Engineering, N325, Engineering Building 1, University of Houston, Houston, TX 77204-4005, USA
[c] Department of Medicine, Abramson Cancer Center, University of Pennsylvania, 421 Curie Boulevard, Philadelphia, PA 19104, USA
* Corresponding author.
E-mail address: demetrisaj@upmc.edu

Clin Liver Dis 14 (2010) 669–685
doi:10.1016/j.cld.2010.07.004
1089-3261/10/$ – see front matter © 2010 Published by Elsevier Inc.

liver.theclinics.com

CURRENT LIMITATIONS OF LIVER AND LIVER ALLOGRAFT BIOPSY INTERPRETATION

Liver biopsies obtained for monitoring inflammatory disease activity and staging, including allograft rejection, play an important role in patient management. However, liver biopsies are invasive, expensive, potentially morbidity- and mortality-producing, and subject to sampling error, and interpretations are prone to subjectivity and inter-observer variability.[1,2] These biopsies are also an unpleasant experience for patients.[1,2] As more advanced imaging and less-invasive monitoring techniques are developed, the value added from histopathologic diagnoses and data, particularly if incomplete, is decreasing. Consequently, the risk-benefit ratio of obtaining biopsies of the liver allograft or native liver is being increasingly questioned because the results of biopsy frequently do not alter patient management strategies.

The First International Conference on Transplantomics and Biomarkers in Organ Transplantation (February 24–26, 2010, San Francisco, CA, USA) highlighted the potential contributions of various emerging technologies, including gene arrays, proteomic and metabolomic tools, and other monitoring mechanisms (A.J. Demetris, personal observation). Specific examples include measurement of urinary levels of granzyme B, perforin messenger RNA, and other molecules[3]; expression array analysis of the peripheral blood for rejection[4,5] and tolerance[6,7]; evaluation of urine and serum proteomics and metabolomics[8-10]; and nucleotide polymorphism analysis for susceptibility to certain disease states and function after transplantation.[11-13] Many presenters at the conference referred to allograft biopsy analysis as the "bronze" standard because of the problems mentioned earlier. Additional examples of legitimate criticisms of routine histopathologic examination of liver and liver allograft biopsies include the following:

1. Subtle reactions, such as sublethal injury and response to low-grade injury, are below the threshold of detection of traditional light microscopy
2. Inability to derive information about molecular signaling pathways from routine tissue examination, such as detection of
    - Myofibroblast activation and transformation before the development of irreversible fibrosis and architectural distortion
    - Predominant signaling mechanisms in liver tumors
    - Subpopulations of cells within inflammatory infiltrates or neoplasms
3. Inability to determine whether subtle low-grade inflammatory infiltrates in the allograft are potentially injurious, beneficial, or neutral
4. Pathologist inadequacies such as failures to assign grading and staging to inflammatory liver diseases and providing only descriptive diagnoses that cannot be translated accurately from center to center.

The recent standardization of protocols for grading and staging of chronic hepatitis[14-16] and allograft rejection[17,18] has encouraged pathologists to increase the amount of information that can be extracted by histopathologic examination by creating protocolized histopathologic features for evaluation and reporting. A variety of immunohistochemical and in situ hybridization stains for viral antigens and IgG4-secreting plasma cells[19] have enabled more precise characterization of necroinflammatory liver diseases. Even more progress has been made in the characterization of dysplastic and neoplastic liver lesions using histochemical and immunohistochemical stains, such as α-fetoprotein, Hep Par 1, glypican-3, glutamine synthetase, β-catenin, heat shock protein 70, Moc-31, Ki-67, CD34, and by immunophenotypic analysis of liver neoplasms.[20-27]

These developments, however, have not kept pace with the revolution in molecular biology and genomics. The newer analytical monitoring tools mentioned earlier are more sophisticated than traditional light microscopy and enable laboratory scientists to extract a tremendous amount of information noninvasively either from the peripheral blood or from small tissue samples. In many, but not all, circumstances, the information provided by these new techniques is exceeding the value added to patient management when compared with that provided by routine morphologic examination.

STRENGTHS OF HISTOPATHOLOGIC EXAMINATION

Routine morphologic examination quickly provides a wealth of information that is often taken for granted and not readily extractable when peripheral blood is analyzed or when liver tissue is homogenized for molecular analyses. The value of information, such as that obtained from the assessment of structural integrity, spatial and temporal relationships between cells and events, and recognition of rare events or cell types, is often not appreciated until it is no longer available. For example, a tangential sample of the liver capsule or a small infarct is easily distinguishable from more-diffuse fibrosis by morphologic analysis. The same might not be true of homogenized tissue examined by a gene expression array. Ceroid-laden macrophages interspersed between the fibers of a collapsed reticulin framework dating a significant insult to a period within the last several weeks also exemplify the utility of morphologic examination.

Pathologists also tend to naturally think and reason in terms of "system science" when evaluating tissue specimens. They routinely deal with the real world complications of tissue biology, in which multiple processes are present, and assign relative values to each process.[28] Examples of coexisting diseases in liver allografts include recurrent hepatitis C virus (HCV) infection and rejection and HCV infection and steatohepatitis or autoimmune hepatitis. Similar difficulties are encountered when evaluating native livers. The ability to think at the systems level also naturally compensates for some of the weaknesses of the monumental amount of data generated from array analyses,[29] especially for validation studies. Examination of particular nucleic acids or proteins or signaling pathways in association with specific events within tissues can quickly validate or refute potentially significant array findings.[29] Notwithstanding the strengths of traditional histopathology, there is a compelling need to extract even more useful information from tissue samples, for reasons described earlier.

At present, liver and liver allograft biopsies are usually (or should be) routinely subjected to standardized grading and staging of chronic hepatitis and allograft rejection, when appropriate. The authors routinely use only hematoxylin-eosin (H&E) stains for liver allograft biopsies and for biopsies evaluating liver masses. Special stains are ordered only after the initial examination. Iron, trichrome, and periodic acid–Schiff with diastase stains are routinely included for native liver biopsies when an inflammatory disease is suspected. Most centers, including those of the authors, routinely use specialized histochemical stains and perform in situ hybridization studies, when appropriate. Some of the most useful stains have been described earlier. There has been little change, however, in the stains used routinely to evaluate liver biopsies during the last several decades.

It would be more ideal to combine routine morphologic analysis with probes for specific proteins of molecular signaling pathways or multiple antigens expressed in tissue sections specific for the disease of interest. Examples would include the routine use of T-cell phenotypes and effector molecules (eg, granzyme, perforin) for chronically inflamed livers. C4d and endothelial cell survival signaling pathways would be ideal for liver allograft biopsies from recipients with circulating donor-specific antibodies (DSAs). Including stains for these molecules would increase the value added to the equation for surgical pathology and empower surgical pathologists in patient management for many disease processes. However, performing such panels using current methods would require multiple tissue sections, each stained for 1 antigen of interest, which in turn would increase the evaluation and turnaround times. In addition, examination of multiple antigens on the same cell and quantification of various events would not be possible.

Colorimetric labeling for in situ hybridization or immunohistochemistry to highlight 2 or more simultaneous targets in a single tissue specimen has been used sparingly in surgical pathology, even though it can rapidly provide useful information. Examples include light chain clonal restriction in plasma cell–rich infiltrates, donor versus recipient phenotype of allograft infiltrative and parenchymal cells using X and Y chromosomes,[30] and characterization of inflammatory cell infiltrates and their relationship with parenchymal tissues.[31–34] However, these more complex staining protocols and analyses have been largely restricted to research laboratories or translational research projects because (1) identification of 3 or more antigens often relies on fluorophores instead of chromogens, which in turn requires inconvenient and expensive fluorescent microscopes and (2) interpretation of stain results is laborious, qualitative, and subjective. Few rigorous validation studies, therefore, have been performed with clinicopathologic correlation, which has significantly limited their use in a routine pathology practice.

PROBLEMATIC AREAS IN LIVER AND LIVER ALLOGRAFT PATHOLOGY

There are numerous circumstances or disease processes in which extraction of additional information from liver or liver allograft biopsies might significantly increase the understanding of the disease processes and influence patient management. Some problematic areas in liver allograft pathology need more sophisticated analyses, including the (1) pathophysiologic significance of minimal infiltrates in long-surviving liver allografts; (2) delineation of underlying CD4$^+$ T-cell polarization pathways in biopsies showing chronic hepatitis; (3) recognition of antibody binding, complement and endothelial activation, and alterations in endothelial cell survival signaling pathways in recipients harboring DSAs; (4) immunologic effector mechanisms in allografts and native livers showing nonalcoholic fatty liver disease; (5) markers of hepatocyte oxidative stress in various disease states; and (6) activation and transdifferentiation pathways in hepatic stellate cells for predicting the development of fibrosis. In addition to the aforementioned pathways, in native livers, the characterization of regenerative, dysplastic, and various neoplastic nodules (discussed earlier) and signaling pathways in hepatocellular carcinomas[35–37] and cholangiocarcinomas[38] would be of significant interest.

For example, many long-surviving allografts contain mild portal-based lymphocytic infiltrates, resembling a low-grade chronic hepatitis (**Fig. 1**)[39,40] but without serologic or molecular biologic evidence of viral infection or typical autoimmunity. A prototypical mock report for such a patient is as follows:

- Liver allograft, needle biopsy
  Negative result for acute and chronic rejection (Rejection Activity Index [RAI] = 0/9)
  Mild chronic portal inflammation with minimal interface activity (see comment)
  Mild portal/periportal fibrosis
- Comment: the underlying cause of the mild portal inflammation with equivocal interface activity is uncertain. Possibilities would include an otherwise unexplained hepatitis, an infiltrate associated with allograft acceptance, or new-onset

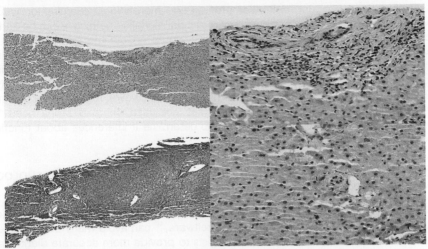

Fig. 1. This biopsy was obtained from a liver allograft recipient who originally underwent liver transplantation for secondary biliary cirrhosis and was immunosuppressive drug–free for a period of 17.3 years before this biopsy was obtained. The surgical report (see text) added some, but not enough, information that might have been useful for patient management. Mild portal/periportal inflammation with minimal interface activity and mild nodular regenerative hyperplasia changes are noted. All panels are stained with hematoxylin and eosin, except for the lower left Masson's Trichrome stained panel. Original maginification of *left panels* ×3.5; *right panels* ×25.

very-low-grade autoimmune hepatitis. Clinical and serologic correlation is suggested.

One could argue that the biopsy was helpful because it documented that the liver allograft was not completely normal, but not cirrhotic, and that otherwise typical acute and chronic rejection were not present. The report, however, provided little insight into the nature of the inflammation or guidance to the clinical physician on whether increased immunosuppressive therapy was indicated or not. Theoretically, if the pathologist was able to easily determine whether these infiltrates were effector memory T cells kept in check by immunosuppression,[41] lowering or removal of immunosuppression might not be advised. Conversely, if the infiltrates were composed of putative adaptive regulatory T cells,[42,43] watchful waiting to determine whether the mildly elevated liver injury test profile would return to normal or baseline spontaneously would be prudent.

Queries regarding inflammatory cell infiltrates, however, often require staining, recognition, and interpretation of 3 or more lymphocyte surface antigens to precisely define inflammatory cell subsets. For example, simply staining for CD4 and the transcription factor FoxP3 is not adequate to identify regulatory T cells in humans.[44] More sophisticated marker analyses are needed. Moreover, the relationship between inflammatory cell subtypes and parenchymal cells (eg, CD8$^+$/granyzme$^+$ T cells inside the bile ducts) provides important information.[32] Characterizing inflammatory infiltrates in tissues using expression arrays without morphologic analysis is infeasible because cell phenotypic analysis requires examination of specific markers on the same cell and some cell types may represent rare events. Nevertheless, cell type–specific expression profiles are being developed, which enable one to infer the composition of leukocyte populations based on their gene expression profiles.[45]

A combination of robust molecular profiling and morphologic examination would provide the most ideal data, particularly if molecular signaling pathways can be attributed to specific cell types. This combination would enable the pathologist to (1) provide specific information about infiltrative cell phenotypes or molecular signaling pathways in parenchymal, stromal, and endothelial cells of allografts with preservation of morphology and (2) build on the disease lexicon already written by examination of H&E-stained slides using traditional light microscopy. However, regardless of whether morphology and/or expression array analyses are used, there is still a need for observing temporal evolution of changes to determine if inferences about function are correct.

ADDRESSING SOME LIMITATIONS OF TRADITIONAL LIGHT MICROSCOPIC PATHOLOGY USING MULTIPLEX TISSUE STAINING

In combination, multiplex quantum dot immunohistochemistry,[46–48] high-resolution digital slide scanning, and image analysis software,[49] can avoid many of the earlier-mentioned limitations and enable pathologists to provide more accurate diagnoses, significantly increase the amount of information extracted from tissue sections, and increase the value added from biopsy interpretation. Nanotechnology and the invention of quantum dots have enabled immunofluorescence labeling for up to 5 antigens on the same tissue section.[46–48] Quantum dots are novel cadmium/selenium-based nanocrystal fluorophores with extremely high fluorescence efficiency and minimal photobleaching.[46,47] Quantum dots also possess a wide excitation band, together with sharp and symmetric emission spectra that can be tuned based on nanoparticle size. Quantum dots have several advantages over conventional fluorophores, including brighter emission signals, less susceptibility to photobleaching, and the ability to permanently mount and store conventionally without significant signal loss.[46,47] These unique optical properties make them near-perfect fluorescent markers, and there has recently been rapid development of their use for bioimaging.[46,47]

The authors have adapted multiplex staining methods for studies on liver and liver allograft tissues, focusing on more precise characterization of leukocyte populations within a single section of inflamed liver tissue[50] and for signaling pathways in biliary epithelium.[51] As described by Fountaine and colleagues,[48] sequential antibody staining (**Fig. 2**) of either frozen or formalin-fixed paraffin-embedded (FFPE) tissues is performed with unconjugated primary antibodies and biotinylated secondary antibodies, followed by addition of streptavidin-conjugated nanoparticles.

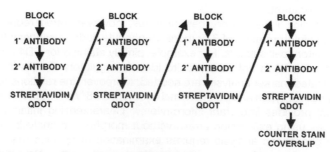

Fig. 2. Representative flow diagram for multiplex immunofluorescent tissue staining. Between each new stain, tissue is reblocked with avidin-biotin and protein blocking. Qdot, quantum dot; 1°, primary; 2°, secondary.

Frozen tissues are sectioned at 4 μm, fixed in cold acetone for 5 minutes, air dried for 1 hour at room temperature, and stored at −80°C until ready to use. FFPE tissues are also sectioned at 4 μm and stored at room temperature until use. Quantum dot–based immunofluorescent staining is performed based on the previously described laboratory protocol using Qdot Streptavidin Conjugate (Invitrogen Corporation, Carlsbad, CA, USA).[48] Briefly, FFPE sections are deparaffinized, hydrated, and treated with various antigen retrieval procedures appropriate to the antigen of interest. Frozen sections are air dried for 30 to 60 minutes and fixed first in cold acetone for 30 minutes and then with 1% paraformaldehyde in phosphate buffer saline (PBS) for 5 minutes at room temperature. This procedure is followed by blocking for 15 minutes each with avidin block (Vector Laboratories Inc, Burlingame, CA, USA), biotin block (Vector Laboratories Inc), and protein block (DAKOCytomation, Carpinteria, CA, USA). After incubation with the first primary antibody, slides are washed thrice in PBS containing 0.05% Tween-20 (PBST), and the biotinylated secondary antibody is applied for 30 minutes at room temperature. After 3 washes with PBST, streptavidin-conjugated 20-nM quantum dots in blocking buffer (PBS + 1% bovine serum albumin + 10% serum from host species producing secondary antibody) is applied and incubated at room temperature for 30 minutes. Before starting on the next antibody, the slides are reblocked with avidin-biotin and protein blocks and all processes are repeated sequentially to complete the panel of antibodies. After staining for all antibodies, 10 μg/mL Hoechst (bisbenzamide) is applied for 1 minute for nuclear staining. Slides are then washed, dehydrated, and coverslipped in Permount mounting medium (Fisher Scientific, Pittsburgh, PA, USA) before microscopic observation.

This sequential staining procedure is labor and time intensive, but primary nanoparticle-conjugated antibodies are becoming increasingly available. These antibodies will greatly simplify the staining protocols and enable automation. At present, the authors have performed nanoparticle multiplex staining to detect up to 5 antigens simultaneously, excluding Hoechst, with optimized antibody panels to detect CD4 helper T-cell subsets, dendritic cell subtypes and maturation, islet hormone production and peri-islet infiltrates,[52] T-cell subtypes (CD3, CD4, CD8, CD56, and PD-1), naive and memory T-cell subsets, and nonconventional T-cell panel (natural killer and γδ T cells). A panel examining the expression of naive (CD45RA) and memory (CD45RO) CD8 T cells and granzyme is shown in **Fig. 3**. In general, panel-staining procedures for frozen tissues are simpler than those for FFPE tissues. The major problem with FFPE tissues is that multiple antigen retrieval techniques, if needed, for various antigens are sometimes not compatible with each other, which in turn preclude their inclusion in a single panel.

IMAGING SOLUTIONS FOR MULTIPLEX STAINING

Novel multiplex staining techniques have the power to unlock significant information from tissue sections. Consideration, however, must be given to the most appropriate method to efficiently capture this information and enable reasonably high throughput that can be incorporated into a routine service pathology workflow. The authors originally used a Nuance multispectral imaging system (CRi, Woburn, MA, USA) that captures the emission spectra of each field of view at every 10 nm over a wide bandwidth (420–720 nm) and combines these into a multispectral image cube. This software enabled the authors to view images contained within a designated spectral range (eg, 500–550 nm to view the emission of a specific quantum dot fluorophore) or to combine the entire range to look at multiple quantum dots. The software also helped to remove or avoid the effects of background autofluorescence typically

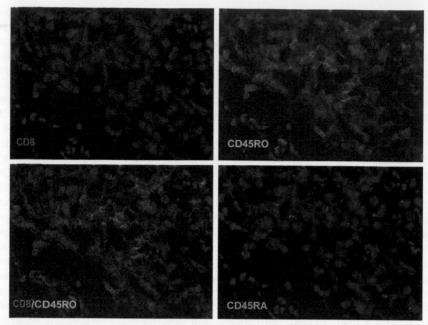

Fig. 3. Screen captures of viewer for WSI using multiplex staining for naive (CD45RA) versus memory (CD45RO) CD8 T cells in a liver allograft biopsy to characterize the infiltrate. The ease of tissue examination using the WSI viewer is difficult to illustrate in print, but each of these screen views are created by simply switching the channels off and on, as desired. Most of the infiltrating lymphocytes are CD8+ (*upper left*) and CD45RO+ (*upper right*) and most cells express both antigens as evidenced by the overlapping red (CD8) and green (CD45RO) signals producing a yellow color in the bottom left panel. Also, the CD45RA stain (*brown, lower right panel*) stains a population of cells distinct from the CD45RO green cells in the upper right panel. Evaluation of the stains, however, becomes complex when using multiple antigens and colors.

present in tissue sections, such as background fluorescence from hepatocytes in FFPE liver sections.[48] However, the major drawbacks to routine use of the Nuance system are as follows: (1) the microscope and system are expensive, (2) slide examination is time consuming, and (3) the combination of the first 2 drawbacks creates a bottleneck in tissue examination, which makes the entire process impractical for routine service work. Therefore, the authors searched for an alternate method that would alleviate these problems.

The current generation of whole-slide imaging (WSI) systems have proven utility for creating high-resolution digital representations of tissue sections for transmitted light and fluorescence applications. Because these scanning units can automate the time-consuming acquisition process, the authors chose to combine the nanoparticle staining protocol with a WSI system to create images for pathology review via computer. This technique offers the added benefit of preservation of the slide image as a permanent photomicrograph and the convenience of review at a computer station that enables use of various morphometric tools. Using nanocrystal fluorophores, which are resistant to photobleaching, enables the combination of multiplex staining and WSI. The Zeiss MIRAX MIDI digital whole-slide scanning system (Carl Zeiss Microlmaging, Jena, Germany) was selected. This system enables scanning in transmitted light for routine use as well as in an epifluorescence mode that can acquire up to 9 individual fluorescence signals and combine them into an image (**Fig. 4**). This image can then be remotely viewed and quantified via image analysis software as discussed later.

The Zeiss MIRAX MIDI scanner combines high-precision robotic slide movement, a high-sensitivity digital charge-coupled device (CCD) camera, and fluorescence excitation and emission filters, all controlled through software via a connected personal computer. The system can hold up to 9 commercially available fluorescence filter cubes, which combine an excitation filter and a dichroic mirror for directing the emission light to the appropriate camera. The filter cubes are selected to match the spectral characteristics of the quantum dots, as well as the other fluorophores in use (eg, Hoechst), and in the authors' case were supplied by Omega Optical Inc (Brattleboro, VT, USA). The scanning process begins by loading the tissue sections, which were prepared as described earlier, into a slide carrier with a capacity of twelve 25 × 75-mm slides. This tray is then loaded into the scanner, and the imaging parameters are selected interactively by the user via the control software. The WSI control software gives the ability to select the fluorescence filters to be used, set the exposure time for each filter independently, and adjust various parameters to ensure that the image produced is in focus. The user then begins the imaging process and selects the specific slides to be scanned as a batch process. The digitization process uses a Zeiss AxioCam MRm (Carl Zeiss MicroImaging GmbH) monochrome digital camera (two-third-inch CCD sensor) with a Zeiss Plan-Apochromat 40x/.95 NA objective (Carl Zeiss Optronics GmbH, Oberkochen, Germany). Fluorescence excitation is provided by an HXP 120 C metal halide illuminator (Carl Zeiss MicroImaging GmbH). As a slide is loaded into the imaging system, the software overlays a grid on the tissue specimen, with each grid box representing a microscopic field of view as produced by the objective lens. In an automated process, each location is robotically positioned under the objective lens by moving the stage holding the slide and the appropriate filter cube is positioned in the optical path via a motorized turret. The field is focused via a software algorithm, an image is acquired from the digital camera, and the process is repeated for the entire tissue area selected for scanning, 1 complete pass per filter.

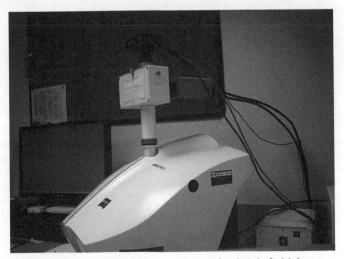

Fig. 4. Setup of Zeiss MIRAX MIDI scanner equipped for brightfield (gray camera on the side) and immunofluorescence microscopy (black camera on top). The camera can be switched using the sliding bar, which deflects the light path.

To minimize photobleaching, the tissue is exposed to the excitation light only when an image is being acquired via an automated shutter on the light source. Fluorescence WSI images are generated by merging the individual captured fields in real time into a file format for storage on the computer hard drive. To minimize space on the disk, image compression can be applied to the data as they are captured by the camera using industry standard methods, such as portable network graphic– or JPEG-encoding algorithms, with user-selectable quality factors.

Once the WSIs are created, they can be viewed on a high-resolution monitor and duplicated and shared using software designed for WSI navigation, zooming, and collaboration. Particularly useful features include the ability to survey structure at very low magnifications and zoom in and out with the mouse wheel and view any individual, any combination, or all fluorophore layers, creating a composite image with overlapping signals (**Fig. 5**). These features are particularly useful for determining the phenotype of infiltrating cells, examining the relationship between various molecular signaling pathways and tissue structure, and for comparison of results of individual liver biopsies from the same patient obtained at separate times.[50,52]

TISSUE EVALUATION TOOLS USING IMAGE ANALYSIS SOFTWARE (FARSIGHT)

The initial excitement of being able to view multiple antigens or molecular components of signaling pathways in a single tissue sample on a computer screen was soon

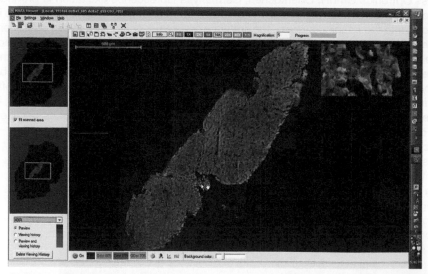

Fig. 5. Screen capture of the slide viewer for a multiplex-stained liver allograft used to characterize the ratio of $\gamma\delta$-1$^+$ to $\gamma\delta$-2$^+$ CD3$^+$ T cells within a liver allograft. This ratio has been associated with an ability to withdraw immunosuppression in 2 separate studies.[7,52] The goal is to determine whether a ratio resembling the tolerance state of a normal pregnancy ($\gamma\delta$-1$^+$>$\gamma\delta$-2$^+$ CD3$^+$ cells) exists in the liver tissue.[62] At the bottom left of the image, the dark blue button controls viewing of the 4',6-diamidino-2-phenylindole (DAPI) channel, $\gamma\delta$-1$^+$ T cells (*green*), $\gamma\delta$-2$^+$ T cells (*red*), and CD3$^+$ T cells (*turquoise*). This multiplex-stained WSI is viewed on the computer screen. Surveying the tissue at low magnification is much easier than using a traditional fluorescent microscope. The small window at the right top corner shows the magnification of the cursor area, which enables one to observe a lower magnification and a higher magnification in the same screen. Any or all individual color channels can be turned off or on, and any individual color can be changed to another for viewing preferences.

dampened by the realization that the information being provided had overwhelmed the capacity to capture, collate, and interpret the data by visual inspection. Counting individual cells by highlighting various combinations of stains led to the realization that manually analyzing the multiplex slides was impractical.[50,52] Tracking individual colors and numerous combinations of overlapping colors and distribution of antigen expression on the same cell type was overwhelming. For example, simply determining a ratio of γδ-1 T cells to γδ-2 T cells in a liver allograft from a potentially tolerant recipient[7,53] can require many hours for each liver biopsy specimen. Therefore, automated analysis of the tissue sections and multiplex staining was done. For further development, the authors collaborated with William M.F. Lee and Dr Roysam, Chair, Electrical & Computer Engineering, University of Houston, and the NIH-funded FARSIGHT image analysis toolkit project (www.farsight-toolkit.org).

The goal of FARSIGHT analysis of a multiplex-labeled specimen is to delineate each cell (or part thereof) in the image field and quantify the amount of fluorescent or chromogenic staining of molecular biomarkers over each cell by spatial association. The first step in the analysis is performing a fully automatic delineation of all cell nuclei in the Hoechst channel.[54] This step generates a rich set of morphologic measurements of cell nuclei including location, size, shape, and chromatin texture. The next step delineates several spatial regions relative to the nuclei, including the intranuclear and perinuclear regions. Although not shown in the examples in this article, FARSIGHT can also delineate cytoplasmic domains of individual cells when the specimen is labeled with cytoplasmic and membrane markers (needed when quantifying cytoplasmic and cell membrane–bound analytes). These regions are used as spatial masks over which molecular biomarkers are quantified by summation. Using these measurements, the system identifies the type of each cell, based on the combination of analytes that are detected over it. Once the type of each cell is known, a variety of determinations become possible. For instance, it is straightforward to quantify the amount of molecular analytes over a chosen cell subpopulation. The resulting data are displayed to the user for visual inspection (any combination of channels can be viewed at a time) and saved to tables for further analysis using a spreadsheet or to a database tool for archiving. Each row of these tables corresponds to a numbered cell in the field that can be referenced specifically. The information in these tables can be summarized into objective scores for the specimen based on any combination of analytes and cell morphologic measurements. These scores, in turn, can also be combined statistically with other forms of data for prognostic, diagnostic, and therapy-planning purposes.

Fig. 6 illustrates FARSIGHT analysis of a specimen that was multiplex labeled and imaged to analyze the CD4+ polarization pathway. Panel A shows the results of the automated nuclear segmentation (delineation) as the first step to automated analysis. The software displays nuclear delineations as outlines and assigns a unique identifier (ID) to each cell nucleus. The ID corresponds to a specific row of a table of measurements (panel F) in which the morphologic and analyte measurements of that cell are stored. Panel B shows an example of cell typing based on CD4. The CD4+ cells detected by FARSIGHT are indicated with color-coded dots for rapid inspection. The corresponding column of the table indicates whether that cell is positive or negative for CD4. Panels C, D, and E show the same analysis applied to GATA3, FoxP3, and T-bet, respectively. Panel F shows a screen view of the software-user interface. When a user clicks on a cell, its outline is highlighted in yellow and the corresponding row of the table of measurements is highlighted in unison. Each row of the table (ie, each cell) also corresponds to a dot on a scatter plot that displays the cellular measurements in much the same fashion as a flow cytometer. In this example, the x-axis of the scatter plot indicates CD4 expression and the y-axis indicates the nuclear

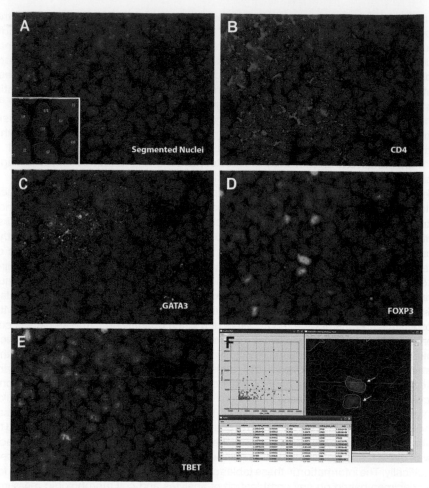

Fig. 6. Screen capture of FARSIGHT image analysis software during analysis of a CD4$^+$ polarization pathway using the following panel. (*A*) Nuclear segmentation. Each nucleus has an identifier as shown in the insert. (*B*) Hoechst (*blue*) and CD4 (*red*). The yellow dot in each nucleus marks the nuclear center; CD4 expression by the cell is determined by the distance from this yellow dot. (*C*) Hoechst (*blue*) and GATA3 (*yellow*), (*D*) Hoechst (*blue*) and FoxP3 (*green*), and (*E*) Hoechst (*blue*) and T-bet (*cyan*), all nuclear transcription factors were detected as a nuclear marker in the FARSIGHT program. (*F*) The graph shows CD4 (x-axis) and FoxP3 (y-axis) expression, and pink points represent CD4$^+$/FoxP3$^+$ double-positive cells. Double-positive cells are highlighted with yellow outline in the screen (*arrows*). The table shows all data for each cells, and the selected cell are highlighted in the table.

expression of FoxP3 signal measured over each cell with respect to CD4 expression. The color of each dot also indicates the cell type (CD4$^+$/FoxP3$^+$). A set of analytical tools are available to the user for data exploration.

POTENTIAL USES AND CHALLENGES

There are innumerable potential applications of this technology in native liver and kidney and transplantation pathology. Areas of specific interest in the authors' laboratory include panels to more precisely characterize leukocyte subsets in inflammatory liver diseases; altered expression of cytokines and major histocompatibility complex antigen expression; C4d binding and subsequent changes in survival and signaling pathways in endothelial cells, such as CD31, CD34, bcl2, pAKT, phospho-S6 ribosomal protein[55]; and various adhesion and complement regulatory molecules. Analysis of potentially neoplastic nodules should also benefit from panel staining for antigens associated with neoplastic transformation of clonal nodules within the liver, as described earlier. In native liver disease, activation and transformation pathways in stellate cells are of particular interest that might influence therapy. Signaling pathways within hepatocellular carcinomas[35-37] and cholangiocarcinomas[38] would be of significant interest and might be used to guide therapy.

There are several challenges, however, before more widespread application can be anticipated. Adoption of WSI and digital pathology is needed first for these staining methods to be incorporated into routine service work. The advantages, disadvantages, and expenses of digital pathology are discussed elsewhere.[56-60] But this inevitable revolution will begin within the next 5 years and expose service pathologists to the power and efficiencies of digital pathology. Continual improvements in image quality, decreased scan time, and participation of major vendors already experienced in creating and managing medical imaging equipment are already hastening this evolution.

Slide scanners will naturally incorporate fluorescent imaging capabilities, considering the power and utility of multiplex staining and the convenience for the pathologist. These technologies will enable pathologists to examine tissue sections on the computer screen with the assistance of tissue algorithms or imaging tools to "query" the tissue sections. Some algorithms, such as for automated estrogen receptor or Her2/neu are already available,[61,62] but nothing comparable exists for inflammatory or neoplastic native liver or transplantation pathology.

Once these digital techniques are introduced into the routine pathology workflow, translational research will be used to optimize multiplex panels appropriate to the disease process. These advances will likely occur at academic and large commercial laboratories. Potentially, these panels will provide guidance on therapy or prognostic information. Before implementing the multiplex digital analysis mode of reporting on tissue samples, however, cost considerations will have to be evaluated, and accuracy and validation studies will be needed before widespread adoption and reimbursement. The cost of reagents will naturally increase, but this should be balanced by the value of the information provided. Validation studies can be more easily accomplished if pathologists are currently evaluating tissue stains using a semiquantitative approach and the scoring has a direct effect on patient management. C4d staining of allograft tissues fits this description. Patients whose biopsies show diffuse C4d staining and evidence of other tissue damage associated with antibody-mediated rejection and circulating DSAs are treated with increased immunosuppression.[63] Automated and standardized staining and scoring have the potential to make this process more accurate and reproducible and provide more information. Comparison to subjective or semiquantitative evaluation by the pathologist and independent verification by measuring circulating DSAs have the potential to quickly validate the completely digital approach.

Regardless, multiplex staining, high-resolution digital imaging, and image analysis software are expected to play a prominent role in the future of liver and anatomic pathology.

REFERENCES

1. Mells G, Mann C, Hubscher S, et al. Late protocol liver biopsies in the liver allograft: a neglected investigation? Liver Transpl 2009;15:931-8.

2. Mells G, Neuberger J. Protocol liver allograft biopsies. Transplantation 2008;85: 1686–92.
3. Muthukumar T, Dadhania D, Ding R, et al. Messenger RNA for FOXP3 in the urine of renal-allograft recipients. N Engl J Med 2005;353:2342–51.
4. Dinu I, Potter JD, Mueller T, et al. Gene-set analysis and reduction. Brief Bioinform 2009;10:24–34.
5. Bunnag S, Einecke G, Reeve J, et al. Molecular correlates of renal function in kidney transplant biopsies. J Am Soc Nephrol 2009;20:1149–60.
6. Martinez-Llordella M, Lozano JJ, Puig-Pey I, et al. Using transcriptional profiling to develop a diagnostic test of operational tolerance in liver transplant recipients. J Clin Invest 2008;118:2845–57.
7. Martinez-Llordella M, Puig-Pey I, Orlando G, et al. Multiparameter immune profiling of operational tolerance in liver transplantation. Am J Transplant 2007;7:309–19.
8. Rush D. Can protocol biopsy better inform our choices in renal transplantation? Transplant Proc 2009;41:S6–8.
9. Schaub S, Nickerson P, Rush D, et al. Urinary CXCL9 and CXCL10 levels correlate with the extent of subclinical tubulitis. Am J Transplant 2009;9:1347–53.
10. Schaub S, Mayr M, Honger G, et al. Detection of subclinical tubular injury after renal transplantation: comparison of urine protein analysis with allograft histopathology. Transplantation 2007;84:104–12.
11. Louvar DW, Li N, Snyder J, et al. "Nature versus nurture" study of deceased-donor pairs in kidney transplantation. J Am Soc Nephrol 2009;20:1351–8.
12. Kamoun M, Holmes JH, Israni AK, et al. HLA-A amino acid polymorphism and delayed kidney allograft function. Proc Natl Acad Sci U S A 2008;105:18883–8.
13. Israni AK, Li N, Cizman BB, et al. Association of donor inflammation- and apoptosis-related genotypes and delayed allograft function after kidney transplantation. Am J Kidney Dis 2008;52:331–9.
14. Ishak K, Baptista A, Bianchi L, et al. Histologic grading and staging of chronic hepatitis. J Hepatol 1995;22:696–9.
15. Batts KP, Ludwig J. Chronic hepatitis. An update on terminology and reporting. Am J Surg Pathol 1995;19:1409–17.
16. Bedossa P, Poynard T. An algorithm for the grading of activity in chronic hepatitis C. The METAVIR Cooperative Study Group. Hepatology 1996;24:289–93.
17. Demetris AJ, Ruppert K, Dvorchik I, et al. Real-time monitoring of acute liver-allograft rejection using the Banff schema. Transplantation 2002;74:1290–6.
18. Demetris A, Adams D, Bellamy C, et al. Update of the International Banff Schema for Liver Allograft Rejection: working recommendations for the histopathologic staging and reporting of chronic rejection. An International Panel. Hepatology 2000;31:792–9.
19. Nakanuma Y, Zen Y. Pathology and immunopathology of immunoglobulin G4-related sclerosing cholangitis: the latest addition to the sclerosing cholangitis family. Hepatol Res 2007;37(Suppl 3):S478–86.
20. Bioulac-Sage P, Laumonier H, Rullier A, et al. Over-expression of glutamine synthetase in focal nodular hyperplasia: a novel easy diagnostic tool in surgical pathology. Liver Int 2009;29:459–65.
21. Di Tommaso L, Destro A, Seok JY, et al. The application of markers (HSP70 GPC3 and GS) in liver biopsies is useful for detection of hepatocellular carcinoma. J Hepatol 2009;50:746–54.
22. Kakar S, Gown AM, Goodman ZD, et al. Best practices in diagnostic immunohistochemistry: hepatocellular carcinoma versus metastatic neoplasms. Arch Pathol Lab Med 2007;131:1648–54.

23. Bioulac-Sage P, Rebouissou S, Thomas C, et al. Hepatocellular adenoma subtype classification using molecular markers and immunohistochemistry. Hepatology 2007;46:740–8.
24. Wang L, Vuolo M, Suhrland MJ, et al. HepPar1, MOC-31, pCEA, mCEA and CD10 for distinguishing hepatocellular carcinoma vs. metastatic adenocarcinoma in liver fine needle aspirates. Acta Cytol 2006;50:257–62.
25. Morrison C, Marsh W Jr, Frankel WL. A comparison of CD10 to pCEA, MOC-31, and hepatocyte for the distinction of malignant tumors in the liver. Mod Pathol 2002;15:1279–87.
26. Minervini MI, Demetris AJ, Lee RG, et al. Utilization of hepatocyte-specific antibody in the immunocytochemical evaluation of liver tumors. Mod Pathol 1997; 10:686–92.
27. Kirimlioglu H, Dvorchick I, Ruppert K, et al. Hepatocellular carcinomas in native livers from patients treated with orthotopic liver transplantation: biologic and therapeutic implications. Hepatology 2001;34:502–10.
28. Banff Working G, Demetris AJ, Adeyi O, et al. Liver biopsy interpretation for causes of late liver allograft dysfunction. Hepatology 2006;44:489–501.
29. Therneau T. The perils and promise of high-dimensional biology. Hepatology 2009;49:1061–2.
30. Wu T, Cieply K, Nalesnik MA, et al. Minimal evidence of transdifferentiation from recipient bone marrow to parenchymal cells in regenerating and long-surviving human allografts. Am J Transplant 2003;3:1173–81.
31. van der Loos CM, Becker AE, van den Oord JJ. Practical suggestions for successful immunoenzyme double-staining experiments. Histochem J 1993;25:1–13.
32. McCaughan GW, Davies JS, Waugh JA, et al. A quantitative analysis of T lymphocyte populations in human liver allografts undergoing rejection: the use of monoclonal antibodies and double immunolabeling. Hepatology 1990;12:1305–13.
33. Krenacs T, Krenacs L, Bozoky B, et al. Double and triple immunocytochemical labelling at the light microscope level in histopathology. Histochem J 1990;22: 530–6.
34. Waiser J, Schwaar S, Bohler T, et al. Immunohistochemical double-staining of renal allograft tissue: critical assessment of three different protocols. Virchows Arch 2002;440:648–54.
35. Wang M, Xue L, Cao Q, et al. Expression of Notch1, Jagged1 and beta-catenin and their clinicopathological significance in hepatocellular carcinoma. Neoplasma 2009;56:533–41.
36. Yang JC, Teng CF, Wu HC, et al. Enhanced expression of vascular endothelial growth factor-A in ground glass hepatocytes and its implication in hepatitis B virus hepatocarcinogenesis. Hepatology 2009;49:1962–71.
37. Suzuki S, Takeshita K, Asamoto M, et al. High mobility group box associated with cell proliferation appears to play an important role in hepatocellular carcinogenesis in rats and humans. Toxicology 2009;255:160–70.
38. Sirica AE. Cholangiocarcinoma: molecular targeting strategies for chemoprevention and therapy. Hepatology 2005;41:5–15.
39. Demetris AJ, Lunz JG 3rd, Randhawa P, et al. Monitoring of human liver and kidney allograft tolerance: a tissue/histopathology perspective. Transpl Int 2009;22:120–41.
40. Evans HM, Kelly DA, McKiernan PJ, et al. Progressive histological damage in liver allografts following pediatric liver transplantation. Hepatology 2006;43:1109–17.
41. Wong T, Nouri-Aria KT, Devlin J, et al. Tolerance and latent cellular rejection in long-term liver transplant recipients. Hepatology 1998;28:443–9.

42. Yoshitomi M, Koshiba T, Haga H, et al. Requirement of protocol biopsy before and after complete cessation of immunosuppression after liver transplantation. Transplantation 2009;87:606–14.

43. Xu Q, Lee J, Jankowska-Gan E, et al. Human CD4+CD25low adaptive T regulatory cells suppress delayed-type hypersensitivity during transplant tolerance. J Immunol 2007;178:3983–95.

44. Kang SM, Tang Q, Bluestone JA. CD4+CD25+ regulatory T cells in transplantation: progress, challenges and prospects. Am J Transplant 2007;7:1457–63.

45. Shen-Orr SS, Tibshirani R, Khatri P, et al. Cell type-specific gene expression differences in complex tissues. Nat Methods 2010;7(4):287–9.

46. Tholouli E, Sweeney E, Barrow E, et al. Quantum dots light up pathology. J Pathol 2008;216:275–85.

47. Sweeney E, Ward TH, Gray N, et al. Quantitative multiplexed quantum dot immunohistochemistry. Biochem Biophys Res Commun 2008;374:181–6.

48. Fountaine TJ, Wincovitch SM, Geho DH, et al. Multispectral imaging of clinically relevant cellular targets in tonsil and lymphoid tissue using semiconductor quantum dots. Mod Pathol 2006;19:1181–91.

49. Bjornsson CS, Lin G, Al-Kofahi Y, et al. Associative image analysis: a method for automated quantification of 3D multi-parameter images of brain tissue. J Neurosci Methods 2008;170:165–78.

50. Isse K, Lunz Iii JG, Specht MS, et al. Combining H&E, multiplex quantum dot immunostaining, and whole slide imaging for liver biopsy evaluation [abstract 1234]. Hepatology 2009;50(Suppl).

51. Isse K, Specht SM, Lunz JG 3rd, et al. Estrogen stimulates female biliary epithelial cell interleukin-6 expression in mice and humans. Hepatology 2009;51: 869–80.

52. Toso C, Isse K, Demetris AJ, et al. Histologic graft assessment after clinical islet transplantation. Transplantation 2009;88:1286–93.

53. Koshiba T, Li Y, Takemura M, et al. Clinical, immunological, and pathological aspects of operational tolerance after pediatric living-donor liver transplantation. Transpl Immunol 2007;17:94–7.

54. Al-Kofahi Y, Lassoued W, Lee W, et al. Improved automatic detection and segmentation of cell nuclei in histopathology images. IEEE Trans Biomed Eng 2009;57(4):841–52.

55. Lepin EJ, Zhang Q, Zhang X, et al. Phosphorylated S6 ribosomal protein: a novel biomarker of antibody-mediated rejection in heart allografts. Am J Transplant 2006;6:1560–71.

56. Weinstein RS, Graham AR, Richter LC, et al. Overview of telepathology, virtual microscopy, and whole slide imaging: prospects for the future. Hum Pathol 2009;40:1057–69.

57. Rocha R, Vassallo J, Soares F, et al. Digital slides: present status of a tool for consultation, teaching, and quality control in pathology. Pathol Res Pract 2009; 205:735–41.

58. Pinco J, Goulart RA, Otis CN, et al. Impact of digital image manipulation in cytology. Arch Pathol Lab Med 2009;133:57–61.

59. Coleman R. Can histology and pathology be taught without microscopes? The advantages and disadvantages of virtual histology. Acta Histochem 2009;111: 1–4.

60. Montalto MC, Cartwright G. From the incandescent light bulb to digital pathology: corporate innovation as an engine for change. Arch Pathol Lab Med 2009;133: 550–2.

61. Minot DM, Kipp BR, Root RM, et al. Automated cellular imaging system III for assessing HER2 status in breast cancer specimens: development of a standardized scoring method that correlates with FISH. Am J Clin Pathol 2009;132:133–8.
62. Gustavson MD, Bourke-Martin B, Reilly D, et al. Standardization of HER2 immunohistochemistry in breast cancer by automated quantitative analysis. Arch Pathol Lab Med 2009;133:1413–9.
63. Colvin RB. Antibody-mediated renal allograft rejection: diagnosis and pathogenesis. J Am Soc Nephrol 2007;18:1046–56.

The Use of Immunohistochemistry in Liver Tumors

Elaine S. Chan, MD, Matthew M. Yeh, MD, PhD

KEYWORDS

• Liver tumors • Hepatocellular carcinoma • Cholangiocarcinoma
• Immunohistochemistry

Characteristic morphologic features on hematoxylin and eosin (H&E)–stained tissue can often guide pathologists in diagnosing different hepatic tumors. In many cases, however, distinction of the different tumors in the liver is not possible on histologic grounds alone. In such cases, immunohistochemical methods become crucial in establishing a definitive diagnosis. In current routine practice, several immunohistochemical markers have been useful in assisting pathologists in the differential diagnosis of hepatic tumors. Each of these markers has its strengths and drawbacks. The well thought-out use of these immunohistochemical markers can greatly aid in differentiating the various types of tumors that are frequently encountered in the liver. This review summarizes the commonly used immunohistochemical stains in the diagnosis of hepatic tumors that clinicians may also encounter by reading the pathology reports or discussing at interdisciplinary conferences.

THE USE OF IMMUNOHISTOCHEMISTRY IN COMMON LIVER TUMORS
Hepatocellular Carcinoma

The use of hepatocyte paraffin 1 in diagnosing hepatocellular carcinoma
Hepatocyte paraffin 1 (Hep Par 1) is a murine monoclonal antibody frequently used to establish the hepatocellular origin of neoplasms. Hep Par 1 was developed in 1993 using an immunogen developed from a failed liver allograft.[1] The antigen of Hep Par 1 has been recently identified as carbamoyl phosphate synthetase 1, a rate-limiting enzyme in urea cycle located in the mitochondria.[2] Hep Par 1 has a diffuse cytoplasmic granular staining pattern in normal and neoplastic hepatocytes (**Fig. 1**).

Hep Par 1 has high sensitivity and high specificity in detecting hepatocellular carcinoma (HCC) (>90% in most studies) (**Table 1**).[3–7] Extrahepatic neoplasms that have similar morphologies as HCC, such as malignant melanoma, mesothelioma, neuroendocrine carcinoma, and renal cell carcinoma, are negative or only focally positive for

Department of Pathology, University of Washington School of Medicine, 1959 North East Pacific Street, NE140D, Box 356100, Seattle, WA 98195-6100, USA
E-mail address: myeh@uw.edu

Clin Liver Dis 14 (2010) 687–703
doi:10.1016/j.cld.2010.10.001
1089-3261/10/$ – see front matter © 2010 Elsevier Inc. All rights reserved.

liver.theclinics.com

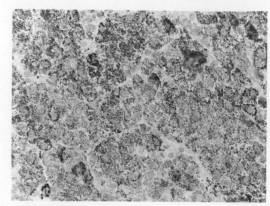

Fig. 1. Hep Par 1 shows strong and diffuse cytoplasmic granular staining in neoplastic hepatocytes of HCC (×400 magnification).

Hep Par 1.[3] In addition, adenocarcinomas from myriad primary sites that often metastasize to the liver, including adenocarcinomas from the biliary tree, colorectum, and pancreas, are also generally negative or only focally positive for Hep Par 1.[4–7]

It is imperative to recognize that Hep Par 1 expression is not entirely specific to HCC. Although most adenocarcinomas are negative for Hep Par 1, gastric, colonic, and pulmonary adenocarcinomas can occasionally demonstrate strong positive staining.[3,4] This can pose a substantial and frequent diagnostic challenge because metastatic adenocarcinomas in the liver are more frequently encountered than HCC in the Western world. Moreover, primary carcinomas of the gastrointestinal tract,

Table 1
Sensitivities of various immunohistochemical markers in detecting HCC, CC, and metastatic adenocarcinoma

	HCC	CC	MA
Hep Par 1	86%,[7] 90%,[5] 92%,[4] 95%,[3] 96%[6]	0%,[5] 0%,[6] 0 %,[7] 7%,[4] 9%,[3] 12.5%[49]	0%,[6] 2%,[7] 6%,[4] 14%[5]
GPC3	75%,[20] 76%,[13] 77%,[17] 79%,[21] 83%,[16] 84%,[12] 88%[15]	0%,[12] 10%,[20] 19%[19]	0%,[18] 6%[16]
pCEA[a]	50%,[28] 69%,[5] 71%,[29] 96%[6]	100%,[5] 100%[6]	93%,[6] 96[5]
MOC 31	0%,[36] 7%,[6] 12%,[5] 14 %[7]	67%,[5] 93%,[6] 100%[36]	66%,[5] 85%,[6] 92 %,[7] 100%[36]
CK7	7%,[42] 20%,[28] 21%[5]	78%,[5] 97%,[42] 100%[28]	3%,[42] 36%,[5]
CK8/18	70%[28]	20%[28]	
CK19	0%,[42] 10 %[5]	44%,[5] 77%,[42] 80%[28]	29%,[5] 64%[42]
CK20	0%,[42] 5 %[5]	10%,[42] 11%[5]	30%,[5] 74%[42]
CD34[b]	94 %,[34] 95%[15]		

Abbreviations: CC, cholangiocarcinoma; MA, metastatic adenocarcinoma.
[a] Positive pCEA staining is regarded as canalicular in HCC and membranous and/or cytoplasmic in CC and MA.
[b] Positive CD34 staining is regarded as a complete/diffuse staining pattern of the sinusoidal endothelial cells.

gallbladder, and pancreas with hepatoid morphology are positive for Hep Par 1, although these tumors are rare.[7–10] In addition, focal Hep Par 1 expression has been reported in a small percentage of cholangiocarcinomas (CCs).[3,4]

The sensitivity of Hep Par 1 is low in poorly differentiated and sclerosing HCC, with sensitivity of approximately 50% or less (**Fig. 2**). Butler and colleagues[2] suggested that this could be due to the suppression of carbamoyl phosphate synthetase 1, which is a highly differentiated cellular protein, at the transcriptional level in more poorly differentiated HCC.

Hep Par 1 expression may be heterogeneous within a given tumor, and patchy staining has been documented in HCC[11]; therefore, needle biopsies can often be negative due to sampling effect.

In addition, because this marker expresses in both non-neoplastic and neoplastic hepatocytes, it is not helpful in discerning benign versus malignant liver tissue.

The use of glypican-3 in diagnosing hepatocellular carcinoma

Glypican-3 (GPC3) is a heparan sulfate proteoglycan that is attached to the cell surface via a glycosyl-phosphatidylinositol anchor. GPC3 is highly expressed in embryonal tissues, and its expression is normally downregulated in adult tissues. GPC3 is expressed at a markedly increased level in HCC.[12] The staining pattern is usually strong and diffusely cytoplasmic, with or without membranous accentuation (**Fig. 3**).

GPC3 has high sensitivity for HCC, with most studies demonstrating sensitivity of approximately 80%.[12–17] It is generally negative in normal and cirrhotic liver tissue adjacent to HCC as well as in benign hepatic neoplasms (see **Fig. 3**). Hence, unlike Hep Par 1, GPC3 is a useful marker in distinguishing benign versus malignant hepatocellular tumors.

Immunohistochemical studies on hepatic fine needle aspirates have shown that GPC3 antibodies provide superb positive predictive value in distinguishing HCC from metastatic malignancies.[16] In several studies, benign hepatic lesions and metastatic carcinomas are negative for GPC3.[15,16,18] Also importantly, the expression of GPC3 is downregulated in both intrahepatic and extrahepatic CC,[12,19,20] making this marker particularly helpful because CC is the second most common primary hepatobiliary malignancy after HCC.

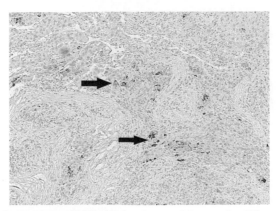

Fig. 2. Hep Par 1 demonstrates focal staining (*arrows*) in poorly differentiated HCC (×100 magnification).

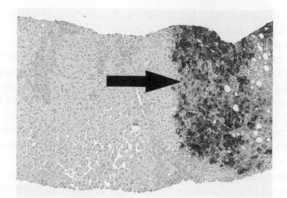

Fig. 3. GPC3 marks the neoplastic hepatocytes in HCC in a granular and cytoplasmic pattern (*arrow*). This is in contrast to the conspicuous absence of GPC3 positivity in the surrounding cirrhotic liver parenchyma (×100 magnification).

GPC3 is also especially useful in detecting poorly differentiated HCC. In a few case series, GPC3 is expressed in 53% to 78% of well-differentiated HCCs, 82% to 93% of moderately differentiated HCCs, and 86% to 100% of poorly differentiated HCCs **(Fig. 4)**.[12,20,21] These findings suggest the higher sensitivity of GPC3 in the poorly differentiated cases, making this stain particularly valuable to pathologists because poorly differentiated neoplasms can pose considerable diagnostic challenges and because Hep Par 1 is often negative in poorly differentiated HCC.

In addition to HCC, GPC3 positivity has been detected to a variable degree in high-grade dysplastic nodules; therefore, GPC3 has limited usefulness in distinguishing the latter from HCC.[12,13,21]

GPC3 is not without limitations. In a study of 60 liver biopsies with chronic hepatitis C, GPC3 positivity in the hepatocytes was seen in 83.6% of cases of high-grade inflammatory activity.[22] This can cause considerable difficulty in the evaluation of liver biopsies when there is significant necrosis and inflammation. Nonetheless, GPC3 expression in hepatitis C tends to be patchy and weak, but focal staining with strong intensity has also been reported. Also, GPC3 expression was only observed in 64% of

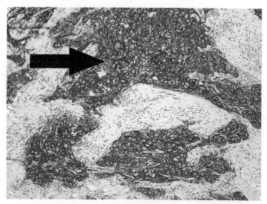

Fig. 4. GPC3 is strongly and uniformly immunoreactive to poorly differentiated HCC (*arrow*) (×100 magnification).

fibrolamellar HCC cases in one study,[21] and, as discussed previously, well-differenti-ated HCCs are often negative for GPC3.

Although GPC3 is a specific marker for HCC, other neoplasms cannot be ruled out on the basis of GPC3 positivity alone. For example, GPC3 was positive in up to 19% of CCs[19,20] and 100% of hepatoblastomas.[12,23] Additionally, GPC3 has had variable positivity in extrahepatic tumors, including extragonadal germ cell tumors (such as yolk sac tumor and choriocarcinoma),[24] squamous cell carcinoma of the lung,[25] mela-noma,[26] and ovarian carcinoma.[27]

Focal GPC3 positivity has also been detected in a small subset of cirrhotic nodules[12,13]; hence, caution is needed when interpreting positive staining with GPC3, and correlation with morphologic findings is essential.

In addition, the expression of GPC3 in HCC can be focal. In one recent study, only 49% of HCCs were labeled by GPC3 on core needle biopsies.[14] Thus, the lack of GPC3 staining, especially in a liver biopsy, should not be regarded as supporting evidence to exclude a diagnosis of HCC.

The use of polyclonal carcinoembryonic antigen in diagnosing hepatocellular carcinoma

In HCC, staining with polyclonal carcinoembryonic antigen (pCEA) produces a canalic-ular staining pattern that has been attributed to cross-reactivity with the biliary glyco-protein on the canalicular surface (**Fig. 5**). This antibody is used less often by pathologists since the development of Hep Par 1; however, this immunohistochemical marker may still provide practical information when used in combination with other well-studied markers.

The canalicular staining pattern is specific for HCC and is not seen in CC and meta-static adenocarcinoma, but its sensitivity has been variably reported, ranging from 50% to 96%.[5,6,28,29] It has high sensitivity for well- to moderately differentiated

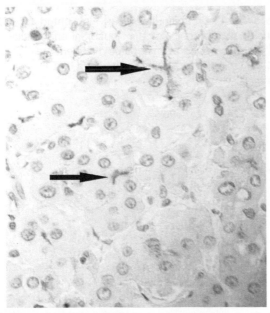

Fig. 5. Immunohistochemical staining of HCC with pCEA yields a canalicular pattern (*arrows*) that is not typically observed in CC or metastatic adenocarcinoma (×40 magnification).

HCC (>80%). In contrast to the canalicular pattern seen in HCC, diffuse cytoplasmic expression of pCEA is seen in a wide variety of metastatic adenocarcinomas to the liver, in which greater than 90% are positive.[5,6] Characteristic cytoplasmic/membranous staining of pCEA is also often identified in CC.[5,6]

HCC is generally nonreactive with monocloncal CEA.[5,30] Monoclonal CEA shows cytoplasmic reactivity in adenocarcinoma, but the sensitivity is only approximately 60% to 70%.[5,30]

Diffuse cytoplasmic and/or membranous staining pattern of pCEA, however, can be seen in approximately 25% of HCCs[5] and decreased immunoreactivity in poorly differentiated HCC has been observed.[31–33] Also, the canalicular pattern can be difficult to interpret in certain cases and may not be readily recognized by untrained eyes, and the marker cannot distinguish between benign and malignant hepatocytic neoplasms.

The use of CD34 in diagnosing hepatocellular carcinoma

Angiogenesis is an important process in hepatocarcinogenesis. The vascular architecture undergoes significant changes in the development of hepatocellular neoplasm. These changes include sinusoidal capillarization and formation of isolated, unpaired arteries,[34] which also underlie the basic concept of the typical hyperenhancement of contrast medium in the arterial phase and washout in the delay phase in four-phase CT image studies of HCC. In normal hepatic parenchyma, arteries are paired with bile ducts within the portal tracts and the sinusoidal endothelial cells are not reactive to endothelial cell marker, such as CD34 or CD31; however, sinusoidal endothelial cells become reactive to these markers in the process of hepatocarcinogenesis, in that immunohistochemical staining with CD34 reveals increasing expression from large regenerative nodules to HCC, in correlation with the proposed stepwise progression of hepatocarcinogenesis. One study has shown that the presence of CD34 expression in greater than 30% of sinusoidal spaces characterizes nodules as at least dysplastic.[35]

In HCC, diffuse sinusoidal capillarization as highlighted by CD34 staining with homogeneous density and intensity of the sinusoidal endothelial cells is frequently observed (**Fig. 6**).[15,35] In comparison, in hepatocytic adenoma (HCA) and focal nodular hyperplasia (FNH), sinusoidal endothelial cell labeling by CD34 is usually not uniform or diffuse.[15]

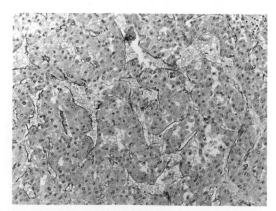

Fig. 6. CD34 labels the diffuse sinusoidal endothelial cells seen in HCC. The staining pattern is uniform and strong in intensity (×200× magnification).

Metastatic Adenocarcinoma in Liver

Although it is not within the scope of this article to extensively discuss the immunohistochemical profiles of the many different neoplasms that can metastasize to the liver, a brief discussion is warranted because metastatic adenocarcinomas are found in the liver at a much higher rate than any primary hepatic neoplasm in the Western world. Metastatic carcinomas typically are not immunoreactive to Hep Par 1.

The use of MOC-31 in diagnosing metastatic adenocarcinoma in liver
MOC-31 is a monoclonal antibody that recognizes an epithelial cell surface glycoprotein of unknown function. It has been a reliable marker in distinguishing HCC from other carcinomas found in the liver. Most HCCs are negative or only weakly positive for MOC-31.[5–7,36] In metastatic adenocarcinoma, however, staining is typically diffuse and intense with only rare exception.[5–7,36] The staining pattern is readily interpretable because the labeling is in the cytoplasmic membranes and is distinct. MOC-31 is expressed in CC as well, with reported sensitivities ranging from 67% to 100%.[5,6,36]

The use of cytokeratin in diagnosing metastatic adenocarcinoma in liver
Cytokeratin (CK) is a marker of epithelial differentiation. Carcinomas tend to express the same CK profiles as the epithelial cells from which they originate; therefore, pathologists commonly use various CKs to explore the primary site of carcinomas when they are observed in the liver.

Non-neoplastic hepatocytes normally express CK8 and CK18. CK7 is typically found in simple epithelia from a variety of sites, including the lung, cervix, upper gastrointestinal epithelium, bile ducts, and mesothelium, among others.[37–39] CK7 is usually not present in hepatocytes but is expressed in the bile duct epithelial cells.[40] CK20 is primarily found in lower intestinal epithelium, gastric foveolar epithelium, and urothelium[41] but is not commonly found in hepatocytes. Correspondingly, HCC is typically immunoreactive to CK8 and CK18[28] but immunonegative for CK7 and CK20.[5,28,42] Nevertheless, HCCs are occasionally CK7+/CK20+ or CK20−, but CK7−/CK20+ in HCC is uncommon. Diffuse CK7 labeling has been described in a modest number of fibrolamellar and classic HCC[5,28,43]; therefore, this stain should be interpreted in correlation with results from other immunohistochemical markers.

In HCC, there is typically strong and distinct CK19 staining of bile duct epithelium in normal and cirrhotic liver parenchyma adjacent to the malignant tumor. The expression of CK19 of bile ducts produces a characteristic pattern, in which CK19+ biliary cells are absent in HCC but present in cirrhotic nodules, a feature that can help to demarcate HCC from cirrhotic tissue, an oftentimes complicated undertaking in H&E–stained sections.[44–46]

A panel of CK7, CK19, and C20 can be helpful in distinguishing metastatic adenocarcinomas from HCC. Depending on the primary site of the metastatic adenocarcinomas, a variety of CK7 and CK20 staining patterns can be found. For example, CK20 positivity is seen in essentially all cases of colorectal carcinomas, whereas the combined staining patterns for CK7 and CK20 show much more variability in gastric adenocarcinomas.[47]

Site- or cell lineage–specific markers, such as CDX-2 for colorectal, TTF-1 for lung and thyroid, and melan-A for melanoma, can be useful in establishing the diagnosis as well.

Cholangiocarcinoma

As discussed previously, CC shows a distinct immunophenotype with coexpression of biliary markers, CK7 and CK19 (**Figs. 7** and **8**),[28] corresponding to the CK7 and CK19 positivity commonly seen in the bile duct epithelial cells.[40] That said, although staining

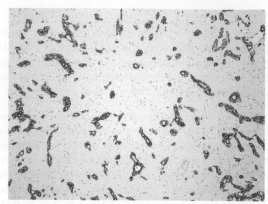

Fig. 7. CK7 distinctly highlights the neoplastic biliary epithelium in an intrahepatic CC (×100 magnification).

for CK7 and CK19 has been classically used to indicate CC differentiation, several studies have observed CK19 staining in morphologically pure HCC.[44–46,48] Hence, CK19 should not be considered a marker specific to CC. The overlap in CK phenotype seen in HCC and CC may be a reflection of their common progenitor cell.

CCs are typically CK20− and thus colorectal cancer is usually immunohistochemically distinguishable from CC by CK7−/CK20+ and CDX-2+ immunostaining profile. On the contrary, there is currently no reliable immunohistochemical marker that can distinguish intrahepatic CC from metastatic adenocarcinomas originating in the upper gastrointestinal sites, such as the stomach, gallbladder, extrahepatic biliary tree, and pancreas.

Hep Par 1 is generally not expressed in CC. In one study, however, 4 of the 32 cases of morphologically pure CC showed staining for Hep Par 1. The staining was seen in the mucin-secreting columnar cells, which displayed the similar granular staining characteristics as that observed in hepatocytes.[49] Although the significance of this observation is uncertain, it emphasizes the importance of morphologic correlation in the pathologic diagnosis of CC, and a diagnosis of CC should not be completely ruled out on the basis of Hep Par 1 positivity.

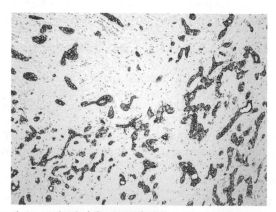

Fig. 8. CK19 marks the neoplastic biliary epithelial cells in an intrahepatic CC. This is the same neoplasm seen in **Fig. 7** (×100 magnification).

The neoplastic cells in CC often show cytoplasmic and luminal positivity for monoclonal and polyclonal CEA. A canalicular pattern is not typically seen, and similar to metastatic adenocarcinoma, MOC-31 is frequently positive in CC.[5,6]

Combined Hepatocellular Carcinoma–Cholangiocarcinoma

There are increasing numbers of published reports of hepatic tumors with mixed features of HCC and CC, also known as combined HCC-CC (C-HCC-CC).[48,50–52] Overall, the staining pattern of C-HCC-CC is a blend of the immunophenotypic profiles of HCC and CC. In C-HCC-CC, Hep Par 1 shows strong and distinct staining of the HCC component, but in general, no marking of the CC component by Hep Par 1 is observed. There is coexpression of CK7 and CK19 in the CC component of C-HCC-CC and it can be identified in cells within the transitional areas of C-HCC-CC.[49] As discussed previously, CK7 and CK19 expressions in HCC are not uncommon from several series[44–46]; thus, a diagnosis of C-HCC-CC solely based on immunohistochemistry may not be fully reliable, and morphologic correlation, including the presence of true glandular structures, is essential, preferably with a positive mucin stain.

Hepatocellular Adenoma, Focal Nodular Hyperplasia, and Telangiectatic Hepatocytic Adenoma

HCAs are strongly linked to excess hormonal exposure. Immunostaining for both estrogen receptor and progesterone receptor was present in a majority of HCAs (approximately 80%), and staining with one hormone receptor has been positively associated with staining for the other receptor.[53]

Morphologically, HCA and FNH can be similar. A combination of CK7 and CK19, along with neuronal cell adhesion molecule (NCAM), was helpful in distinguishing the two entities.[54] In HCA, hepatocytes are strongly immunoreactive with CK7 in a patchy fashion. There is a gradual reduction in the staining intensity of CK7 as the hepatocytes become more differentiated and more mature (ie, non-neoplastic). Because bile ducts are normally absent in HCA, CK7 only highlights occasional bile ductules. In FNH, alternatively, CK7 expression is weak and focal in hepatocytes, but bile ductules within the fibrous septa display strong CK7 staining. CK19 and NCAM show patchy and moderate staining in the biliary epithelium of the ductules in FNH. Contrasting to FNH, in the HCA, CK19 is only rarely positive in occasional cells within ductules, and NCAM highlights occasional isolated cells in the tumor.

CD34 marks sinusoids in periportal areas in both FNH and HCA. These staining patterns have been confirmed in biopsy specimens as well.[55] As discussed previously, this staining pattern is different from the diffuse sinusoidal labeling by CD34 typically seen in HCC.

Telangiectatic hepatocytic Adenoma (T-HCA) was formerly referred to as telangiectatic variant of FNH, but recent molecular studies and protein profiling have demonstrated that these lesions are more similar to HCA than FHN, hence the reclassification of these lesions as a subtype of HCA (inflammatory subtype).[56,57]

Recently, Bioulac-Sage and colleagues[58–60] classified HCA into four subgroups according to their genotypic/phenotypic features. In their study, they found that in cases of β-catenin–mutated HCA, there was aberrant cytoplasmic and nuclear staining with β-catenin antibody. In normal hepatocytes, β-catenin expression is localized to the cytoplasmic membranes. Inflammatory/telangiectatic HCA with activation of β-catenin also behaves like β-catenin–mutated HCA, with abnormal cytoplasmic and nuclear β-catenin staining.

Glutamine synthetase (GS) has been investigated as a possible marker in distinguishing HCA from FNH and from normal liver.[61,62] The staining pattern of GS was different in normal liver, FNH, HCA expressing wild-type β-catenin (hepatocyte nuclear factor 1α [HNF1α]–mutated or inflammatory/telangiectatic HCA), and HCA expressing β-catenin mutations. (1) In normal liver, GS staining is limited to 1 or 2 centrilobular plates. (2) In FNH, GS expression is strong and cytoplasmic, and the pattern of staining has been described as anastomosing and continuous or map-like, involving large hepatoctyic areas. GS is not expressed in hepatocytes close to fibrotic bands containing arteries and ductules, and the staining tends to be more intense at the periphery than in the center of FNH. (3) In HCA expressing wild-type β-catenin (HNF1α–mutated or inflammatory/telangiectatic HCA), GS staining is largely absent, and, when present, GS labeling is restricted to the periphery of HCA and in a few hepatocytes around the veins (**Fig. 9**). (4) In HCA and well-differentiated HCC showing β-catenin mutations, the distribution of GS labeling is diffuse and does not display the anastomosing or map-like pattern seen in FNH.

THE USE OF IMMUNOHISTOCHEMISTRY IN OTHER LESS COMMON LIVER TUMORS
Hepatic Angiomyolipoma

Angiomyolipoma (AML) is a rare mesenchymal neoplasm speculated to arise from perivascular epithelioid cells. AML consists of an intimate mixture of three components, namely, mature adipose tissue, tortuous thick-walled vessels, and bundles of smooth muscle.

The neoplastic cells express several melanocytic markers, including HMB-45, melan-A, and microphthalmia transcription factor.[63,64] Of these three markers of melanocytic differentiation, HMB-45 is the most sensitive, followed by melan-A and lastly by microphthalmia transcription factor.[63,64] The extent of staining of these melanocytic markers in AML ranges from focal to diffuse. Other melanocytic markers, including tyrosinase and NK1-C3, have strikingly low sensitivities and are of limited use in the diagnosis of AML.[64,65] The usefulness of CD117 (also known as CKIT), another melanocytic marker, is less clear, with one study demonstrating 100% sensitivity in hepatic and renal AMLs[66] and a different study showing only 40% sensitivity in renal AMLs.[65] Because HMB-45 and melan-A stains complement each other,[65] it is recommended starting with these two markers in the work-up of AML.

In addition, muscle-specific actin and smooth muscle actin are two established immunohistochemical markers for AML, with respective sensitivities of 100% and

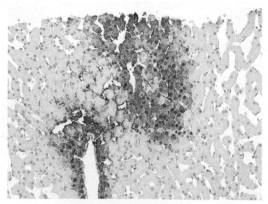

Fig. 9. GS staining surrounds terminal hepatic veins in a telangiectatic HCA (×200 magnification).

94%.[64,67] The neoplastic cells are negative for CK (CAM 5.2 and AE1/AE3) and Hep Par 1.[68,69] Mature adipose cells are mostly positive for S100, and the angiomatous components exhibit positivity for vascular markers, including CD34 and factor VIII.[67,70]

Lymphangioma

Hepatic lymphangiomas are benign lesions that could be solitary or may be associated with multiple liver lesions (hepatic lymphangiomatosis), characterized by cystic dilatation of the lymphatic vessels in the liver parenchyma.

Because lymphangioma and peritoneal cystic mesothelioma can be morphologically similar, the use of immunohistochemical markers becomes important in differentiating the two entities. Neoplastic cells of peritoneal cystic mesothelioma are positive for CK and epithelial membrane antigen, whereas the endothelial lining of lymphangioma stains positively with factor VIII–related antigen and CD31.

D2-40 is a monoclonal antibody that recognizes human podoplanin, a transmembrane mucoprotein that is expressed in lymphatic endothelial cells.[71–73] This immunohistochemical marker is selectively expressed in lymphatic endothelial cells and differs from other endothelial markers that highlight both lymphatic and vascular endothelial cells. D2-40 has been useful in the identification of lymphangiomas.[74] This marker, however, was also positive in 93% of peritoneal mesotheliomas in one study.[75] Hence, D2-40 should be interpreted with caution in cases where lymphangioma and peritoneal cystic mesothelioma are in the differential.

Epithelioid Hemangioendothelioma

Epithelioid hemangioendothelioma (EHE) is a rare neoplasm of vascular origin and can be confused with angiosarcoma. The absence of marked nuclear atypia, high mitotic rate, and anastomosing vascular architecture, however, argues against a diagnosis of angiosarcoma when a vascular tumor is under consideration.

In the largest series of EHE of the liver reported to date,[76] several immunohistochemical markers were reliable in distinguishing EHE from other hepatic tumors. Of the three endothelial cell markers, factor VIII–related antigen was the most frequently positive (99%), followed by CD34 (94%), and then by CD31 (86%), supporting the vascular endothelial origin of this neoplasm. In the majority of these cases (>88%), the neoplastic cells were surrounded by a thin, continuous basement membrane that stained strongly positive for type IV collagen and laminin. The stroma in the highly cellular area consisted of a large amount of type IV collagen. In contrast, in the dense sclerotic areas, laminin and type IV collagen expressions were negative or only weakly positive. There were a few cases in which the epithelioid cells showed cytoplasmic expression of laminin.

Immunostaining with Hep Par 1 usually highlights surrounding reactive hepatocytes and individual hepatocytes overrun by the neoplasm, but Hep Par 1 should not mark the neoplastic cells in EHE.

Recently, D2-40 has been a useful immunohistochemical marker in differentiating EHE from other vascular neoplasms within the liver.[77] In normal liver parenchyma, podoplanin is expressed in mesothelial cells of the hepatic capsule, lymphatic endothelial cells, and nerve fibers but is not usually detected in any other cells within the liver. In a recent study, the presence of podoplanin expression was identified in seven of nine cases (78%) of EHE but not in other hepatic tumors, including angiosarcoma. Importantly, the intensity of podoplanin expression was inversely correlated with the expression of CD34 and factor VIII, markers deemed useful in identifying EHE. Therefore, an immunohistochemical panel consisting of D2-40, factor VIII, CD34, and CD31 can be potentially helpful in the diagnosis of EHE.

Angiosarcoma

In angiosarcoma, the neoplastic cells usually stain strongly and diffusely positive for CD34 and von Willebrand factor, confirming vascular differentiation of the malignant neoplasm. CD31 is a specific stain for vascular endothelial cells but is less sensitive compared with CD34. Therefore, it is not unusual to encounter an angiosarcoma with absent CD31 staining. Stains for the cytokeratins and Hep Par 1 often highlight entrapped non-neoplastic bile ducts and hepatocytes, respectively.

EHE is frequently in the differential diagnosis when a malignant vascular neoplasm in the liver is encountered. A diffuse, sinusoidal pattern, however, favors angiosarcoma. Also, as discussed previously, the immunohistochemical marker D2-40 is useful in distinguishing between the two.

Hepatobiliary Cystadenomas

Hepatobiliary cystadenomas (HBCs) are lined by a single layer of columnar to cuboidal mucinous epithelium with basal nuclei and apical mucin. The tumor typically shows underlying spindle cells reminiscent of the ovarian-type stroma. Therefore, morphologically, HBCs and pancreatic mucinous cystic neoplasms are similar, because the latter also has ovarian-type stroma underlying mucinous epithelium.

Immunohistochemically, the epithelium of HBC shows positive cytoplasmic staining for CK7, CK8, CK18, and CK19, typical of biliary-type epithelium. Nuclear staining of the mesenchymal stromal cells for ER and PR, as well as strong cytoplasmic staining of stromal cells for smooth muscle actin, is seen. A subset of HBC stroma also stains positively for inhibin.[78,79] Similarly, the ovarian-type stromal cells in pancreatic mucinous cystic neoplasms also express inhibin, smooth muscle actin, progesterone receptor, and estrogen receptor.[80]

SUMMARY

This review summarizes the up-to-date immunohistochemical markers commonly used in the pathologic diagnosis of liver tumors.

In the work-up of liver tumors in which the differential diagnosis includes HCC, CC, and metastatic adenocarcinoma, a useful initial antibody panel could include Hep Par 1, GPC3, pCEA, and MOC-31 (see **Table 1**). Cytoplasmic staining of Hep Par 1 is usually seen in HCC but not in CC or metastatic adenocarcinoma. GPC3 is also typically positive in HCC, with lower sensitivity in well-differentiated HCC and higher sensitivity in poorly differentiated HCC. A canalicular staining pattern with pCEA is generally seen in HCC, whereas a cytoplasmic/membranous staining pattern with pCEA is often present in CC and metastatic adenocarcinoma. MOC-31 is frequently negative in HCC but positive in CC and metastatic adenocarcinoma.

A second panel of useful stains could include CK7, CK19, and CK20. Overall, HCCs are usually negative for CK7, CK19, and CK20. CCs are typically positive for CK7 and CK19 but negative for CK20. For metastatic adenocarcinoma, the staining pattern is dependent on the various primary sites. Also, when metastatic adenocarcinomas are suspected, site- or cellular-specific immunohistochemical markers can be used to further determine the site of origin.

In the work-up of hepatic tumors in which HCC, HCA, FNH, and T-HCA are in the differential diagnosis, the following panel can be used: Hep Par 1, GPC3, and CD34. Hep Par 1 can confirm the hepatocellular origin of the tumor. GPC3 typically only marks HCC and is generally negative in benign lesions, such as HCA, FNH, and T-HCA. A diffuse and uniform labeling of the sinusoidal endothelial cells by CD34 is often observed in HCC, whereas labeling of the sinusoidal endothelial cells by CD34 is usually incomplete or focal in HCA and FNH. Additionally, CK7, CK19, NCAM, and GS have been reliable immunohistochemical markers in differentiating HCA from FNH.

Finally, it cannot be overemphasized, as stated by the late Hans Popper, that "The best tool in liver disease is an H&E slide that is connected to the human brain". A careful morphologic examination with clinical and image correlation should be made first to guide the selection of immunohistochemical stains in the diagnosis of liver tumors.

REFERENCES

1. Wennerberg AE, Nalesnik MA, Coleman WB. Hepatocyte paraffin 1: a monoclonal antibody that reacts with hepatocytes and can be used for differential diagnosis of hepatic tumors. Am J Pathol 1993;143(4):1050–4.
2. Butler SL, Dong H, Cardona D, et al. The antigen for Hep Par 1 antibody is the urea cycle enzyme carbamoyl phosphate synthetase 1. Lab Invest 2008;88(1): 78–88.
3. Fan Z, van de Rijn M, Montgomery K, et al. Hep par 1 antibody stain for the differential diagnosis of hepatocellular carcinoma: 676 tumors tested using tissue microarrays and conventional tissue sections. Mod Pathol 2003;16(2):137–44.
4. Chu PG, Ishizawa S, Wu E, et al. Hepatocyte antigen as a marker of hepatocellular carcinoma: an immunohistochemical comparison to carcinoembryonic antigen, CD10, and alpha-fetoprotein. Am J Surg Pathol 2002;26(8):978–88.
5. Lau SK, Prakash S, Geller SA, et al. Comparative immunohistochemical profile of hepatocellular carcinoma, cholangiocarcinoma, and metastatic adenocarcinoma. Hum Pathol 2002;33(12):1175–81.
6. Morrison C, Marsh W Jr, Frankel WL. A comparison of CD10 to pCEA, MOC-31, and hepatocyte for the distinction of malignant tumors in the liver. Mod Pathol 2002;15(12):1279–87.
7. Geramizadeh B, Boub R, Rahsaz M. Histologic differentiation of hepatocellular carcinoma from adenocarcinoma by a simple panel: evaluation of the pitfalls. Indian J Pathol Microbiol 2007;50(3):507–10.
8. Maitra A, Murakata LA, Albores-Saavedra J. Immunoreactivity for hepatocyte paraffin 1 antibody in hepatoid adenocarcinomas of the gastrointestinal tract. Am J Clin Pathol 2001;115(5):689–94.
9. Villari D, Caruso R, Grosso M, et al. Hep Par 1 in gastric and bowel carcinomas: an immunohistochemical study. Pathology 2002;34(5):423–6.
10. Augustin G, Jelincic Z, Tentor D, et al. Hepatoid adenocarcinoma of the stomach: case report and short notes on immunohistochemical markers. Acta Gastroenterol Belg 2009;72(2):253–6.
11. Senes G, Fanni D, Cois A, et al. Intratumoral sampling variability in hepatocellular carcinoma: a case report. World J Gastroenterol 2007;13(29):4019–21.
12. Yamauchi N, Watanabe A, Hishinuma M, et al. The glypican 3 oncofetal protein is a promising diagnostic marker for hepatocellular carcinoma. Mod Pathol 2005; 18(12):1591–8.
13. Wang HL, Anatelli F, Zhai QJ, et al. Glypican-3 as a useful diagnostic marker that distinguishes hepatocellular carcinoma from benign hepatocellular mass lesions. Arch Pathol Lab Med 2008;132(11):1723–8.
14. Anatelli F, Chuang ST, Yang XJ, et al. Value of glypican 3 immunostaining in the diagnosis of hepatocellular carcinoma on needle biopsy. Am J Clin Pathol 2008;130(2):219–23.

15. Coston WM, Loera S, Lau SK, et al. Distinction of hepatocellular carcinoma from benign hepatic mimickers using Glypican-3 and CD 34 immunohistochemistry. Am J Surg Pathol 2008;32(3):433–44.

16. Ligato S, Mandich D, Cartun RW. Utility of glypican-3 in differentiating hepatocellular carcinoma from other primary and metastatic lesions in FNA of the liver: an immunocytochemical study. Mod Pathol 2008;21(5):626–31.

17. Libbrecht L, Severi T, Cassiman D, et al. Glypican-3 expression distinguishes small hepatocellular carcinomas from cirrhosis, dysplastic nodules, and focal nodular hyperplasia-like nodules. Am J Surg Pathol 2006;30(11):1405–11.

18. Kandil D, Leiman G, Allegretta M, et al. Glypican-3 immunocytochemistry in liver fine-needle aspirates: a novel stain to assist in the differentiation of benign and malignant liver lesions. Cancer 2007;111(5):316–22.

19. Man XB, Tang L, Zhang BH, et al. Upregulation of Glypican-3 expression in hepatocellular carcinoma but downregulation in cholangiocarcinoma indicates its differential diagnosis value in primary liver cancers. Liver Int 2005;25(5):962–6.

20. Wang XY, Degos F, Dubois S, et al. Glypican-3 expression in hepatocellular tumors: diagnostic value for preneoplastic lesions and hepatocellular carcinomas. Hum Pathol 2006;37(11):1435–41.

21. Shafizadeh N, Ferrell LD, Kakar S. Utility and limitations of glypican-3 expression for the diagnosis of hepatocellular carcinoma at both ends of the differentiation spectrum. Mod Pathol 2008;21(8):1011–8.

22. Abdul-Al HM, Makhlouf HR, Wang G, et al. Glypican-3 expression in benign liver tissue with active hepatitis C: implications for the diagnosis of hepatocellular carcinoma. Hum Pathol 2008;39(2):209–12.

23. Zynger DL, Gupta A, Luan C, et al. Expression of glypican 3 in hepatoblastoma: an immunohistochemical study of 65 cases. Hum Pathol 2008;39(2):224–30.

24. Zynger DL, Everton MJ, Dimov ND, et al. Expression of glypican 3 in ovarian and extragonadal germ cell tumors. Am J Clin Pathol 2008;130(2):224–30.

25. Aviel-Ronen S, Lau SK, Pintilie M, et al. Glypican-3 is overexpressed in lung squamous cell carcinoma, but not in adenocarcinoma. Mod Pathol 2008;21(7):817–25.

26. Nakatsura T, Kageshita T, Ito S, et al. Identification of glypican-3 as a novel tumor marker for melanoma. Clin Cancer Res 2004;10(19):6612–21.

27. Stadlmann S, Gueth U, Baumhoer D, et al. Glypican-3 expression in primary and recurrent ovarian carcinomas. Int J Gynecol Pathol 2007;26(3):341–4.

28. Stroescu C, Herlea V, Dragnea A, et al. The diagnostic value of cytokeratins and carcinoembryonic antigen immunostaining in differentiating hepatocellular carcinomas from intrahepatic cholangiocarcinomas. J Gastrointestin Liver Dis 2006;15(1):9–14.

29. Ma CK, Zarbo RJ, Frierson HF Jr, et al. Comparative immunohistochemical study of primary and metastatic carcinomas of the liver. Am J Clin Pathol 1993;99(5):551–7.

30. Rishi M, Kovatich A, Ehya H. Utility of polyclonal and monoclonal antibodies against carcinoembryonic antigen in hepatic fine-needle aspirates. Diagn Cytopathol 1994;11(4):358–61 [discussion: 361–2].

31. Balaton AJ, Nehama-Sibony M, Gotheil C, et al. Distinction between hepatocellular carcinoma, cholangiocarcinoma, and metastatic carcinoma based on immunohistochemical staining for carcinoembryonic antigen and for cytokeratin 19 on paraffin sections. J Pathol 1988;156(4):305–10.

32. Christensen WN, Boitnott JK, Kuhajda FP. Immunoperoxidase staining as a diagnostic aid for hepatocellular carcinoma. Mod Pathol 1989;2(1):8–12.

33. Borscheri N, Roessner A, Röcken C. Canalicular immunostaining of neprilysin (CD10) as a diagnostic marker for hepatocellular carcinomas. Am J Surg Pathol 2001;25(10):1297–303.
34. Nascimento C, Bottino A, Nogueira C, et al. Analysis of morphological variables and arterialization in the differential diagnosis of hepatic nodules in explanted cirrhotic livers. Diagn Pathol 2007;2:51.
35. Nascimento C, Caroli-Bottino A, Paschoal J, et al. Vascular immunohistochemical markers: contributions to hepatocellular nodule diagnosis in explanted livers. Transplant Proc 2009;41(10):4211–3.
36. Proca DM, Niemann TH, Porcell AI, et al. MOC31 immunoreactivity in primary and metastatic carcinoma of the liver. Report of findings and review of other utilized markers [review]. Appl Immunohistochem Mol Morphol 2000;8(2):120–5.
37. Lagendijk JH, Mullink H, Van Diest PJ, et al. Tracing the origin of adenocarcinomas with unknown primary using immunohistochemistry: differential diagnosis between colonic and ovarian carcinomas as primary sites. Hum Pathol 1998; 29(5):491–7.
38. Chhieng DC, Cangiarella JF, Zakowski MF, et al. Use of thyroid transcription factor 1, PE-10, and cytokeratins 7 and 20 in discriminating between primary lung carcinomas and metastatic lesions in fine-needle aspiration biopsy specimens. Cancer 2001;93(5):330–6.
39. Tot T. Adenocarcinomas metastatic to the liver: the value of cytokeratins 20 and 7 in the search for unknown primary tumors. Cancer 1999;85(1):171–7.
40. Yabushita K, Yamamoto K, Ibuki N, et al. Aberrant expression of cytokeratin 7 as a histological marker of progression in primary biliary cirrhosis. Liver 2001;21(1):50–5.
41. Moll R, Löwe A, Laufer J, et al. Cytokeratin 20 in human carcinomas. A new histodiagnostic marker detected by monoclonal antibodies. Am J Pathol 1992; 140(2):427–47.
42. Maeda T, Kajiyama K, Adachi E, et al. The expression of cytokeratins 7, 19, and 20 in primary and metastatic carcinomas of the liver. Mod Pathol 1996;9(9):901–9.
43. Górnicka B, Ziarkiewicz-Wróblewska B, Wróblewski T, et al. Carcinoma, a fibrolamellar variant–immunohistochemical analysis of 4 cases. Hepatogastroenterology 2005;52(62):519–23.
44. Durnez A, Verslype C, Nevens F, et al. The clinicopathological and prognostic relevance of cytokeratin 7 and 19 expression in hepatocellular carcinoma. A possible progenitor cell origin. Histopathology 2006;49(2):138–51.
45. Klein WM, Molmenti EP, Colombani PM, et al. Primary liver carcinoma arising in people younger than 30 years. Am J Clin Pathol 2005;124(4):512–8.
46. Wu PC, Fang JW, Lau VK, et al. Classification of hepatocellular carcinoma according to hepatocellular and biliary differentiation markers. Clinical and biological implications. Am J Pathol 1996;149(4):1167–75.
47. Chu P, Wu E, Weiss LM. Cytokeratin 7 and cytokeratin 20 expression in epithelial neoplasms: a survey of 435 cases. Mod Pathol 2000;13(9):962–72.
48. Yeh MM. Immunohistochemical analysis in hepatocellular carcinoma: does age matter? Am J Clin Pathol 2005;124(4):491–3.
49. Leong AS, Sormunen RT, Tsui WM, et al. Hep Par 1 and selected antibodies in the immunohistological distinction of hepatocellular carcinoma from cholangiocarcinoma, combined tumours and metastatic carcinoma. Histopathology 1998; 33(4):318–24.
50. Aoki K, Takayasu K, Kawano T, et al. Combined hepatocellular carcinoma and cholangiocarcinoma: clinical features and computed tomographic findings. Hepatology 1993;18(5):1090–5.

51. Maeda T, Adachi E, Kajiyama K, et al. Combined hepatocellular and cholangio-carcinoma: proposed criteria according to cytokeratin expression and analysis of clinicopathologic features. Hum Pathol 1995;26(9):956–64.
52. Goodman ZD, Ishak KG, Langloss JM, et al. Combined hepatocellular-cholangio-carcinoma. A histologic and immunohistochemical study. Cancer 1985;55(1): 124–35.
53. Torbenson M, Lee JH, Choti M, et al. Hepatic adenomas: analysis of sex steroid receptor status and the Wnt signaling pathway. Mod Pathol 2002;15(3):189–96.
54. Iyer A, Robert ME, Bifulco CB, et al. Different cytokeratin and neuronal cell adhe-sion molecule staining patterns in focal nodular hyperplasia and hepatic adenoma and their significance. Hum Pathol 2008;39(9):1370–7.
55. Ahmad I, Iyer A, Marginean CE, et al. Diagnostic use of cytokeratins, CD 34, and neuronal cell adhesion molecule staining in focal nodular hyperplasia and hepatic adenoma. Hum Pathol 2009;40(5):726–34.
56. Bioulac-Sage P, Rebouissou S, Sa Cunha A, et al. Clinical, morphologic, and molecular features defining so-called telangiectatic focal nodular hyperplasias of the liver. Gastroenterology 2005;128(5):1211–8.
57. Paradis V, Benzekri A, Dargère D, et al. Telangiectatic focal nodular hyperplasia: a variant of hepatocellular adenoma. Gastroenterology 2004;126(5):1323–9.
58. Bioulac-Sage P, Rebouissou S, Thomas C, et al. Hepatocellular adenoma subtype classification using molecular markers and immunohistochemistry. Hep-atology 2007;46(3):740–8.
59. Bioulac-Sage P, Blanc JF, Rebouissou S, et al. Genotype phenotype classification of hepatocellular adenoma. World J Gastroenterol 2007;13(19):2649–54. review.
60. Bioulac-Sage P, Balabaud C, Bedossa P, et al. Pathological diagnosis of liver cell adenoma and focal nodular hyperplasia: Bordeaux update [review]. J Hepatol 2007;46(3):521–7.
61. Bioulac-Sage P, Laumonier H, Rullier A, et al. Over-expression of glutamine synthetase in focal nodular hyperplasia: a novel easy diagnostic tool in surgical pathology. Liver Int 2009;29(3):459–65.
62. Gebhardt R, Baldysiak-Figiel A, Krügel V, et al. Hepatocellular expression of glutamine synthetase: an indicator of morphogen actions as master regulators of zonation in adult liver [review]. Prog Histochem Cytochem 2007;41(4):201–66.
63. Makhlouf HR, Ishak KG, Shekar R, et al. Melanoma markers in angiomyolipoma of the liver and kidney: a comparative study. Arch Pathol Lab Med 2002;126(1):49–55.
64. Zavala-Pompa A, Folpe AL, Jimenez RE, et al. Immunohistochemical study of mi-crophthalmia transcription factor and tyrosinase in angiomyolipoma of the kidney, renal cell carcinoma, and renal and retroperitoneal sarcomas: comparative eval-uation with traditional diagnostic markers. Am J Surg Pathol 2001;25(1):65–70.
65. Roma AA, Magi-Galluzzi C, Zhou M. Differential expression of melanocytic markers in myoid, lipomatous, and vascular components of renal angiomyolipo-mas. Arch Pathol Lab Med 2007;131(1):122–5.
66. Makhlouf HR, Remotti HE, Ishak KG. Expression of KIT (CD117) in angiomyolipoma. Am J Surg Pathol 2002;26(4):493–7.
67. Jungbluth AA, Iversen K, Coplan K, et al. Expression of melanocyte-associated markers gp-100 and Melan-A/MART-1 in angiomyolipomas. An immunohisto-chemical and rt-PCR analysis. Virchows Arch 1999;434(5):429–35.
68. Xu PJ, Shan Y, Yan FH, et al. Epithelioid angiomyolipoma of the liver: cross-sectional imaging findings of 10 immunohistochemically-verified cases. World J Gastroenterol 2009;15(36):4576–81.

69. Petrolla AA, Xin W. Hepatic angiomyolipoma. Arch Pathol Lab Med 2008;132(10): 1679–82. review.
70. Suster S, Fisher C. Immunoreactivity for the human hematopoietic progenitor cell antigen (CD 34) in lipomatous tumors. Am J Surg Pathol 1997;21(2):195–200.
71. Breiteneder-Geleff S, Soleiman A, Kowalski H, et al. Angiosarcomas express mixed endothelial phenotypes of blood and lymphatic capillaries: podoplanin as a specific marker for lymphatic endothelium. Am J Pathol 1999;154(2):385–94.
72. Kahn HJ, Bailey D, Marks A. Monoclonal antibody D2-40, a new marker of lymphatic endothelium, reacts with Kaposi's sarcoma and a subset of angiosarcomas. Mod Pathol 2002;15(4):434–40.
73. Kahn HJ, Marks A. A new monoclonal antibody, D2-40, for detection of lymphatic invasion in primary tumors. Lab Invest 2002;82(9):1255–7.
74. Fukunaga M. Expression of D2-40 in lymphatic endothelium of normal tissues and in vascular tumours. Histopathology 2005;46(4):396–402.
75. Ordóñez NG. The diagnostic utility of immunohistochemistry and electron microscopy in distinguishing between peritoneal mesotheliomas and serous carcinomas: a comparative study. Mod Pathol 2006;19(1):34–48.
76. Makhlouf HR, Ishak KG, Goodman ZD. Epithelioid hemangioendothelioma of the liver: a clinicopathologic study of 137 cases. Cancer 1999;85(3):562–82.
77. Fujii T, Zen Y, Sato Y, et al. Podoplanin is a useful diagnostic marker for epithelioid hemangioendothelioma of the liver. Mod Pathol 2008;21(2):125–30.
78. Abdul-Al HM, Makhlouf HR, Goodman ZD. Expression of estrogen and progesterone receptors and inhibin-alpha in hepatobiliary cystadenoma: an immunohistochemical study. Virchows Arch 2007;450(6):691–7.
79. Lam MM, Swanson PE, Upton MP, et al. Ovarian-type stroma in hepatobiliary cystadenomas and pancreatic mucinous cystic neoplasms: an immunohistochemical study. Am J Clin Pathol 2008;129(2):211–8.
80. Yeh MM, Tang LH, Wang S, et al. Inhibin expression in ovarian-type stroma in mucinous cystic neoplasms of the pancreas. Appl Immunohistochem Mol Morphol 2004;12(2):148–52.

Hepatic Progenitor Cells: An Update

Tania Roskams, MD, PhD*, Aezam Katoonizadeh, MD,
Mina Komuta, MD, PhD

KEYWORDS

- Hepatic progenitor cells • Liver stem cells • Cancer stem cells
- Wnt pathway • Notch pathway • Regeneration

The liver is located in a toxic-rich environment, and consequently is required to tolerate frequent exposure to toxins. In addition, the liver can be affected by a wide variety of toxins, infections, tumors, and disorders, such as viral diseases, genetic, or immunologic disorders. Therefore, the liver has evolutionary adapted to cope well with these insults.[1] The liver has an amazing capacity to regenerate after different types of injury. Liver regeneration is an extremely complex process.[2] Cell types and mechanisms involved depend on the extent of liver damage (mild to severe), the type of damage (with or without necrosis, inflammation), the underlying liver disease (acute or chronic), and the capacity of the whole body to respond (eg, affected by age). This restitutive response requires the activation of multiple complex pathways that do not act independent of each other and involves, based on the type of the injury, different cell types, including stem cells.[2-5]

WHAT IS A STEM CELL?

A stem cell is an undifferentiated cell capable throughout life of renewing itself and generating one or more types of differentiated cells.[6-8] The ultimate stem cells are those of the early embryo, which are totipotential. Farther down along the line, in the fetus and also the adult, multipotential (pluripotential) stem cells are found. Those closer to final differentiation are called *progenitor, committed*, or *transit* cells. In continuously renewing lining epithelia, such as the epidermis, stem cells are easy to find because they squat against the basement membrane. The liver is normally a quiescent organ, but contains different cell types with stem cell properties: hepatocytes and progenitor cells in the most peripheral branches of the biliary tree.[9-13] Stem cells in continuously renewing systems are embedded in a niche, consisting of mesenchymal cells, extracellular matrix, and soluble factors released by the niche cells to help to

Liver Research Unit, Department of Morphology and Molecular Pathology, University of Leuven, Minderbroederstraat 12, Leuven, Belgium
* Corresponding author.
E-mail address: tania.roskams@uz.kuleuven.ac.be

Clin Liver Dis 14 (2010) 705–718
doi:10.1016/j.cld.2010.08.003

liver.theclinics.com

maintain the "stemness" state of the stem cell. In the liver, the stem/progenitor cell niche is now being characterized.

HEPATOCYTES HAVE STEM CELL PROPERTIES

Hepatocyte-mediated liver regeneration is the quickest and the most efficient way to generate hepatocytes and is typically achieved through the repeated division of the remaining healthy hepatocytes. The adult liver is normally quiescent. Quiescent hepatocytes are in a state known as G0, indicating that the cells are not cycling. Hepatocytes in normal adult liver have a life span of more than a year. After partial hepatectomy, however, proliferation of the main epithelial compartments (hepatocytes and cholangiocytes), followed by proliferation of the mesenchymal cells (hepatic stellate cells and endothelial cells), quickly restores the liver. In rodents, the liver can restore its original volume after two-thirds hepatectomy in approximately 10 days.[14]

After mild acute injury or after partial hepatectomy, which is a classic model of hepatocyte-mediated liver regeneration, hepatocytes enter the cell cycle (G1 phase), progress to DNA replication (S phase), and then undergo mitosis (M phase), with cell division completing the sequence. This highly regulated process is simultaneously mediated by different growth factors and cytokines. Gut-derived factors, such as lipopolysaccharide, or the other molecules that are crucial for the innate immunity, such as C3a and C5a, activate Kupffer cells and stellate cells and increase the production of tumor necrosis factor (TNF)-α and interleukin (IL)-6, which prime hepatocytes to respond to growth factors such as hepatocyte growth factor and epidermal growth factor receptor. Other factors are released from the pancreas (insulin), duodenum or salivary gland (epidermal growth factor), adrenal gland (norepinephrine), thyroid gland (triodothronine; T3), and stellate cells (hepatocyte growth factor). Cooperative signals from these factors allow the hepatocytes to move from G0, through G1, to the S phase of the cell cycle. This progression leads to DNA synthesis and hepatocyte proliferation. Transforming growth factor signaling, which inhibits hepatocyte DNA synthesis, is blocked during the proliferative phase but is restored at the end of the regeneration process through helping to return hepatocytes to the quiescent state.[2]

Serial transplantation experiments have shown that hepatocytes have a near infinite capacity to proliferate.[15,16] The fact that at least 69 doublings can occur confirms the clonogenic potential of hepatocytes, one of the crucial properties of a stem cell. Hepatic stellate cells play a crucial role in the hepatocyte regeneration process because they produce not only mitogens for hepatocytes (eg, hepatocyte growth factor, TGF-α, insulin growth factor) but also inhibiting growth factors such as TGF-β, to stop the regeneration process.[1,2] This process and their close anatomic relationship with hepatocytes suggests that they are part of the local stem cell niche for hepatocytes.[17]

HEPATIC PROGENITOR CELLS

Hepatocytes are the cells that normally shoulder the burden of regeneration after liver damage. However, when loss of hepatocytes is massive (eg, in acute liver failure, characterized by massive necrosis of hepatocytes), or combined with inhibition of proliferative capacity of mature hepatocytes (eg, in cirrhosis caused by diverse etiologies), activation of a dormant compartment of intrahepatic progenitor cells occurs.[18–20] Therefore, it is not surprising that proliferation of these adult progenitor cells has been identified in a wide variety of human liver diseases, because they are all characterized by a certain degree of hepatocyte loss and damage, with impaired regeneration of remaining hepatocytes or bile duct epithelial cells.[18,19]

These cells, referred to as *hepatic progenitor cells* (HPCs), or *oval cells* in rodents, in the nondiseased human liver are located in the bile ductules and the Hering canals that are localized in the portal tract and the periportal parenchyma.[12,21] Because HPCs are hardly recognizable on routine histochemical stainings such as hematoxylin-eosin, immunohistochemistry or electron microscopy is required to detect these cells. HPCs are small epithelial cells (8–18 μm) with a relatively large oval nucleus and scanty cytoplasm, which is immunoreactive for rat oval cell marker OV-6, neural cell adhesion molecule (NCAM), CD133, and tumor-associated calcium signal transducer 1 (TACSTD1/epithelial cell adhesion molecule [EpCAM]).[21] HPCs also express markers of both biliary epithelial cells (keratin [K] 7, K19, K14) and hepatocytes lineages (K8, K18, C-met, albumin) and are able to differentiate into both cholangiocytes and hepatocytes, depending on the epithelial cell type that is damaged the most.[22]

When activated to proliferate/differentiate, HPCs form tortuous duct-like structures (pseudoducts), emanating from the portal zone and expanding into the parenchyma. Hepatocytic differentiation of these cells leads to the formation of intermediate hepatocytes (**Figs. 1–4**), which are polygonal cells with a size and phenotype intermediate between those of progenitor cells and mature hepatocytes.[12,23–25] Intermediate hepatocytes in very early stages of differentiation are positive for K19 and K7 in a submembranous pattern, but they lose immunoreactivity for K19 much earlier than for K7. Finally, the full maturation of intermediate hepatocytes into hepatocytes is characterized by disappearance of these biliary markers.

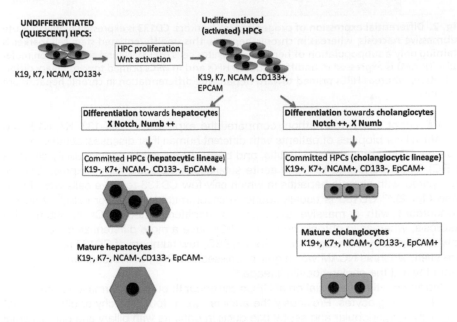

Fig. 1. Liver stem/progenitor cells can differentiate into hepatocytes and cholangiocytes, both during embryogenesis and regeneration after injury. After injury the differentiation of stem/progenitor cells depends on the site of injury: after hepatocytes loss, progenitor cells differentiate into hepatocytes; after bile duct loss, they form new cholangiocytes. Expansion of the stem/progenitor cells depend on Wnt pathway activation. Activation of the Notch pathway is necessary for biliary differentiation, whereas its inhibition/blockage induces hepatocyte differentiation. On the way to the differentiated cell type, intermediate cell types are formed.

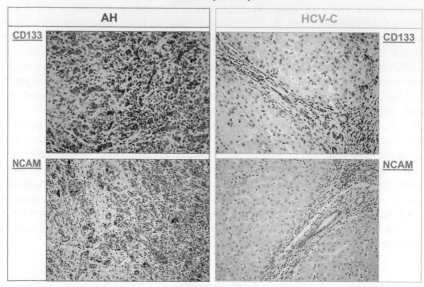

RESULTS: HPC markers

CD133 and NCAM are Up-regulated in Acute disease (AH) compared with chronic disease (HCV-C)

Fig. 2. Differential expression of progenitor cell markers. CD133 is expressed highly in acute submassive necrosis, whereas in chronic hepatitis, this undifferentiated stem cell marker is staining only a subpopulation of hepatic progenitor cells (HPCs). Neural cell adhesion molecule (NCAM) is expressed in undifferentiated HPCs and in HPCs primed toward biliary differentiation, whereas HPCs primed toward hepatocytic differentiation in chronic hepatitis are negative.

In a recent study, the authors compared the expression of CD133, K7, K19, and NCAM in liver biopsies of patients with different human liver diseases: acute submassive necrosis, chronic viral hepatitis, and biliary diseases like primary biliary cirrhosis (PBC). They found that HPCs in acute submassive necrosis highly express CD133, compared with chronic hepatitis in which only few CD133 reactive cells were found (see **Fig. 2**).[26] CD133 is usually found in uncommitted progenitor cells,[27] which is concordant with a massive expansion of undifferentiated HPCs in submassive necrosis, whereas in chronic hepatitis, HPCs have a more differentiated (committed toward hepatocytic lineage) state. Also in PBC, few numbers of CD133 reactive cells are seen, whereas NCAM was highly expressed in HPCs, concordant with a commitment toward the cholangiocytic lineage.[26]

Cholangiocytic differentiation of HPCs can occur through the formation of immature (small) cholangiocytes. Previously the authors' group found patchy or diffuse NCAM positivity in interlobular and septal bile ducts in patients with biliary and parenchymal cirrhosis, with a higher proportion of NCAM-positive bile ducts in biliary cirrhosis than in parenchymal (posthepatitic) cirrhosis.[28] The NCAM-positive biliary cells sometimes appeared smaller than the surrounding NCAM-negative biliary epithelial cells in the same bile duct.

Because in the liver NCAM is a marker of immature cells that are committed to the biliary lineage,[29] the patchy and diffuse presence of NCAM-positive biliary cells in septal and interlobular bile ducts in both biliary and parenchymal cirrhosis suggests

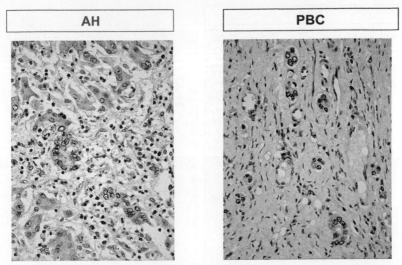

Fig. 3. Lymphoid enhancer binding factor 1 is part of the Wnt pathway and is expressed in the nucleus of activated hepatic progenitor cells.

that immature biliary cells may contribute to the repair of damaged bile ducts in chronic liver diseases. In this way, HPCs represent a dynamic cellular compartment that continuously changes its morphology and phenotype in relation to its differentiation state, which is why no universal HPC marker specific to this cell compartment has been identified.

Mechanisms of Hepatic Progenitor Cell Activation

The mechanisms controlling the behavior of human HPCs are not fully understood. Most current knowledge in this field was gained from animal models. A central role of inflammatory cytokines has been suggested in rodents.[30] In both acute and chronic human liver diseases, the extent of HPC activation correlates with the severity of liver disease.[31–34] Studies have also shown that the severity and localization of the inflammatory infiltrate in chronic viral hepatitis correlates with the activation and localization of HPCs.[33] These findings suggest that cytokines produced by the inflammatory infiltrate may function as a growth or chemotactic factor for HPCs to initiate the response; for instance, TNF-like weak inducer of apoptosis (TWEAK), a member of the proinflammatory TNF super family, plays an important role in HPC activation. In addition to the other members of the TNF super family, such as TNF-α and lymphotoxin, which play important roles in both HPC- and hepatocyte-mediated liver regeneration, TWEAK has shown effects only on progenitor cell compartment and not on the mature hepatocytes.[35] TWEAK, produced by monocytes and T cells, is up-regulated in various human liver diseases, and can stimulate HPC proliferation directly through its specific receptor Fn14.[35] Therefore, TWEAK is an important intercellular signal for inducing the hepatic HPC response.

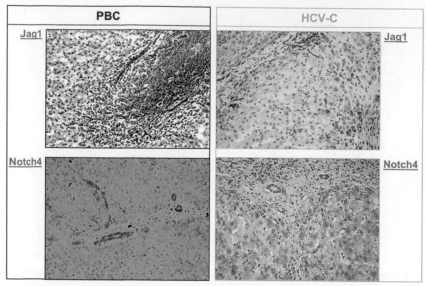

Fig. 4. Jagged1 and Notch2 and -4 are highly expressed in hepatic progenitor cells in biliary diseases, compared with hepatocytic diseases. Inhibition of the Notch pathway is necessary for hepatocyte differentiation.

Other elements of the inflammatory response that may stimulate oval cells include IL-6 family (leukemia inhibitory factor and oncostatin M), lymphotoxin–β, interferon gamma (IFN-γ), and TNF-α.[2,36–38] Another important chemokine is stromal cell–derived factor 1 (SDF-1), which is up-regulated during human chronic liver disease[39] and uniquely binds to the chemokine (C-X-C motif) receptor 4 (CXCR4) and plays various roles, including cell trafficking, proliferation, and organogenesis. CXCR4 is expressed by various progenitor cells, SDF-1 attracts CXCR4+ T cells, and these cells express TWEAK.[40]

Hedgehog (Hh) signaling, acting through the receptor Patched on oval cells/HPCs, is required for their survival.[41] Studies have recently shown that in patients with alcoholic steatohepatitis and primary biliary cirrhosis, HPCs and hepatic stellate cells, as a part of the HPC niche, are capable of both producing and responding to Hh ligands, which are required for optimal viability and growth of these cells.[42]

The study of other well-described stem cell niches in other organs (intestinal, hair follicle, and hematopoietic stem cell compartment) has indicated that Wnt and Notch signaling pathways are important for the regulation of stem cell proliferation and differentiation toward committed lineages.[43–46] Wnt and Notch signaling pathways have also been shown to play a key role during embryonic liver development.[47–53] Whether these signaling pathways also play a role during human adult diseases is hardly studied. Therefore, the authors recently used laser microdissection to generate gene expression profiles from microdissected K7-positive cells in different liver diseases: acute hepatitis, post–hepatitis C virus liver cirrhosis, and PBC. Immunohistochemistry and immunofluorescence were used to confirm the obtained gene expression profile (see **Figs. 1–4**).[26]

In acute hepatitis, activated HPCs predominantly proliferate rather than differentiate.[44,54,55] HPC activation plays a key role in the prognosis of this pathology, as indicated by Katoonizadeh et al.[34] Although HPCs massively proliferate in acute hepatitis, the differentiation toward hepatocytes occurs only after 1 week from the initial liver injury. This delay in differentiation then affects the outcome of the patients with acute hepatitis.[34] The Wnt pathway, which has a key role in stimulating stem cell proliferation,[56] was more pronounced in the authors' study in acute hepatitis compared with hepatitis C virus or PBC (see **Fig. 3**). The important role of the Wnt pathway in HPC activation/proliferation was described previously in several in vitro assays and in murine HPC proliferation models.[57–60] The similar activation of Wnt in human acute hepatitis and murine models underlines the importance of this pathway in human liver diseases.

In the hematopoietic, intestinal, and neuronal stem cell niche, the modulation of Notch activity is fundamental in influencing the fate of progenitor cells.[56] The role of the Notch pathway in bile duct development first became apparent in the Alagille syndrome, in which mutations in the Jagged1 gene (*JAG1*) were identified as the cause of the Alagille syndrome, causing bile duct paucity. In general, Notch 2 is responsible for the morphogenesis of bile duct structures.[47] Notch1 and -3 play an important role in biliary differentiation and maintenance in murine models.[61] The authors' recent study[26] measured lower *JAG1* encoding mRNA in hepatocytic diseases (hepatitis C virus and acute hepatitis) than in PBC. This finding could therefore be related to commitment towards the hepatocytic lineage. The increased values of *JAG1* in PBC could be linked with fate choice towards cholangiocytes, which is in agreement with the observation that immature and mature cholangiocytes express members of the Notch pathway in vivo.[62] In rodent models, Notch was found to play an important role in biliary differentiation of HPCs in a model of biliary ductopenia.[47,49,63] The authors' data show that Notch plays a similar role in biliary differentiation of human HPCs (see **Fig. 4**).[26] In most conditions, the Notch signal requires physical contact between cells.[64] The observation that desmin- and Notch1-positive myofibroblasts are mostly present around HPCs in PBC indicates that these cells might be responsible for the (Notch) cell–cell communication between progenitor cells and mesenchymal cells regulating their bipotential cell fate.

Controlled manipulation of the HPC niche holds great promise for therapeutic intervention in currently untreatable liver diseases.[65–67] Although some of these treatments (such as γ-secretase inhibitors) mostly rely on Wnt or Notch inhibition in neoplastic diseases,[68] these treatments might be used to stimulate the patients' own progenitor cell compartment.

POSSIBLE ROLE OF PROGENITOR CELLS IN CARCINOGENESIS

In adult life, the two major primary liver cancers are hepatocellular carcinoma (HCC) and cholangiocellular carcinoma (CC). Mixed forms of HCC and CC are also described. When more detailed immunohistochemical phenotyping is performed, a whole range of phenotypical traits of hepatocytes, cholangiocytes, and progenitor cells can be seen in tumors, which is consistent with a progenitor cell origin (**Figs. 5** and **6**).[69]

In humans, chronic viral hepatitis B and C, alcoholic and non–alcoholic steatohepatitis, metabolic diseases, and mutagens such as aflatoxins (toxic metabolites of the food mould *Aspergillus* sp) are the most important risk factors for the development of HCC. Chronic inflammatory biliary diseases, such as primary sclerosing cholangitis, hepatolithiasis (gall stones), and liver fluke infection by *Opisthorchis viverrini* and *Clonorchis sinensis*, are known risk factors for the development of

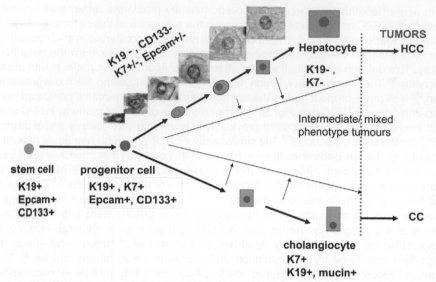

Fig. 5. Hepatic progenitor cells can differentiate into cholangiocytes and hepatocytes through intermediate cell types. Each of these intermediate cell types can become a cancer stem cell according to the maturation arrest theory. This finding explains the huge diversity of phenotypes within a tumor. A whole range of phenotypes with traits of progenitor cells, hepatocytes, and cholangiocytes can be formed. Furthermore, mature hepatocyte or cholangiocytes can act as cancer stem cells, because these cells also have stem cell properties. They then form mature hepatocellular carcinomas or cholangiocellular carcinomas.

cholangiocarcinomas, underscoring that oxidative stress and chronic inflammation are common carcinogenic risk factors in all primary liver cancers.

As in rodents, HCC and CC evolve from focal precursor lesions that reflect the stages of multistep carcinogenesis.[70,71]

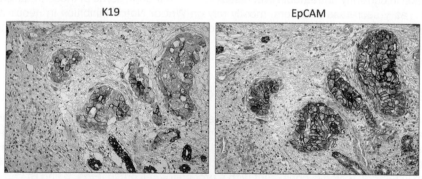

Fig. 6. Hepatocellular carcinoma with progenitor cell features expressing keratin (K) 19 and epithelial cell adhesion molecule (EpCAM). K19 and EpCAM stain showing invasive strands of a hepatocellular carcinoma with small undifferentiated progenitor cells and a range of intermediate phenotypes in between hepatocytes and progenitor/biliary cells. Several studies show that a cutoff of 5% of cytokeratin 19–reactive cells already influences the outcome of the patient. These hepatocellular carcinomas with progenitor cell features have faster and greater incidence of recurrence of disease after surgical treatment.

Because progenitor cells are activated in most chronic liver diseases, which are known risk factors for the development of hepatocellular carcinoma and CC, progenitor cells are potential target cells for carcinogenesis.

Most tumors show still phenotypical features of their cell of origin, and the histopathologic classification of tumors is largely based on these features. Several studies using detailed immunophenotyping of HCCs showed that a substantial number (approximately 15%) of human HCCs express markers of progenitor/biliary cells such as cytokeratins 7 and 19, and OV6 (see **Fig. 6**).[72-76]

Morphologically, these tumors consist of cells with a very immature phenotype, and a range of cells with intermediate phenotypes in between progenitor cells and hepatocytes. In particular, expression in HCC of K19, a marker for intrahepatic bile duct cells, activated hepatic progenitor cells, and hepatoblasts (see **Fig. 6**), has been associated with a worse prognosis and faster and greater incidence of recurrence after surgical treatment.[69,73,77-83] Up-regulation of KRT19 has been reported in several subclasses of HCCs that have already been linked to poor prognosis or progenitor cell phenotype (see **Fig. 6**).[84-86]

Integrated gene expression data from rat fetal hepatoblasts and adult hepatocytes, with HCC from human and mouse models, identified a novel group of HCCs, called the *hepatoblast* subtype, suggesting a progenitor cell origin.[86] A distinct signature based on the expression of EpCAM (also known as TACSTD1 or TROP1), a biliary/hepatic progenitor cell marker, combined with elevated α-fetoprotein serum levels, has been described as a novel subtype of HCCs with an increased tumor-initiating capacity.[87,88]

According to the cancer stem cell concept, HCC consists of a hierarchy of cell populations, of which the very small cancer stem cell population is the one that has the growth and metastatic potential of the tumor. The other neoplastic cells are offspring of the cancer stem cells and each can differentiate a little differently, according to the local microenvironment in each part of the tumor, hence explaining the enormous phenotypic heterogeneity of a neoplasm (see **Fig. 5**).

Current therapeutic strategies mostly target rapidly growing differentiated tumor cells, using drugs like sorafenib, erlotinib, and bevacizumab.[89] However, the results are often unsatisfactory because of the chemoresistance of HCC. New therapies targeting cancer stem cells should therefore be developed. A prerequisite is a good understanding of the mechanisms of activation and differentiation of normal stem/progenitor cells in normal and diseased liver. Hepatocytes and cholangiocytes have stem cell features, but also progenitor cells, located in the smallest branches of the biliary tree. These cells are especially activated in the cirrhotic stage of chronic liver diseases, the stage in which HCC develops. HCC with progenitor cell features, possibly reflecting a progenitor cell origin, have a very bad prognosis and therefore should be recognized and treated accordingly.

The identification of liver cancer stem cell markers and their related pathways is one of the most important goals of liver cancer research. Understanding the mechanisms of activation and differentiation of non–neoplastic stem/progenitor cells, and especially the differences with their malignant counterparts, should therefore be a top priority. New therapies should ideally target cancer stem cells and not normal stem/progenitor cells, because these are very important in regeneration and repair mechanisms.

SUMMARY

Liver progenitor cells are activated in most human liver diseases. The dynamics, and therefore subpopulations, of progenitor cells are, however, different in acute versus chronic hepatocytic diseases and in biliary diseases (see **Fig. 3**). The role of Wnt and Notch signaling pathways in activation and differentiation of human HPCs holds great promise because they can be manipulated by drugs. Hepatocytic differentiation requires inhibition of Notch (numb switched on), whereas cholangiocytic differentiation requires Notch activation. In this way, the patients' own regenerative response could be supported, which could eventually even avoid the need for transplantation in several patients.

The role of progenitor cells in carcinogenesis is being increasingly accepted. Because these cells can therefore function as cancer stem cells, they should form a target for future treatment strategies.

REFERENCES

1. Taub R. Liver regeneration: from myth to mechanism. Nat Rev Mol Cell Biol 2004; 5(10):836–47.
2. Fausto N, Campbell JS, Riehle KJ. Liver regeneration. Hepatology 2006;43(2 Suppl 1):S45–53.
3. Sell S. The role of progenitor cells in repair of liver injury and in liver transplantation. Wound Repair Regen 2001;9(6):467–82.
4. Alison M. Liver stem cells: a two compartment system. Curr Opin Cell Biol 1998; 10(6):710–5.
5. Alison M, Golding M, Lalani el-N, et al. Wound healing in the liver with particular reference to stem cells. Philos Trans R Soc Lond B Biol Sci 1998;353(1370): 877–94.
6. Watt FM, Hogan BL. Out of Eden: stem cells and their niches. Science 2000; 287(5457):1427–30.
7. Alison M, Sarraf C. Hepatic stem cells. J Hepatol 1998;29:676–82.
8. Hall PA. What are stem cells and how are they controlled? J Pathol 1989;158: 275–7.
9. Kuwahara R, Kofman AV, Landis CS, et al. The hepatic stem cell niche: identification by label-retaining cell assay. Hepatology 2008;47(6):1994–2002.
10. Theise ND, Kuwahara R. The tissue biology of ductular reactions in human chronic liver disease. Gastroenterology 2007;133(1):350–2.
11. Roskams TA, Libbrecht L, Desmet VJ. Progenitor cells in diseased human liver. Semin Liver Dis 2003;23(4):385–96.
12. Roskams TA, Theise ND, Balabaud C, et al. Nomenclature of the finer branches of the biliary tree: canals, ductules, and ductular reactions in human livers. Hepatology 2004;39(6):1739–45.
13. Yang L, Jung Y, Omenetti A, et al. Fate-mapping evidence that hepatic stellate cells are epithelial progenitors in adult mouse livers. Stem Cells 2008;26(8): 2104–13.
14. Fausto N. Liver regeneration and repair: hepatocytes, progenitor cells, and stem cells. Hepatology 2004;39(6):1477–87.
15. Overturf K, Al-Dhalimy M, Finegold M, et al. The repopulation potential of hepatocyte populations differing in size and prior mitotic expansion. Am J Pathol 1999;155(6):2135–43.
16. Overturf K, Al-Dhalimy M, Manning K, et al. Ex vivo hepatic gene therapy of a mouse model of Hereditary Tyrosinemia Type I. Hum Gene Ther 1998;9(3): 295–304.
17. Roskams T. Relationships among stellate cell activation, progenitor cells, and hepatic regeneration. Clin Liver Dis 2008;12(4):853–60, ix.

18. Roskams T. Different types of liver progenitor cells and their niches. J Hepatol 2006;45(1):1–4.
19. Roskams T. Progenitor cell involvement in cirrhotic human liver diseases: from controversy to consensus. J Hepatol 2003;39(3):431–4.
20. Theise ND, Saxena R, Portmann BC, et al. The canals of Hering and hepatic stem cells in humans. Hepatology 1999;30(6):1425–33.
21. Bird TG, Lorenzini S, Forbes SJ. Activation of stem cells in hepatic diseases. Cell Tissue Res 2008;331(1):283–300.
22. Xiao JC, Ruck P, Adam A, et al. Small epithelial cells in human liver cirrhosis exhibit features of hepatic stem–like cells: immunohistochemical, electron microscopic and immunoelectron microscopic findings. Histopathology 2003;42(2): 141–9.
23. Falkowski O, An HJ, Ianus IA, et al. Regeneration of hepatocyte 'buds' in cirrhosis from intrabiliary stem cells. J Hepatol 2003;39(3):357–64.
24. Fujita M, Furukawa H, Hattori M, et al. Sequential observation of liver cell regeneration after massive hepatic necrosis in auxiliary partial orthotopic liver transplantation. Mod Pathol 2000;13:152–7.
25. Demetris A, Seaberg EC, Wennerberg A, et al. Ductular reaction after submassive necrosis in humans. Special emphasis on analysis of ductular hepatocytes. Am J Pathol 1996;149:439–48.
26. Spee B, Carpino G, Schotanus BA, et al. Characterisation of the activated liver progenitor cell niche, potential involvement of Wnt and Notch signalling. Gut 2009;59(2):247–57.
27. Yovchev MI, Grozdanov PN, Joseph B, et al. Novel hepatic progenitor cell surface markers in the adult rat liver. Hepatology 2007;45(1):139–49.
28. Libbrecht L, Cassiman D, Desmet V, et al. Expression of neural cell adhesion molecule in human liver development and in congenital and acquired liver diseases. Histochem Cell Biol 2001;116(3):233–9.
29. Fabris L, Strazzabosco M, Crosby HA, et al. Characterization and isolation of ductular cells coexpressing neural cell adhesion molecule and Bcl-2 from primary cholangiopathies and ductal plate malformations. Am J Pathol 2000; 156(5):1599–612.
30. Knight B, Matthews VB, Akhurst B, et al. Liver inflammation and cytokine production, but not acute phase protein synthesis, accompany the adult liver progenitor (oval) cell response to chronic liver injury. Immunol Cell Biol 2005;83(4):364–74.
31. Roskams T, Desmet V. Ductular reaction and its diagnostic significance. Semin Diagn Pathol 1998;15(4):259–69.
32. Lowes KN, Brennan BA, Yeoh GC, et al. Oval cell numbers in human chronic liver diseases are directly related to disease severity. Am J Pathol 1999;154(2):537–41.
33. Libbrecht L, Desmet V, Van Damme B, et al. Deep intralobular extension of human hepatic 'progenitor cells' correlates with parenchymal inflammation in chronic viral hepatitis: can 'progenitor cells' migrate? J Pathol 2000;192(3):373–8.
34. Katoonizadeh A, Nevens F, Verslype C, et al. Liver regeneration in acute severe liver impairment: a clinicopathological correlation study. Liver Int 2006;26(10): 1225–33.
35. Jakubowski A, Ambrose C, Parr M, et al. TWEAK induces liver progenitor cell proliferation. J Clin Invest 2005;115(9):2330–40.
36. Streetz KL, Wüstefeld T, Klein C, et al. Lack of gp130 expression in hepatocytes promotes liver injury. Gastroenterology 2003;125(2):532–43.
37. Streetz KL, Tacke F, Leifeld L, et al. Interleukin 6/gp130–dependent pathways are protective during chronic liver diseases. Hepatology 2003;38(1):218–29.

38. Znoyko I, Sohara N, Spicer SS, et al. Expression of oncostatin M and its receptors in normal and cirrhotic human liver. J Hepatol 2005;43(5):893–900.
39. Terada R, Yamamoto K, Hakoda T, et al. Stromal cell–derived factor-1 from biliary epithelial cells recruits CXCR4–positive cells: implications for inflammatory liver diseases. Lab Invest 2003;83(5):665–72.
40. Hatch HM, Zheng D, Jorgensen ML, et al. SDF-1alpha/CXCR4: a mechanism for hepatic oval cell activation and bone marrow stem cell recruitment to the injured liver of rats. Cloning Stem Cells 2002;4(4):339–51.
41. Sicklick JK, Li YX, Melhem A, et al. Hedgehog signaling maintains resident hepatic progenitors throughout life. Am J Physiol Gastrointest Liver Physiol 2006;290(5): G859–70.
42. Jung Y, McCall SJ, Li YX, et al. Bile ductules and stromal cells express hedgehog ligands and/or hedgehog target genes in primary biliary cirrhosis. Hepatology 2007;45(5):1091–6.
43. Barker N, van de Wetering M, Clevers H. The intestinal stem cell. Genes Dev 2008;22(14):1856–64.
44. Moore KA, Lemischka IR. Stem cells and their niches. Science 2006;311(5769): 1880–5.
45. Scoville DH, Sato T, He XC, et al. Current view: intestinal stem cells and signaling. Gastroenterology 2008;134(3):849–64.
46. Waters JM, Richardson GD, Jahoda CA. Hair follicle stem cells. Semin Cell Dev Biol 2007;18(2):245–54.
47. Geisler F, Nagl F, Mazur PK, et al. Liver-specific inactivation of Notch2, but not Notch1, compromises intrahepatic bile duct development in mice. Hepatology 2008;48(2):607–16.
48. Kodama Y, Hijikata M, Kageyama R, et al. The role of notch signaling in the development of intrahepatic bile ducts. Gastroenterology 2004;127(6):1775–86.
49. Lozier J, McCright B, Gridley T. Notch signaling regulates bile duct morphogenesis in mice. PLoS One 2008;3(3):e1851.
50. Micsenyi A, Tan X, Sneddon T, et al. Beta-catenin is temporally regulated during normal liver development. Gastroenterology 2004;126(4):1134–46.
51. Ober EA, Verkade H, Field HA, et al. Mesodermal Wnt2b signalling positively regulates liver specification. Nature 2006;442(7103):688–91.
52. Thompson MD, Monga SP. Wnt/beta-catenin signaling in liver health and disease. Hepatology 2007;45(5):1298–305.
53. Flynn DM, Nijjar S, Hubscher SG, et al. The role of Notch receptor expression in bile duct development and disease. J Pathol 2004;204(1):55–64.
54. Zhang L, Theise N, Chua M, et al. The stem cell niche of human livers: symmetry between development and regeneration. Hepatology 2008;48(5):1598–607.
55. Naveiras O, Daley GQ. Stem cells and their niche: a matter of fate. Cell Mol Life Sci 2006;63(7–8):760–6.
56. Crosnier C, Stamataki D, Lewis J. Organizing cell renewal in the intestine: stem cells, signals and combinatorial control. Nat Rev Genet 2006;7(5):349–59.
57. Apte U, Thompson MD, Cui S, et al. Wnt/beta-catenin signaling mediates oval cell response in rodents. Hepatology 2008;47(1):288–95.
58. Hu M, Kurobe M, Jeong YJ, et al. Wnt/beta-catenin signaling in murine hepatic transit amplifying progenitor cells. Gastroenterology 2007;133(5):1579–91.
59. Yang W, Yan HX, Chen L, et al. Wnt/beta-catenin signaling contributes to activation of normal and tumorigenic liver progenitor cells. Cancer Res 2008;68(11): 4287–95.

60. Zhang Y, Li XM, Zhang FK, et al. Activation of canonical Wnt signaling pathway promotes proliferation and self-renewal of rat hepatic oval cell line WB-F344 in vitro. World J Gastroenterol 2008;14(43):6673–80.
61. Jensen CH, Jauho EI, Santoni-Rugiu E, et al. Transit-amplifying ductular (oval) cells and their hepatocytic progeny are characterized by a novel and distinctive expression of delta-like protein/preadipocyte factor 1/fetal antigen 1. Am J Pathol 2004;164(4):1347–59.
62. Nijjar SS, Wallace L, Crosby HA, et al. Altered Notch ligand expression in human liver disease: further evidence for a role of the Notch signaling pathway in hepatic neovascularization and biliary ductular defects. Am J Pathol 2002;160(5):1695–703.
63. McCright B, Lozier J, Gridley T. A mouse model of Alagille syndrome: Notch2 as a genetic modifier of Jag1 haploinsufficiency. Development 2002;129(4):1075–82.
64. Fortini ME. Notch signaling: the core pathway and its posttranslational regulation. Dev Cell 2009;16(5):633–47.
65. Alison MR, Choong C, Lim S. Application of liver stem cells for cell therapy. Semin Cell Dev Biol 2007;18(6):819–26.
66. Prockop DJ, Olson SD. Clinical trials with adult stem/progenitor cells for tissue repair: let's not overlook some essential precautions. Blood 2007;109(8):3147–51.
67. Shafritz DA, Oertel M, Menthena A, et al. Liver stem cells and prospects for liver reconstitution by transplanted cells. Hepatology 2006;43(2 Suppl 1):S89–98.
68. van Es JH, Clevers H. Notch and Wnt inhibitors as potential new drugs for intestinal neoplastic disease. Trends Mol Med 2005;11(11):496–502.
69. Roskams T. Liver stem cells and their implication in hepatocellular and cholangiocarcinoma. Oncogene 2006;25(27):3818–22.
70. Libbrecht L, Desmet V, Roskams T. Preneoplastic lesions in human hepatocarcinogenesis. Liver Int 2005;25(1):16–27.
71. Roskams T, Kojiro M. Pathology of early hepatocellular carcinoma: conventional and molecular diagnosis. Semin Liver Dis 2010;30(1):17–25.
72. Hsia CC, Evarts RP, Nakatsukasa H, et al. Occurrence of oval-type cells in hepatitis B virus–associated human hepatocarcinogenesis. Hepatology 1992;16(6):1327–33.
73. Uenishi T, Kubo S, Yamamoto T, et al. Cytokeratin 19 expression in hepatocellular carcinoma predicts early postoperative recurrence. Cancer Sci 2003;94(10):851–7.
74. Van Eyken P, Sciot R, Paterson A, et al. Cytokeratin expression in hepatocellular carcinoma: an immunohistochemical study. Hum Pathol 1988;19:562–8.
75. Yoon DS, Jeong J, Park YN, et al. Expression of biliary antigen and its clinical significance in hepatocellular carcinoma. Yonsei Med J 1999;40(5):472–7.
76. Wu PC, Lai VC, Fang JW, et al. Hepatocellular carcinoma expressing both hepatocellular and biliary markers also expresses cytokeratin 14, a marker of bipotential progenitor cells. J Hepatol 1999;31(5):965–6.
77. Roskams T, Desmet V. Embryology of extra- and intrahepatic bile ducts, the ductal plate. Anat Rec (Hoboken) 2008;291(6):628–35.
78. Durnez A, Verslype C, Nevens F, et al. The clinicopathological and prognostic relevance of cytokeratin 7 and 19 expression in hepatocellular carcinoma. A possible progenitor cell origin. Histopathology 2006;49(2):138–51.
79. Zhuang PY, Zhang JB, Zhu XD, et al. Two pathologic types of hepatocellular carcinoma with lymph node metastasis with distinct prognosis on the basis of CK19 expression in tumor. Cancer 2008;112(12):2740–8.

80. Yang XR, Xu Y, Shi GM, et al. Cytokeratin 10 and cytokeratin 19: predictive markers for poor prognosis in hepatocellular carcinoma patients after curative resection. Clin Cancer Res 2008;14(12):3850–9.
81. Ding SJ, Li Y, Tan YX, et al. From proteomic analysis to clinical significance: over-expression of cytokeratin 19 correlates with hepatocellular carcinoma metastasis. Mol Cell Proteomics 2004;3(1):73–81.
82. Wee A. Diagnostic utility of immunohistochemistry in hepatocellular carcinoma, its variants and their mimics. Appl Immunohistochem Mol Morphol 2006;14(3):266–72.
83. Aishima S, Nishihara Y, Kuroda Y, et al. Histologic characteristics and prognostic significance in small hepatocellular carcinoma with biliary differentiation: subdivision and comparison with ordinary hepatocellular carcinoma. Am J Surg Pathol 2007;31(5):783–91.
84. Lee JS, Chu IS, Heo J, et al. Classification and prediction of survival in hepatocellular carcinoma by gene expression profiling. Hepatology 2004;40(3):667–76.
85. Hoshida Y, Nijman SM, Kobayashi M, et al. Integrative transcriptome analysis reveals common molecular subclasses of human hepatocellular carcinoma. Cancer Res 2009;69(18):7385–92.
86. Lee JS, Heo J, Libbrecht L, et al. A novel prognostic subtype of human hepatocellular carcinoma derived from hepatic progenitor cells. Nat Med 2006;12(4):410–6.
87. Yamashita T, Forgues M, Wang W, et al. EpCAM and alpha-fetoprotein expression defines novel prognostic subtypes of hepatocellular carcinoma. Cancer Res 2008;68(5):1451–61.
88. Yamashita T, Ji J, Budhu A, et al. EpCAM-positive hepatocellular carcinoma cells are tumor-initiating cells with stem/progenitor cell features. Gastroenterology 2009;136(3):1012–24.
89. Siegel A. Moving targets in hepatocellular carcinoma: hepatic progenitor cells as novel targets for tyrosine kinase inhibitors. Gastroenterology 2008;135(3):733–5.

Benign Liver Tumors: An update

Valérie Paradis, MD, PhD[a,b]

KEYWORDS

- Hepatocellular adenoma • Focal nodular hyperplasia
- Hepatocellular carcinoma

One of the consequences of extensive use of abdominal imaging, and especially liver ultrasonography, is the detection of asymptomatic liver tumors. In the absence of underlying chronic liver disease, the vast majority of these lesions correspond to benign liver tumors including solid and cystic lesions. Solid benign lesions encompass a broad spectrum of regenerative and true neoplastic processes, arising from either epithelial or nonepithelial cells of the liver. Epithelial lesions include hepatocellular (focal nodular hyperplasias [FNHs] and hepatocellular adenomas [HCAs]) and biliary tumors (biliary adenomas). Among the nonepithelial tumors, hemangiomas are the most common.

The vast majority of solid benign liver lesions, including the most frequent, such as hemangioma and FNH, remain asymptomatic, do not increase in volume, and therefore do not require any treatment or follow-up. By contrast, HCAs may be associated with serious complications justifying surgical resection in most cases. The knowledge of the molecular mechanisms underlying the pathogenesis of each lesion may contribute to their accurate diagnosis but also indicate their potential behavior, to propose the appropriate management. In recent years, especially thanks to combined genotypic and phenotypic molecular approaches, significant advances have been performed in the characterization of HCAs, showing a great heterogeneity of these tumors associated with specific morphologic, phenotypical, and evolutive features. Therefore, diagnosis of benign hepatocellular tumors is becoming a multidisciplinary approach based on clinics, imaging, and pathomolecular analysis. This article is dedicated to hepatocellular tumors and also addresses hemangiomas as the most common benign liver tumors, and angiomyolipomas as a rare tumor often misdiagnosed.

HEPATOCELLULAR TUMORS
Focal Nodular Hyperplasias

FNH accounts for the second most common benign liver process, following hemangioma. It is a benign, tumorlike condition predominantly diagnosed in women of 30

a Pathology Department, Beaujon Hospital, 100 bd du Général Leclerc, 92118 Clichy Cedex, France
b INSERM U773, CRB3 Bichat-Beaujon, 100 bd du Général Leclerc, 92118 Clichy Cedex, Paris, France
E-mail address: vparadis@teaser.fr

Clin Liver Dis 14 (2010) 719–729
doi:10.1016/j.cld.2010.07.008
1089-3261/10/$ – see front matter © 2010 Elsevier Inc. All rights reserved.
liver.theclinics.com

to 50 years of age, noninfluenced by oral contraceptives.[1-3] FNH is considered as a hyperplastic reaction resulting from arterial malformation.[4] This hypothesis, suggesting that increased arterial flow hyperperfuses the local liver parenchyma leading to secondary hepatocellular hyperplasia, has been reinforced by molecular data showing that FNHs are polyclonal regenerative processes.[5,6] This regenerative process induced in a specific vascular territory could explain the absence of significant changes in size over time. The vast majority of FNHs are asymptomatic and are discovered incidentally during liver ultrasound examination. In addition, complications of FNH, such as rupture or bleeding, are exceptional, and no evidence of malignant transformation has been reported so far.

FNH displays a typical morphologic pattern for both radiologists and pathologists. Grossly, FNH is a well-circumscribed, unencapsulated, usually solitary mass, characterized by a central fibrous scar that radiates into the liver parenchyma (**Fig. 1**A). Histologically, FNH is composed of benign-appearing hepatocytes arranged in nodules that are partly or completely delineated by fibrous septa originating from the central scar. In the fibrous septa, large and dystrophic vessels are observed, associated with ductular proliferation and inflammatory cells in varied intensity (see **Fig. 1**B, C). The hepatocytes are hyperplastic, arranged in liver plates of normal or slightly increased thickness with a well-preserved reticulin framework. Hepatocytes may be hydropic, related to cholestatic changes. Presence of steatosis inside the lesion may be observed.

Besides this typical form of FNH, several variant lesions are described with increased frequency, and commonly classified as "atypical FNH" by radiologists.

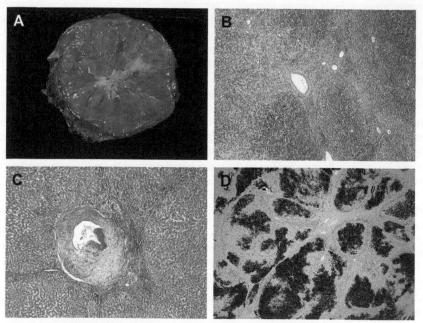

Fig. 1. Focal nodular hyperplasia. (*A*) Macroscopic view showing a well-limited lesion of nodular appearance containing a central fibrous scar. (*B*) Histologically, hepatocellular nodules are delineated by fibrous septa (trichrome, original magnification ×100). (*C*) A large dystrophic vessel inside the central scar (H&E, original magnification ×200). (*D*) Glutamine synthetase immunostaining revealing focal hepatocellular positivity ("maplike pattern," original magnification ×25).

This group is somehow heterogeneous, including mainly FNHs without central fibrous scar, FNH with prominent steatosis, or lesions displaying telangiectatic changes or with adenomatous features.[7] On histologic examination, FNH without macroscopic central fibrous scar exhibits all the pathologic elementary features of classic FNH, with few, thin and short fibrous septa. Importantly, pathologic diagnosis of FNH, even typical, may be difficult on biopsy specimen where thick abnormal arteries are usually missing.[8] In addition to the presence of ductular reaction at the border between fibrous septa and hepatocellular component, immunostaining with glutamine synthetase showing focal positive hepatocellular areas usually centered by hepatic veins, described as a maplike pattern, is highly consistent with the diagnosis of FNH (see **Fig. 1**D).[8,9] Interestingly, molecular studies demonstrated that in this group of "atypical FNHs," lesions displaying telangiectatic changes and initially so-called "telangiectatic form of FNH" are clonal processes and should be rather regarded as variant form of HCA than FNH.[10–12] Since then, their specific characteristics have been further well described in terms of clinics, imaging, and genotyping. Pathologic features of this entity will be detailed in the section "hepatocellular adenomas."

Given that FNHs are regenerative lesions with exceptional occurrence of complications, no treatment for asymptomatic FNH is required, whatever the size and the number of lesions, when the diagnosis is firmly established. Finally, surgical resection is indicated in doubtful cases or in symptomatic cases, such as a large FNH located in the left liver and pedunculated lesions.

Hepatocellular Adenomas

HCA is a rare, benign liver neoplasm strongly associated with oral contraceptive (OC) use and androgen steroid therapy.[13,14] Its incidence is estimated to be 0.1 per year per 100,000 in non-OC users, and reaches 3 to 4 per 100,000 in long-tem OC users.[15] HCA can also occur spontaneously or be associated with underlying metabolic diseases, including type 1 glycogen storage disease, iron overload related to betathalassemia, and diabetes mellitus.[16] HCAs are usually solitary, sometimes pedunculated, with a diameter that can reach 30 cm. Large subcapsular vessels are commonly found on macroscopic examination. On cut sections, the tumor is well delineated, sometimes encapsulated, of fleshy appearance, and ranging in color from white to brown. Heterogeneous areas of necrosis and/or hemorrhage may be observed, preferentially in tumors of large size. Histologically, HCA consists of a proliferation of benign hepatocytes arranged in a trabecular pattern, without any residual portal tracts. Small thin and unpaired vessels are usually found throughout the tumor (**Fig. 2**). Hepatocytes may have intracellular fat or increased glycogen. A certain degree of cellular atypias can be detected, especially in patients who have taken steroids for many years. In that context, differential diagnosis with hepatocellular carcinoma (HCC) may be difficult.

Compared with FNH, patients with HCA are more likely to present with symptoms, especially if they have large tumors. HCA is of clinical importance because of its potential serious complications. Among them, spontaneous bleeding and hemorrhage concern 20% to 40% of patients, with an increased risk for tumors larger than 5 cm in diameter.[17,18] About 10% of patients present acutely with severe abdominal pain attributable to intra-peritoneal rupture and hemoperitoneum, which may be associated with hypovolemic shock. The risk for malignant transformation of HCA ranges between 4% and 10%.[16,18,19] Recent studies confirmed that this risk is higher in males and in patients with large HCAs.[18] It also recently appears that metabolic syndrome, the incidence of which is increasing worldwide, may favor development of HCC in

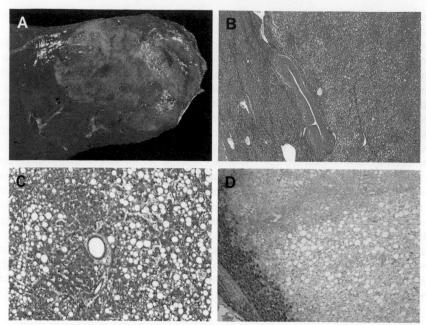

Fig. 2. Steatotic LFABP-negative hepatocellular adenoma (HNF1α-inactivated). (*A*) Macroscopic view showing a large yellowish unencapsulated tumor developing on a normal liver. (*B*) Steatotic hepatocellular adenoma is well-limited, unencapsulated (H&E, original magnification ×25). (*C*) Well-differentiated hepatocellular proliferation with prominent steatosis (note the small unpaired artery inside the tumor, H&E, original magnification ×200). (*D*) LFABP immunostaining demonstrating absence of labeling in the tumor compared with the positive staining of the surrounding normal hepatocytes (H&E, original magnification ×100).

a preexisting HCA.[20] In most cases, HCC is restricted to the HCA and discovered on the analysis of the surgical specimen.[16,18]

By contrast to FNH, and because of the potential risk for complications, surgical resection is required for HCAs larger than 5 cm in diameter and all HCAs in males whatever their size. Small lesions with a low risk of complication could be initially observed after cessation of OC. Importantly, long-term follow-up of patients with unresected HCA showed a relative stability for most of them and even a significant regression in a small proportion of cases after interruption of OC.[18,19]

Pathomolecular classification of hepatocellular adenomas

Molecular comprehensive studies have recently gained further insights into the knowledge of HCA showing a great heterogeneity in that group of tumors, resulting in the description of 3 main subtypes associated with specific phenotypical and molecular features.[21] Thus, based on morphologic and molecular characteristics, one initially recognized the hepatocyte nuclear factor 1α (HNF1α)-mutated steatotic, the telangiectatic/inflammatory (Tel/Infl), and the β-catenin-mutated HCA. Finally, a small group of HCAs remain "unclassified," because they do not display any specific morphologic or genotypical features.

The first group of HCAs displays biallelic mutations of the *TCF1* gene inactivating the HNF1α transcription factor, and is phenotypically characterized by marked steatosis, absence of cytologic abnormalities, and inflammatory infiltrates (see **Fig. 2**C).[21,22] Whereas, HNF1α mutations are somatic in most cases of these HCAs, patients with inherited mutation in one allele of HNF1α may develop maturity-onset diabetes of the young type 3 (MODY3) and are predisposed to have familial liver adenomatosis, classically defined by the presence of at least 10 HCAs, when the second allele is inactivated in hepatocytes by somatic mutation or chromosome deletion.[23,24] The second group of HCAs displays β-catenin-activating mutations and is characterized by increased risk for malignant transformation into HCC. These HCAs are mostly encountered in male patients and frequently show significant cell atypias and pseudo-glandular formations on hematoxylin and eosin (H&E) staining (**Fig. 3**). The third group of HCAs corresponds mainly to the initially called "telangiectatic form of FNH," appearing as well-delineated, unencapsulated tumors showing significant areas of vascular changes, without any fibrous scar (**Fig. 4**A).[10] Histologically, the hepatocellular proliferation contains few and short fibrous septa around clusters of small vessels, sometimes accompanied by inflammatory infiltrates (mainly composed of lymphocytes and macrophages) and a relatively low ductular reaction (see **Fig. 4**B). In addition, foci of sinusoidal dilation and peliotic changes are usually present (see **Fig. 4**C). Notably, significant steatosis may be observed inside and outside the lesion, with various degrees of intensity.[25] Although commonly observed in women using OP contraception for OC use, Tel/Infl HCA are reported in patients with increased body mass index and are associated with inflammatory syndrome (increased C reactive protein [CRP] or fibrinogen serum levels).[25] Interestingly, in approximately 60% of Tel/Inf HCAs, interleukin (IL)-6 signaling pathway has been shown to be activated in relation to mutations in the *IL6ST* gene that encodes the signaling coreceptor gp130. As a matter of fact, the

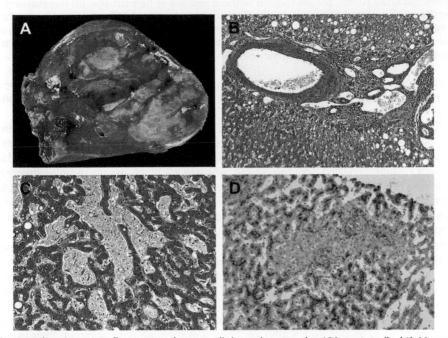

Fig. 3. Telangiectatic/Inflammatory hepatocellular adenoma (gp130-mutated). (*A*) Macroscopic view showing an 8-cm well-limited tumor, heterogeneous with extensive vascular changes without fibrous scar. (*B*) Hepatocellular proliferation containing clusters of vessels surrounding by extracellular matrix (H&E, original magnification ×100). (*C*) Foci of vascular dilatation inside the tumor (H&E, original magnification ×200). (*D*) SAA immunostaining showing cytoplasmic positivity of the tumoral hepatocytes (original magnification ×200).

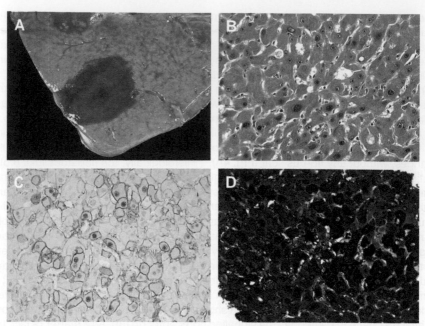

Fig. 4. β-catenin-mutated hepatocellular adenoma. (*A*) Macroscopic view showing a 2-cm unencapsulated tumor, brown-colored without necrosis or hemorrhage. (*B*) Hepatocellular proliferation with cell atypias and pseudoglandular formations (H&E, original magnification ×400). (*C*) β-catenin immunostaining showing aberrant nuclear and cytoplasmic staining in few tumoral hepatocytes (original magnification ×400). (*D*) Strong and diffuse glutamine synthetase immunostaining in tumor cells (original magnification ×200).

gain-of-function somatic mutations in gp130 may result in the inflammatory phenotype of HCA and explain activation of the acute inflammatory phase observed in tumoral hepatocytes (see **Fig. 4**D).[26]

Surrogate immunophenotypical markers related to the genetic abnormalities may be used in the classification of the 3 main subtypes of HCA.[27] Indeed, expression of liver fatty acid binding protein (LFABP), a protein positively regulated by HNF1α, is absent in steatotic HNF1α-mutated HCA, whereas it is highly expressed in nontumoral liver (see **Fig. 2**D). Similarly, Tel/Infl HCAs display positive immunostaining with acute phase inflammatory proteins such as serum amyloid A (SAA) and CRP. Most of β-catenin-mutated HCAs present abnormal and nuclear staining of β-catenin in tumoral hepatocytes, usually with a focal positivity restricted to few isolated tumoral hepatocytes. Immunostaining with glutamine synthetase, a β-catenin-targeted gene, showing a strong homogeneous or heterogeneous cytoplasmic staining, increases the sensibility for diagnosis of β-catenin-mutated HCA. Last, β-catenin mutations may be observed in some SAA-positive Tel/Infl HCAs, whereas gp130 activation (Tel/Infl subtype) and HNF1α inactivation (steatotic subtype) are mutually exclusive.[26,27] Overall, although diagnostic value of the different phenotypical markers is very good to excellent on paraffin sections, it is mandatory to compare their tissue expression in the tumor and its nontumoral liver in parallel. Finally, the fourth group of HCAs includes the lesions without any specific morphologic features or the genetic abnormalities previously described. In surgical series of HCAs, steatotic and Tel/Inf subtypes appear to be equally distributed, accounting for 85% of overall HCAs, when β-catenin-mutated HCAs are reported in 10% to 15%.

Although significant advances have been made in the subtyping of HCAs, some tumors remain difficult to classify and usually difficult to differentiate from well-differentiated HCCs. For instance, using comparative genomic analysis, HCAs displaying some clinical and/or morphologic atypias but not sufficient for an unequivocal diagnosis of HCC showed chromosomal abnormalities similar to HCC, suggesting that some of these tumors may represent the earliest form of well-differentiated HCC.[28] Differential diagnosis between HCA and HCC may also rely on surrogate immunophenotypical markers. Among them, Glypican-3, an oncofetal protein, appears to be the most performant so far, with no HCA positive for GPC-3 when more than 50% of well-differentiated HCCs are stained.[29,30]

Multiple Adenomas and Liver Adenomatosis

Review of the literature reporting patients with multiple HCAs, including the so-called adenomatosis, does not support an arbitrary classification based on clinical and imaging characteristics.[16,31] Patients with multiple HCAs are predominantly females but the use of OC appears to be less prevalent.[23] Patients with glycogen storage disease type I are also at risk of developing multiple HCA.[32] Recent study confirmed that risk of complications, including bleeding and malignant transformation, is similar to that in patients with solitary HCA, and is not influenced by the number of tumors.[16,18,31] Except for the number of lesions, no difference is observed between imaging features of adenomatosis and solitary HCA. Interestingly, on imaging, 3 main morphologic patterns of liver adenomatosis have been described: the steatotic form, the peliotic/telangiectatic form, and the mixed form.[33] To note, the proportion of steatotic HCA is higher and presence of micro-adenomatous foci in the "nontumoral liver" is more often observed in patients with liver adenomatosis.[18] As proposed for patients in solitary HCA, surgical treatment should be restricted to HCA associated with higher risk for complications.

HEMANGIOMAS

Hepatic hemangiomas, belonging to the group of nonepithelial lesions, are probably the most common of all liver tumors, with a prevalence ranging from 1% to 20%.[34] As the other main benign tumors of the liver, hemangiomas are more prevalent in women with a 5:1 female:male ratio with a mean age of 50 years.[35] They are usually incidentally observed by imaging without significant complications.[35] However, hemangiomas measuring 10 cm or more, referred to "giant hemangiomas," may be symptomatic, with pain and also signs and symptoms of an inflammatory process that may include a coagulopathy syndrome named Kasabach-Merritt syndrome. Such complication is rare, initially localized in the liver but may progress to secondary increased systemic fibrinolysis and thrombocytopenia,[36] leading to a fatal outcome in 20% to 30% of patients. Macroscopic examination demonstrates well-delineated, flat lesions of red-blue color that may partially collapse on sectioning (**Fig. 5**A). Some degrees of fibrosis, calcification, and thrombosis may be observed, most commonly on the largest lesions. Microscopically, hemangiomas are made of cavernous vascular spaces lined by flattened endothelium underlying fibrous septa of various width (see **Fig. 5**B). Small hemangiomas may become entirely fibrous, appearing as "a solitary fibrous nodule."

The pathogenesis of hemangioma is not well understood, even though hormonal dependence has been suggested.[35] Whatever the size, there is no treatment for asymptomatic hemangioma. Indications for treatment, usually surgical resection, include severe symptoms, complications, and inability to exclude malignancy.[37,38]

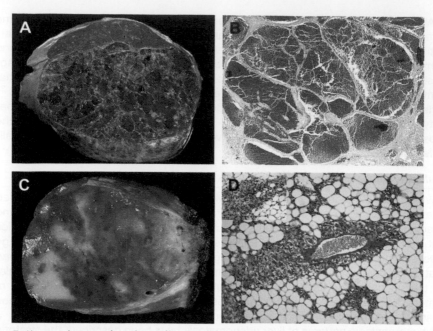

Fig. 5. Hemangioma and angiomyolipoma. (*A*) Macroscopic view of a hemangioma showing a well-delineated lesion of red-blue color. (*B*) Hemangioma made of cavernous vascular spaces lined by flattened endothelium underlying fibrous septa (H&E, original magnification ×100). (*C*) Macroscopic view of an angiomyolipoma as a circumscribed lesion with red (vascular component), yellow (fat tissue), and brown (smooth muscle component) areas. (*D*) The tumor is composed of 3 different components: fat tissue, vessels, and smooth muscle cells with epithelioid shape (H&E, original magnification ×200). HMB45 immunostaining is strongly positive in myoid component (*inset*).

ANGIOMYOLIPOMAS

Hepatic angiomyolipoma is a rare mesenchymal tumor belonging to the group of tumors derived from the "perivascular epithelioid cell," referred to as perivascular epithelial cell tumors or PEComas.[39] This tumor may occur as a solitary mass or as an associated finding with tuberous sclerosis where renal angiomyolipomas are much more frequent.[40] These lesions predominantly affect females at any age and are found incidentally by imaging. Tumors are often larger than 5 cm in diameter and well circumscribed from red to yellow color (see **Fig. 5**C). They are composed of smooth muscle, fat, and vessels in various combinations (see **Fig. 5**D). The fatty component, which may vary between 10% and 90%, is usually mature. Vessels are tortuous, thick walled, and often surrounded by smooth muscle cells. The myoid component may be prominent, composed of epithelioid, intermediate, or spindle cells. Many morphologic variants, reflecting degree of differentiation of the perivascular endothelial cells, have been recognized, certainly contributing to the difficulty of diagnosis.[39] Therefore, the accuracy of preoperative diagnosis is low as a result of variable imaging and morphologic appearances, owing to the varying content of the 3 components and the rarity of the lesion. Fortunately, immunoreactivity of the myoid component, with melanocytic antigens (HMB45, Melan-A) in addition to smooth muscle markers, is a key diagnostic (see **Fig. 5**D inset).[41] More recently, it has been shown that angiomyolipomas may express KIT (CD117) in the myoid compartment with focal staining of fat cells.[42]

Although monoclonality of these tumors has been clearly demonstrated, both in renal and liver localizations, its potential to malignancy is usually considered with skepticism.[43,44] Nevertheless, very few cases of malignant angiomyolipomas of the liver have been reported so far.[43,44] Large size (>10 cm) and presence of coagulative necrosis are almost consistently observed in malignant angiomyolipomas, whereas invasive growth around the tumor and cellular atypias may be shared by benign angiomyolipomas. Although rare, diagnosis of angiomyolipoma is a major issue in the characterization of liver tumors, because in case of such diagnosis, conservative management is recommended, with follow-up in asymptomatic patients.[45–47]

SUMMARY

Diagnosis of benign liver tumors is becoming a challenge for pathologists as a consequence of the extensive use of abdominal imaging leading to the detection of asymptomatic liver tumors. Most of these lesions occur on a background normal liver and, except for hemangiomas, are subjected to pathologic analysis. Among hepatocellular tumors, differential diagnosis between FNH and HCA is crucial in order to propose the adequate management (abstention for FNH and surgical resection in most HCA). In addition, recent years have seen major advances in the description of HCAs, which are now considered as a heterogeneous entity based on molecular and morphologic features. From this new pathomolecular classification, it appears that some subtypes are at higher risk for complications, including progression to HCC for few of them. Interestingly, diagnosis and management of patients with HCAs require a multidisciplinary approach, including radiologists, clinicians, and pathologists.

REFERENCES

1. Edmondson HA. Tumors of the liver and intrahepatic bile ducts. Atlas of Tumor Pathology section 7, part 25. Washington, DC: Armed Forces Institute of Pathology; 1958.
2. International Working Party. Terminology of nodular hepatocellular lesions. Hepatology 1995;22:983–93.
3. Ishak KG. Hepatic neoplasms associated with contraceptive and anabolic steroids. Carcinogenesis hormones. Recent results. Cancer Res 1979;66:73–128.
4. Wanless IR, Mawdsley C, Adams R. On the pathogenesis of focal nodular hyperplasia. Hepatology 1985;5:1194–200.
5. Gaffey MJ, Iezzoni JC, Weiss LM. Clonal analysis of focal nodular hyperplasia of the liver. Am J Pathol 1996;148:1089–96.
6. Paradis V, Laurent A, Fléjou JF, et al. Evidence for the polyclonal nature of focal nodular hyperplasia of the liver by the study of X chromosome inactivation. Hepatology 1997;26:891–5.
7. Nguyen BN, Fléjou JF, Terris B, et al. Focal nodular hyperplasia of the liver. A comprehensive pathologic study of 305 lesions and recognition of new histologic forms. Am J Surg Pathol 1999;23:1441–54.
8. Makhlouf HR, Abdul-Al HM, Goodman ZD. Diagnosis of focal nodular hyperplasia of the liver by needle biopsy. Human Pathol 2005;36:1210–6.
9. Bioulac-Sage P, Laumonier H, Rullier A, et al. Over-expression of glutamine synthetase in focal nodular hyperplasia: a novel easy diagnostic tool in surgical pathology. Liver Int 2009;29:459–65.
10. Wanless IR, Albrecht S, Bilbao J. Multiple focal nodular hyperplasia of the liver associated with vascular malformations of various organs and neoplasia of the brain. Mod Pathol 1989;2:456–62.

11. Paradis V, Benzekri A, Dargère D, et al. Telangiectatic focal nodular hyperplasia: a variant of hepatocellular adenoma. Gastroenterology 2004;126:1323–9.
12. Bioulac-Sage P, Rebouissou S, Sa Cunha A, et al. Clinical morphologic, and molecular features defining so-called telangiectatic focal nodular hyperplasias of the liver. Gastroenterology 2005;128:1211–8.
13. Nime F, Pickren JW, Vana J, et al. The histology of liver tumors in oral contraceptive users observed during a national survey by the American College of Surgeons Commission on Cancer. Cancer 1979;44:1481–9.
14. Coombes GB, Reiser J, Paradinas FJ, et al. An androgen associated hepatic adenoma in a trans-sexual. Br J Surg 1978;65:869–70.
15. Wittekind C. Hepatocellular carcinoma and cerholangiocarcinoma. In: Hermanek P, Gospodarowicz MK, Henson DE, editors. Prognostic factors in cancer. Berlin: Springer; 1995. p. 88–93.
16. Barthelemes L, Tait IS. Liver cell adenomas and liver cell adenomatosis. HBP (Oxford) 2005;7:186–96.
17. Terkivatan T, De Wilt JH, De Man RA, et al. Treatment of ruptured hepatocellular adenoma. Br J Surg 2001;88:207–9.
18. Dokmak S, Paradis V, Vilgrain V, et al. A single-center surgical experience of 122 patients with single and multiple hepatocellular adenomas. Gastroenterology 2009;137:1698–705.
19. Bioulac-Sage P, Laumonnier H, Couchy G, et al. Hepatocellular adenoma management and phenotypic classification: the Bordeaux experience. Hepatology 2009;50:481–9.
20. Paradis V, Zalinski S, Chelbi E, et al. Hepatocellular carcinomas in patients with metabolic syndrome often develop without significant fibrosis: a pathological analysis. Hepatology 2009;49:851–9.
21. Zucman-Rossi J, Jeannot E, Van Nhieu JT, et al. Genotype-phenotype correlation in hepatocellular adenoma: new classification and relationship with HCC. Hepatology 2006;43:515–24.
22. Bluteau O, Jeannot E, Bioulac-Sage P, et al. Bi-allelic inactivation of TCF1 in hepatic adenomas. Nat Genet 2002;32:312–5.
23. Flejou JF, Barges J, Menu Y, et al. Liver adenomatosis: an entity distinct from liver adenoma? Gastroenterology 1985;89:1132–8.
24. Bacq Y, Jaquemin E, Balabaud C, et al. Familial liver adenomatosis associated with hepatocyte nuclear factor 1 alpha inactivation. Gastroenterology 2003;125:1470–5.
25. Paradis V, Champault A, Ronot M, et al. Telangiectatic adenomas: an entity associated with increased body mass index and inflammation. Hepatology 2007;46:140–6.
26. Rebouissou S, Amessou M, Thomas C, et al. Frequent in-frame somatic deletions activate gp130 in inflammatory hepatocellular tumors. Nature 2009;457:2000–4.
27. Bioulac-Sage P, Rebouissou S, Thomas C, et al. Hepatocellular adenoma subtype classification using molecular markers and immunohistochemistry. Hepatology 2007;46:740–8.
28. Kakar S, Chen X, Ho C, et al. Chromosomal abnormalities determined by comparative genomic hybridation are helpful in the diagnosis of atypical hepatocellular neoplasms. Histopathology 2009;55:197–205.
29. Wang XY, Degos F, Dubois S, et al. Glypican-3 expression in hepatocellular tumors: diagnostic value for preneoplastic lesions and hepatocellular carcinomas. Human Pathol 2006;37:1435–41.
30. Shafizadeh N, Ferrell LD, Kakar S. Utility and limitations of glypican-3 expression for the diagnosis of hepatocellular carcinoma at both ends of the differentiation spectrum. Modern Pathol 2008;21:1011–8.

31. Ribeiro A, Burgart LJ, Nagorney DM, et al. Management of liver adenomatosis: results with a conservative surgical approach. Liver Transpl Surg 1998;4:388–98.
32. Labrune P, Trioche P, Duvaltier I, et al. Hepatocellular adenomas in glycogen storage disease type I and III: a series of 43 patients and review of the literature. J Pediatr Gastroenterol Nutr 1997;24:276–9.
33. Lewin M, Handra-Luca A, Arrivé L, et al. Liver adenomatosis: classification pf MR imaging features and comparison with pathologic findings. Radiology 2006;241: 433–40.
34. Semelka RC, Sofka CM. Hepatic hemangiomas. Magn Reson Imaging Clin N Am 1997;5:241–53.
35. Trotter JF, Everson GT. Benign focal lesions of the liver. Clin Liver Dis 2001;5: 17–42.
36. Maceyko RF, Camisa C. Kasabach-Merritt syndrome. Pediatr Dermatol 1991;8: 113–36.
37. Yoon SS, Charny CK, Fong Y, et al. Diagnosis, management and outcomes of 115 patients with hepatic hemangioma. J Am Coll Surg 2003;197:392–402.
38. Herman P, Costa MLV, Machado MAC, et al. Management of hepatic hemangiomas: a 14-year experience. J Gastrointest Surg 2005;9:853–9.
39. Tsui WM, Colombari R, Portmann BC, et al. Hepatic angiomyolipoma: a clinicopathologic study of 30 cases and delineation of unusual morphologic variants. Am J Surg Pathol 1999;23:34–48.
40. Hooper LD, Mergo PJ, Ros PR. Multiple hepatorenal angiomyolipomas: diagnosis with fat suppression, gadolinium-enhanced MRI. Abdom Imaging 1994;19: 549–51.
41. Sturtz CL, Dabbs DJ. Angiomyolipomas: the nature and expression of the HMB45 antigen. Mod Pathol 1994;7:842–5.
42. Makhlouf HR, Remotti HE, Ishak KG. Expression of KIT (CD117) in angiomyolipoma. Am J Surg Pathol 2002;26:493–7.
43. Paradis V, Laurendeau I, Vieillefond A, et al. Clonal analysis of renal sporadic angiomyolipomas. Hum Pathol 1998;29:1063–7.
44. Xu AM, Zhang SH, Zheng WQ, et al. Pathological and molecular analysis of sporadic hepatic angiomyolipoma. Human Pathol 2006;37:735–41.
45. Nguyen TT, Gorman B, Shields D, et al. Malignant hepatic angiomyolipoma: report of a case and review of the literature. Am J Surg Pathol 2008;32:793–8.
46. Deng Y-F, Lin Q, Zhang S-H, et al. Malignant angiomyolipoma in the liver: a case report with pathological and molecular analysis. Pathol Res Pract 2008;204:911–8.
47. Sawai J, Manabe T, Yamanaka Y, et al. Angiomyolipoma of the liver: case report and collective review of cases diagnosed from fine needle aspiration biopsy specimens. J Hepatobiliary Pancreat Surg 1998;5:333–8.

Hepatic Neoplasia and Metabolic Diseases in Children

Angshumoy Roy, MD, PhD[a], Milton J. Finegold, MD[b],*

KEYWORDS

• Cirrhosis • Tyrosinemia • α_1-Antitrypsin • Hemochromatosis
• Reversion • NTBC • Hepatocellular cancer

Hepatic involvement in metabolic diseases is a natural corollary to the central and pivotal role of the liver in metabolism. Most childhood metabolic liver diseases are classical mendelian single-gene disorders affecting key enzymes and proteins in diverse metabolic pathways.[1,2] Other disorders, such as the metabolic syndrome and its hepatic manifestation, nonalcoholic fatty liver disease, are multifactorial (genetic dyslipidemias, insulin resistance, and diet),[3–5] and increasingly prevalent in the pediatric age group in association with childhood obesity.[6] Yet others (eg, idiopathic copper toxicosis and Indian childhood cirrhosis) are postulated to be multifactorial, with contribution from as yet unresolved genetic and environmental risk factors.[7–9]

Metabolic liver disease is often studied within the paradigm of "toxic metabolite" accumulation and chronic injury. In this model of pathogenesis, metabolic disorders initially present with characteristic histologic and ultrastructural patterns on liver biopsy,[10,11] but chronic injury over months or years leads to cirrhosis or hepatic neoplasia. Prototypes of such a model are the endoplasmic reticulum retention of α_1-antitrypsin (AAT) in AAT deficiency, increased levels of succinylacetone in hereditary tyrosinemia, and increased glycogen in glycogen storage disease (GSD). Accordingly, the most frequently diagnosed hepatic neoplasm in children with inherited metabolic disorders is hepatocellular carcinoma (HCC),[10,12] a tumor otherwise rare in the pediatric population[13] but the most common to arise in a cirrhotic liver. Cholangiocarcinoma, combined cholangio-hepatocellular carcinoma, hepatic adenoma, and focal nodular hyperplasia are less frequently encountered (**Table 1**). In contrast, hepatoblastoma, the most common pediatric liver malignancy, is not usually associated with cirrhosis or metabolic disease but rather with other heritable defects.[10,12]

[a] Department of Pathology, Baylor College of Medicine, One Baylor Plaza, Houston, TX 77030, USA
[b] Department of Pathology, Baylor College of Medicine, Texas Children's Hospital, 6621 Fannin Street, Houston, TX 77030, USA
* Corresponding author.
E-mail address: mjfinego@texaschildrens.org

Clin Liver Dis 14 (2010) 731–746
doi:10.1016/j.cld.2010.07.002
1089-3261/10/$ – see front matter © 2010 Elsevier Inc. All rights reserved.

liver.theclinics.com

Table 1
List of metabolic disorders associated with hepatocellular carcinoma

Disorder	Gene	Inheritance	Neoplasia	Background Cirrhosis	RR
Hereditary tyrosinemia	FAH	AR	HCC	++	ND
AAT deficiency	SERPINA1	ACoD	HCC, CC, CHCC	±	5
Hereditary hemochromatosis	HFE	AR	HCC	++	20
Wilson disease	ATP7B	AR	HCC, CC	+	ND
Acute intermittent porphyria	HMBS	AD	HCC	+	>30
PFIC-2	ABCB11 (MDR3)	AR	HCC, CC, CHCC	±	ND
Mitochondrial ETC disorders	Multiple	AR	HCC	+	ND
GSD-I	G6PC, G6PT	AR	HA, HCC	-	ND
GSD-III	AGL	AR	HCC, HA	+	ND
GSD-IV	GBE1	AR	HCC	+	ND
NASH	Multiple	Complex	HCC	+	ND

Abbreviations: AAT, α_1-antitrypsin; ABCB11, ATP-binding cassette, subfamily B, member 11; ACoD, autosomal codominant; AD, autosomal dominant; AGL, amylo-1,6-glucosidase, 4-α-glucanotransferase (glycogen debrancher enzyme); AR, autosomal recessive; ATP7B, ATPase, Cu++ transporting, beta polypeptide; CC, cholangiocarcinoma; CHCC, mixed cholangio-hepatocellular carcinoma; FAH, fumarylacetoacetate hydrolase; G6PC, glucose-6-phosphatase, catalytic subunit; G6PT, glucose-6-phosphatase transporter; GBE1, glucan (1,4-α-), branching enzyme 1 (glycogen branching enzyme); GSD, glycogen storage disease; HCC, hepatocellular carcinoma; HFE, hemochromatosis; HMBS, hydroxymethylbilane synthase; NASH, nonalcoholic steatohepatitis; ND, not determined; PFIC, progressive familial intrahepatic cholestasis; RR, relative risk; SERPINA1, serine protease inhibitor, alpha 1.

A few counterpoints deserve special mention. First, cirrhosis is not a prerequisite for developing HCC in metabolic disorders, the most prominent example being malignant transformation of hepatic adenomas in type I glycogenosis.[14] De novo HCC in AAT deficiency[15] and hereditary hemochromatosis (HH)[16] have also been reported. Second, even in the presence of cirrhosis, HCC and other cancers develop in only a minority of patients with metabolic disease, underscoring the crucial role played by environmental and other genetic modifiers in tumorigenesis. Third, modifiers must also be involved in the latency of progression to cirrhosis or HCC; although the molecular defects are present since conception in AAT deficiency, HH, Wilson disease (WD), and acute hepatic porphyrias, tumors rarely occur before adulthood.[1] In contrast, cirrhosis and hepatic carcinogenesis in untreated hereditary tyrosinemia occurs in early childhood.[17]

A comprehensive review of all aspects of metabolic diseases is beyond the scope of this article and the reader is referred to several exhaustive references.[1,2,10] This article focuses on hepatic neoplasia as a complication of metabolic liver disease in the pediatric population with emphasis on recent advances in the molecular mechanisms of tumorigenesis in tyrosinemia, AAT deficiency, and GSD (see **Table 1** for a list of disorders). Hepatic tumors not associated with metabolic disease (eg, hepatoblastoma and mesenchymal hamartoma)[12] or arising in developmental disorders (eg, Alagille syndrome and Caroli disease)[18,19] are not included. Also excluded are the cancer predisposition syndromes (Fanconi anemia, ataxia telangiectasia, familial adenomatous polyposis, Li-Fraumeni syndrome, and Beckwith-Wiedemann syndrome) in which hepatic and extrahepatic tumorigenesis is driven by germ-line mutations and epimutations activating oncogenic pathways.[20,21]

HEREDITARY TYROSINEMIA (OMIM 276700)

Hereditary tyrosinemia type 1 is an autosomal-recessive metabolic disorder caused by deficiency of fumarylacetoacetate hydrolase (FAH), the last enzyme of tyrosine degradation. The disease is quite common in Quebec, Canada (1 in 16,786 live births),[17] and is especially prevalent in the French Canadian population of Saguenay-Lac-St-Jean, Quebec, because of a complex founder effect.[22] Worldwide more than 30 mutations have been reported in the FAH gene,[23] but the IVS12+5G→A allele is responsible for more than 90% of mutant alleles in Saguenay-Lac-St-Jean, Quebec.[24] The mutational spectrum in FAH in different ethnic groups has been reviewed elsewhere.[23] An elevated succinylacetone level in blood or urine is confirmatory for the diagnosis.[17]

Before 1992, when Lindstedt and colleagues[25] published the first report of successful treatment of tyrosinemic children with 2-(nitro-4-trifluoromethylbenzoyl)–1,3 cyclohexanedione (NTBC), two major clinical presentations of tyrosinemia were recognized. An acute form with hepatic decompensation (hepatomegaly, ascites, and coagulopathy) and neurologic crises (painful paresthesias and autonomic signs) led to death in more than 80% of patients before age 2 years.[17] Liver biopsy of the acute stage typically shows a hepatitic pattern with necrosis, steatosis, and sometimes giant cell transformation.[10] Patients who survive the acute phase develop chronic hepatic disease (cirrhosis or hepatosplenomegaly). Liver histopathology of the chronic stage usually shows mixed micronodular and macronodular cirrhosis with bile duct proliferation and, most significantly, foci of dysplasia or HCC (**Fig. 1**).[26]

In cirrhotic livers, the remarkable phenomenon of "reversion" was first reported by Kvittingen and colleagues,[27,28] in which rare discrete regenerative nodules were found to be immunoreactive for FAH protein interspersed with most FAH-negative nodules.

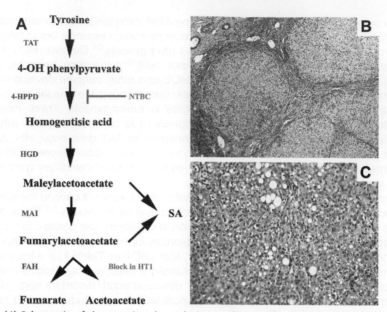

Fig. 1. (*A*) Schematic of the tyrosine degradation pathway. FAH deficiency in hereditary tyrosinemia type I (HT1) leads to accumulation of fumarylacetoacetate and maleylacetoacetate, with production of succinylacetone (SA) that becomes detectable in the urine and plasma. NTBC (nitisinone) is a potent inhibitor of the 4-HPPD enzyme. Photomicrograph of liver from a patient with HT1 showing typical micronodular and macronodular cirrhosis (*B*) and a focus of hepatocellular cancer (*C*) (hematoxylin and eosin stain, original magnificatons: *B* - 40x and *C* - 200x). FAH, fumarylacetoacetate hydrolase; HGD, homogentisate deoxygenase; 4-HPPD, 4-OH phenylpyruvate dioxygenase; MAI, maleylacetoacetate isomerase; TAT, tyrosine aminotransferase.

DNA analyses of these "revertant nodules" have showed heterozygous correction of the *FAH* gene sequence for at least three separate mutations in different populations.[28,29] There seems to be an inverse correlation between the extent of revertant nodules and clinical severity.[29] More importantly, dysplasia and HCC was found to develop only within nonrevertant nodules,[29] indicating the cell-autonomous nature of the oncogenic transformation. Reversion to wild-type sequence in these nodules cannot be explained by gene conversion because it occurs in patients homozygous for the mutations. Rather, the high mutation rates induced by the toxic metabolites fumarylacetoacetate, maleylacetoacetate, and succinylacetone (SA)[30] seem to cause spontaneous reversion of the mutant allele back to wild-type.[31] If so, it will be interesting to compare the mutation rates at other genetic loci between revertant and nonrevertant nodules.

The risk of developing HCC in tyrosinemia is considered the highest among all metabolic disorders.[31] Earlier reports of a 37% incidence of HCC[26] may have been overestimated,[17] but current estimates of a 13% to 17% risk[17,23,32] is extremely high. In contrast to other metabolic disorders, tyrosinemic individuals are also at risk of developing HCC earlier, often before age 5 years,[17,33] and as early as 1 year[34] (see later). Typically, dysplastic changes within regenerative nodules with or without discrete foci of HCC (see **Fig. 1**) are evident. Such findings promote regular screening for serum alpha fetoprotein elevation and ultrasonography and intervention by orthotopic liver transplantation in affected children The introduction of NTBC (nitisinone) has dramatically altered the nonsurgical management and the short- and medium-term outlook in these patients. NTBC is a potent inhibitor of 4-hydroxyphenylpyruvate dioxygenase,[35] an upstream enzyme in the tyrosine catabolism pathway (see **Fig. 1**). Over 300 patients have been enrolled in the International NTBC study[34] and the incidence of acute tyrosinemia (liver failure and neurologic crises) has been reduced to 10%, a remarkable outcome with very few adverse effects.[23,34] Given that most patients in the pre-NTBC era succumbed to acute symptoms, these results are hugely promising.

NTBC has also been reported to decrease the short- and medium-term risk of HCC development when patients are started on therapy at less than 2 years of age.[34,36] In the smaller Quebec trial, only 1 (2.85%) of 35 patients on NTBC was transplanted for suspected cirrhosis and had hepatocellular dysplasia at 51 months of follow-up.[23] In an interim report on the international NTBC study by Holme and Lindstedt,[34] only 1 (1.25%) out of 80 patients placed on therapy at less than 2 years of age was identified with proved HCC at 5 to 7 years follow-up. In a longer-term follow-up of French patients, none of 41 patients started on NTBC at less than 2 years of age developed HCC.[37] Although these figures are encouraging, other statistics give one pause; HCC developed in 8 (13.3%) out of 60 patients in the international study,[34] and in 2 out of 5 patients in the French study[37] when NTBC treatment was started after 2 years of age. Furthermore, HCC has been reported in patients as late as 6 years[38] and 10 years[39] after starting NTBC therapy, suggesting that the long-term risk assessment of HCC in patients on NTBC awaits further studies.

The molecular mechanisms of hepatic carcinogenesis in tyrosinemia have been the focus of many studies. Several lines of evidence point toward a major role of fumarylacetoacetate, maleylacetoacetate, and SA, metabolites upstream of the block in tyrosine degradation, in the development of HCC. First, NTBC treatment targets the 4-hydroxyphenylpyruvate dioxygenase enzyme upstream of FAH (see **Fig. 1**) leading to a marked decrease in plasma SA levels in responsive patients.[25] Second, although FAH knockout ($Fah^{-/-}$) mice on NTBC develop HCC by 7 to 10 months,[40] $Fah^{-/-}$ $Hppd^{-/-}$ double knockout mice are protected from hepatic carcinogenesis even at 18 months of age.[41] Third, and perhaps most telling, is the observation that HCC develops only in FAH-negative nodules (see previously) in livers with spontaneous reversion.[29] Fourth, fumarylacetoacetate has been shown to be a mutagen in cultured cell lines[42] inducing mitotic abnormalities and genomic instability. Fifth, SA may have a direct inhibitory effect on DNA repair mechanisms.[43] Finally, the activation of the AKT survival signaling pathway and inhibition of apoptosis in $Fah^{-/-}$ mice with discontinuation of NTBC may provide a mechanistic basis for the carcinogenesis in tyrosinemia.[44]

AAT DEFICIENCY (OMIM 107400)

AAT deficiency is an autosomal-recessive disorder caused by mutations in the *SERPINA1* gene that primarily affects the lungs and the liver. It is a relatively common condition affecting 1:1600 to 1:2000 live births and AAT-deficiency liver disease is the most common inherited metabolic cause of liver transplantation in childhood. AAT is a glycoprotein synthesized and secreted by the liver and its principal physiologic role is to inhibit neutrophil serine proteases. Although lung disease in AAT deficiency is the result of decreased levels of circulating AAT, liver disease, the focus of this section, is caused by toxicity from the retention of the mutant protein within the endoplasmic reticulum of hepatocytes. Abnormal migration of mutant AAT proteins on serum isoelectric focusing constitutes the confirmatory test for diagnosing the disease.

The most common AAT variant associated with clinical disease (protease inhibitor Z [PiZ]) is caused by a missense mutation (Glu342Lys) that produces a conformationally altered unstable protein prone to homomeric aggregation. Such aggregates are retained within the endoplasmic reticulum (hence the deficiency in the plasma); can be identified on routine histologic sections with periodic acid–Schiff (PAS) stains after diastase digestion; lead to intracellular toxicity and cellular injury (mitochondrial dysfunction and autophagy); activate the NF-κB pathway; and are believed to underlie the molecular pathogenesis of liver disease. The current state of knowledge regarding the pathogenesis of AAT deficiency liver disease has been reviewed.[45]

Liver disease is primarily seen with homozygous PiZZ AAT deficiency. Long-term follow-up studies of PiZZ newborns in Scandinavian populations indicate only 10% to 15% develop any biochemical evidence (without clinical signs) of liver dysfunction at 25 years of age, suggesting that AAT-deficiency liver disease is a low penetrance disorder dependent on additional host or environmental risk factors. In skin fibroblasts from individuals with AAT-deficiency liver disease, constitutively expressed PiZ protein were found to be degraded less efficiently than in PiZZ individuals without liver disease,[46] confirming the presence of additional host factors in modifying disease phenotype. One such host factor involved in the degradation of endoplasmic reticulum–retained and misfolded glycoproteins is mannosidase I, the translation and protein levels of which are suppressed by a variant allele in its 3'UTR that is more prevalent in symptomatic PiZZ infants, providing evidence for the role of genetic modifiers in AAT-deficiency liver disease.[47]

AAT deficiency should be considered in any newborn with liver dysfunction and biopsy showing neonatal cholestasis with or without giant cells. Bile duct proliferation mimicking extrahepatic biliary atresia is a common finding. Uncommonly, a ductopenic pattern mimicking Alagille syndrome can be seen.[10] Characteristic eosinophilic cytoplasmic globules of AAT may be seen in periportal hepatocytes, most prominent in older children with the PAS stain after diastase digestion (PASD), and can be diagnosed earlier with anti-AAT monoclonal antibodies. Chronic liver disease with hepatitis or cirrhosis usually occurs only in older children and adults.

Hepatic neoplasia arising in AAT-deficiency liver disease has been well-documented. An autopsy study from Sweden first showed a strong association between AAT deficiency and cirrhosis and liver cancer, the risk for liver cancer greater than explained by cirrhosis alone.[48] The life-time relative risk of developing HCC in a PiZZ individual is increased (relative risk = 5)[49,50] and with few exceptions,[51] hepatic tumors develop in adults.[15] Unlike tyrosinemia, hepatic neoplasia in AAT deficiency often develops in noncirrhotic livers, and cholangiocarcinoma or mixed cholangio-hepatocellular carcinomas, in addition to HCC, have been reported.[15] The development of HCC and cholangiocarcinomas in PiMZ (heterozygous for Z) individuals has also been reported,[52] although the incidence of liver disease in PiMZ individuals remains controversial.

Hepatic carcinogenesis in AAT deficiency is incompletely understood but Perlmutter[53] advanced an interesting cell nonautonomous model.[45] Using a transgenic mouse model for AAT deficiency (PiZ mice), Rudnick and colleagues[54] demonstrated two distinct hepatocyte populations: a globule-containing compartment with PASD-positive AAT aggregates and another globule-devoid compartment negative for PASD. Furthermore, using double labeling with the DNA proliferation marker BrdU, the proliferating hepatocytes were found to be within the globule-devoid compartment. These findings have led to a model whereby the globule-devoid hepatocytes are considered to have a selective proliferation advantage and respond to proliferation signals emanating from the globule-containing hepatocytes.[45] However, conclusive evidence for such a "trans" signal awaits further studies.

HH (OMIM 235200)

HH is an autosomal-recessive disorder of iron metabolism, in most cases caused by mutations in the *HFE* gene. Before the identification of the gene, a diagnosis of HH on liver biopsy was based on documentation of iron overloading (hepatic iron index >2 and iron content >4500 μg/g dry weight). Current screening and confirmatory strategies for HH diagnosis include fasting transferrin-iron saturation and ferritin levels, and if abnormal, genotyping for the C282Y and H63D alleles in *HFE* for confirmation.[16] Homozygosity for the C282Y allele has a prevalence of 1 in 200 to 400 in white populations and accounts for 85% to 90% of all cases of HH. The molecular mechanisms of HFE-mediated regulation of iron metabolism have been reviewed elsewhere.[16,55]

HH is one of the most common inherited disorders in descendants of northern European ancestry. In a comprehensive population-based study on 1847 Swedish individuals, Elmberg and colleagues[56] reported a 20-fold increased risk of HCC in patients with HH. With few exceptions, HCC arises in cirrhotic livers.[55] Although the defect in iron metabolism may be detected in utero, clinical symptoms in HH rarely develop before adulthood. The long-term complications of HH (cirrhosis and HCC) are prime examples of the aforementioned hypothesis of cumulative chronic injury through childhood. Therefore, children of affected parents should be screened annually with transferrin saturation and phlebotomy should be initiated with the first abnormal result.

The mechanism of chronic injury is presumed to be related to iron overload. Excess iron has been shown to cause liver injury through generation of free radicals and lipid peroxidation, leading to mitochondrial dysfunction and cell death.[57] Furthermore, iron has been shown to activate hepatic stellate cells to promote fibrosis. Beyond the role of cirrhosis itself in predisposing to HCC, several observations support a direct role for iron in promoting hepatic carcinogenesis. First, there are several reports of HCC in noncirrhotic livers of patients with HH.[55] Second, stainable iron can be found in more than 50% of patients with HCC without HH.[55] Third, as reported by Lehmann and colleagues,[58] epigenetic alterations commonly encountered in HCC are more frequently identified in liver biopsies of HH individuals without HCC. Finally, iron-mediated carcinogenesis is associated with increased frequency of mutations at the p53 locus.[59,60]

TYPE I GSD (OMIM 232200 AND 232220)

Type I GSD (GSD-I), or von Gierke disease, is an autosomal-recessive disorder caused by mutations in the glucose-6-phosphatase complex. It is the most common of the hepatic glycogenoses, representing approximately 25% of all cases.[14] GSD-I has been further subdivided based on the molecular defect: type Ia (the classic form) is caused by mutations in the catalytic subunit of glucose-6-phosphatase, and type Ib is caused by mutations in the transporter (G6PT). More than 80 allelic variants in the *G6PC* gene have been reported in the literature[61] and sequence analysis of the gene is now offered commercially (www.genetests.org) and is especially useful for prenatal diagnosis.[62] Stringent genotype-phenotype correlations do not exist, however,[61] and the gold standard for diagnosis is measurement of enzyme activity on fresh liver tissue.[14]

GSD-I is characterized by protean metabolic derangements,[62] chief being profound hypoglycemia and hyperlipidemia. The clinical manifestations and laboratory findings have been thoroughly reviewed.[2,14,62] Patients can present in the newborn period but typically present within the first 6 months of life with hypoglycemia and hepatomegaly. Liver biopsy shows swollen, pale hepatocytes with cytoplasmic PAS-positive storage material completely sensitive to diastase digestion (**Fig. 2**). Monoparticulate glycogen can be seen on electron microscopy.

Between 16% and 75% of patients with GSD-I develop hepatic adenomas detectable by ultrasonography.[63,64] In several series, the prevalence of adenomas was found to increase with age, developing first around puberty. The pathogenesis of adenomas in GSD-I is incompletely understood. The fact that maintenance of glycemic control through dietary therapy since childhood (with frequent meals, uncooked corn starch, or continuous nocturnal nasogastric drip feeding) has reduced the incidence of adenomas[65] and that some adenomas have been reported to regress with dietary therapy[66] has led to the suggestion that increased glucagon levels are hepatotrophic.[14] However, documented glucagon levels are usually normal.[63] A recent study comparing genomic alterations in hepatic adenomas arising in GSD-I with adenomas in the general population did not identify specific changes in any group.[67] Further studies are necessary to resolve the mechanism of adenoma formation (and neoplasia in general) in this disorder.

Ominously, adenomas have been reported to undergo malignant transformation to HCC in several case series.[68–70] However, the pathogenesis of malignant transformation remains elusive. In a recent case series of eight patients with GSD-I and hepatic adenomas, the age of diagnosis of HCC ranged from 19 to 49 years of age.[68] Because of the risk of HCC in patients with GSD-I, current recommendations propose imaging with regular monitoring of serum alpha fetoprotein levels. However, six of eight patients with HCC had normal alpha fetoprotein levels,[68] highlighting the need for other surveillance mechanisms in these patients.

TYPE III GSD (OMIM 232400)

Type III GSD (GSD-III or Cori disease) is caused by deficiency of the glycogen debranching enzyme (amylo-1,6-glucosidase, 4-α-glucanotransferase). It is an autosomal-recessive disorder caused by mutations in the *AGL* gene. Affected patients typically present in infancy with hepatomegaly and hypoglycemia with or without myopathy. Liver biopsy at this stage depicts distended hepatocytes with diastase-resistant PAS-positive cytoplasmic material that on ultrastructural examination reveal abnormal glycogen with short outer chains. Periportal fibrosis is common but progressive cirrhosis is a rare complication of long-term disease in patients.[71] Hepatic neoplasia is a rare complication of GSD-III in adults. Adenomas are seen in 5% to 25% of patients.[71,72] There are only six reports of HCC in GSD-III, all arising in cirrhosis,[71] the earliest at 32 years age.[73]

TYPE IV GSD (OMIM 232500)

Type IV GSD (GSD-IV or Andersen disease) is an extremely rare (0.3% of glycogenoses) autosomal-recessive disorder caused by deficiency of the glycogen branching enzyme.[14] More than 15 alleles have been reported in the *GBE1* gene to cause this clinically heterogeneous disorder that in the classic form presents with cirrhosis in infancy. The liver biopsy is remarkable for swollen hepatocytes with amphophilic cytoplasmic material that is PAS positive but partially resistant to diastase digestion. The amylopectin-like material also stains with colloidal iron. Cirrhosis develops very early in patients with GSD-IV, often at presentation. Development of HCC in GSD-IV has been rarely reported.[74,75]

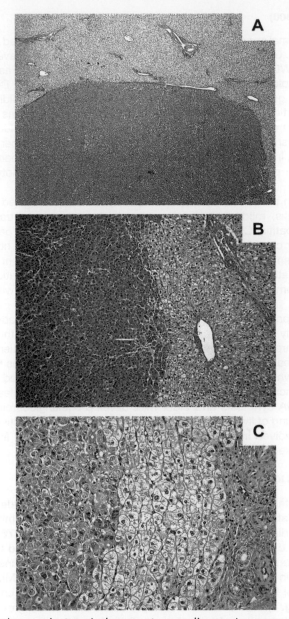

Fig. 2. Hepatic adenoma in type I glycogen storage disease. Low-power (*A*) and higher magnification (*B*) hematoxylin and eosin-stained sections show the interface between the adenoma and surrounding liver tissue. Note the pale swollen hepatocytes in the adjacent liver that are sensitive to diastase, in contrast to the adenoma (*C*) PAS-diastase. (Original magnifications: *A* - 40x, *B* - 200x, *C* - 400x.)

WD (OMIM 277900)

WD is an autosomal-recessive disorder of copper metabolism caused by mutations in the *ATP7B* gene. Greater than 250 different mutations in the gene have been reported in patients with WD.[7] The gene encodes a copper-transporting ATPase protein in the trans-Golgi complex that is essential for copper secretion into bile. Deficiency of the protein leads to gradual copper accumulation in the liver over childhood, and then within extrahepatic sites leading to the typical clinical manifestations of the disease. Diagnosis of WD depends on a combination of several tests, including decreased serum ceruloplasmin levels (<20 mg/dL); increased hepatic copper content (>250 μg/g dry weight); increased 24-hour urinary copper excretion post–penicillamine challenge (>25 μmol per 24 hours); *ATP7B* genotyping; or DNA haplotype analysis in affected families.[7]

Liver biopsy in patients may reveal an acute phase characterized by hepatocyte swelling, steatosis, mild cholestasis, and portal lymphocytic infiltrates, mimicking autoimmune hepatitis. Chronic stages typically show steatosis with periportal fibrosis or macronodular cirrhosis.[10] Stainable copper is characteristic but not detectable in the younger patient or in regenerative nodules; hepatic copper content measurements are more informative. Treatment consists of life-long copper chelation therapy and dietary zinc to compete for copper absorption from the diet, without which the disease is fatal.[7]

The risk of hepatic neoplasia in patients with WD has not been adequately determined but is likely to be low because there are very few reports. In the largest series, two HCCs and three cholangiocarcinomas were identified in 159 patients with WD followed over 10 years.[76] The pathophysiology of elevated copper has been studied in $Atp7b^{-/-}$ mice where it has been shown that liver damage is related to the duration of exposure to increased copper. In mice, elevated hepatocyte nuclear copper leads to increased DNA synthesis and older mice develop cholangiocarcinomas.[77] Gene expression profiling of livers from knockout mice has revealed selective down-regulation of genes involved in cholesterol biosynthesis,[78] an interesting finding given the potential for altered cell-cell interactions.

OTHER METABOLIC CONDITIONS

A few other metabolic conditions are associated with a low incidence of hepatic neoplasia (see **Table 1**). The mechanisms of carcinogenesis are similarly not understood in these disorders. Acute intermittent porphyria (OMIM 176000), an autosomal-dominant disorder of heme biosynthesis, has been reported to have relative risk of greater than 30 of developing HCC.[49,79] Defective bile salt transport and resultant cytotoxicity in progressive familial intrahepatic cholestasis-2 (OMIM 601847) may form the basis for the HCC and cholangiocarcinomas seen even in children less than 10 years age (**Fig. 3**).[80,81] Of late in developed countries, with the growing prevalence of pediatric obesity, various forms of nonalcoholic fatty liver disease, including nonalcoholic steatohepatitis, have become common causes of chronic liver disease in children. Nonalcoholic fatty liver disease, the histologic manifestation of the metabolic syndrome, is characterized by insulin resistance and oxidative stress, and is often associated with "cryptogenic cirrhosis."[82,83] A prospective cohort study in a Japanese population has revealed an approximately 7% incidence of HCC in patients with nonalcoholic steatohepatitis.[84] Studies on the molecular pathogenesis of cirrhosis and hepatic neoplasia in these disorders are essential, because this epidemic seems destined to replace hepatitis B viral infection as the leading antecedent of HCC in the world.

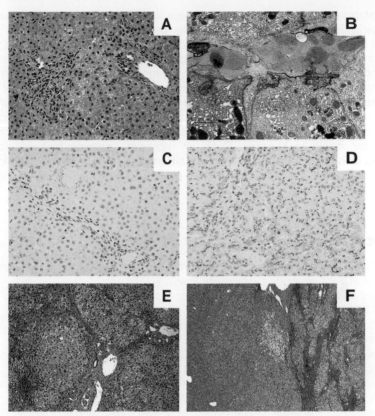

Fig. 3. Liver pathology in progressive familial intrahepatic cholestasis-2. (*A*) Mild periportal inflammation and canalicular bile stasis seen in the liver biopsy of an 8-month-old child. (*B*) Ultrastructural demonstration of amorphous canalicular bile. (*C*) Immunohistochemistry for bile salt export protein (ABCB11) shows complete lack of canalicular staining in the patient (*C*) as compared with the control (*D*) (Immunochemistry performed by Alex Knisely, King's College Hospital Liver Unit). (*E*) Eight years later, the patient presented with cirrhosis and cholestasis. (*F*) Liver adenoma in the resected specimen. (*A, E, F*: hematoxylin and eosin stain, original magnifications: *A, C-D* - 200x, *E* - 100x, *F* - 40x.)

DISCUSSION

Neoplasia in metabolic liver disease is a relatively rare complication of a group of individually rare disorders. For instance, homozygous PiZZ AAT deficiency, the most common genetic cause of liver disease in children, has an incidence of 1:1600 to 1:2000 in newborns.[85,86] In long-term follow-up studies by Sveger and others, only 10% to 15% had any biochemical evidence of liver disease at 25 years age[87,88]; even if all were eventually to develop HCC, this translates roughly to an incidence of 1:20,000 affected individuals. Similarly, the rate of children affected with tyrosinemia in Quebec[17] is approximately 1:17,000, the highest in the world. Nevertheless, the relative risk of developing HCC with the PiZZ genotype is significantly increased[50] (relative risk = 5)[49] and warrants close surveillance of affected individuals. By the estimated 15% incidence of HCC in tyrosinemic livers,[17] the risk of HCC is approximately 1:190,000 births.

Understanding of the molecular pathways involved in disease progression and carcinogenesis in metabolic disorders has benefited tremendously from studies in model organisms. Although the physiology of humans differs somewhat, several useful mouse knockouts (eg, $Fah^{-/-}$, $Atp7b^{-/-}$) have provided significant insight into pathogenic mechanisms.[40,89] One of the most significant advances in hereditary tyrosinemia over the past two decades has been the introduction of NTBC, a triketone herbicide that was first tested in rats before introduction in humans.[35] More recently, high-throughput approaches in genomics, transcriptomics, and metabolomics are currently making it possible to investigate these rare disorders with greater depth in humans. Such an unbiased "systems biology" approach has the added advantage of uncovering hitherto unknown or silent genetic modifiers that are likely to explain the variable penetrance seen in virtually all metabolic disorders.

REFERENCES

1. Suchy FJ, Sokol RJ, Balistreri WF. Liver disease in children. 3rd edition. Cambridge (UK): Cambridge University Press; 2007.
2. Scriver CR. The metabolic & molecular bases of inherited disease. 8th edition. New York: McGraw-Hill; 2001.
3. Speliotes EK. Genetics of common obesity and nonalcoholic fatty liver disease. Gastroenterology 2009;136(5):1492–5.
4. Schwimmer JB, Celedon MA, Lavine JE, et al. Heritability of nonalcoholic fatty liver disease. Gastroenterology 2009;136(5):1585–92.
5. Malaguarnera M, Di Rosa M, Nicoletti F, et al. Molecular mechanisms involved in NAFLD progression. J Mol Med 2009;87(7):679–95.
6. Roberts EA. Pediatric nonalcoholic fatty liver disease (NAFLD): a "growing" problem? J Hepatol 2007;46(6):1133–42.
7. O'Connor JA, Sokol RJ. Copper metabolism and copper storage disorders. In: Suchy FJ, Sokol RJ, Balistreri WF, editors. Liver disease in children. 3rd edition. Cambridge (UK): Cambridge University Press; 2007. p. 626–60.
8. Muller T, Schafer H, Rodeck B, et al. Familial clustering of infantile cirrhosis in Northern Germany: a clue to the etiology of idiopathic copper toxicosis. J Pediatr 1999;135(2 Pt 1):189–96.
9. Muller T, Feichtinger H, Berger H, et al. Endemic tyrolean infantile cirrhosis: an ecogenetic disorder. Lancet 1996;347(9005):877–80.
10. Jevon G, Dimmick J. Metabolic disorders in childhood. In: Russo P, Ruchelli ED, Piccoli DA, editors. Pathology of pediatric gastrointestinal and liver disease. 1st edition. New York: Springer-Verlag; 2004. p. 270–99.
11. Ishak KG. Inherited metabolic diseases of the liver. Clin Liver Dis 2002;6(2):455–79.
12. Finegold MJ. Hepatic tumors in childhood. In: Russo P, Ruchelli ED, Piccoli DA, editors. Pathology of pediatric gastrointestinal and liver disease. 1st edition. New York: Springer-Verlag; 2004. p. 300–46.
13. Emre S, McKenna GJ. Liver tumors in children. Pediatr Transplant 2004;8(6): 632–8.
14. Ghishan FK, Zawaideh M. Inborn errors of carbohydrate metabolism. In: Suchy FJ, Sokol RJ, Balistreri WF, editors. Liver disease in children. 3rd edition. Cambridge (UK): Cambridge University Press; 2007. p. 595–625.
15. Zhou H, Fischer HP. Liver carcinoma in PiZ alpha-1-antitrypsin deficiency. Am J Surg Pathol 1998;22(6):742–8.

16. Knisely AS, Narkewicz MR. Iron storage disorders. In: Suchy FJ, Sokol RJ, Balistreri WF, editors. Liver disease in children. 3rd edition. Cambridge (UK): Cambridge University Press; 2007. p. 661–76.
17. Mitchell G, Russo PA, Dubois J, et al. Tyrosinemia. In: Suchy FJ, Sokol RJ, Balistreri WF, editors. Liver disease in children. 3rd edition. Cambridge (UK): Cambridge University Press; 2007. p. 694–713.
18. Kamath BA, Spinner NB, Piccoli DA. Alagille syndrome. In: Suchy FJ, Sokol RJ, Balistreri WF, editors. Liver disease in children. 3rd edition. Cambridge (UK): Cambridge University Press; 2007. p. 326–45.
19. Jonas MM, Perez-Atayde AR. Fibrocystic liver disease. In: Suchy FJ, Sokol RJ, Balistreri WF, editors. Liver disease in children. 3rd edition. Cambridge (UK): Cambridge University Press; 2007. p. 928–42.
20. Litten JB, Tomlinson GE. Liver tumors in children. Oncologist 2008;13(7):812–20.
21. Fearon ER. Human cancer syndromes: clues to the origin and nature of cancer. Science 1997;278(5340):1043–50.
22. Laberge C. Hereditary tyrosinemia in a French Canadian isolate. Am J Hum Genet 1969;21(1):36–45.
23. Mitchell GA, Grompe M, Lambert M. Hypertyrosinemia. In: Scriver CR, Sly WS, Childs B, et al, editors. New York: McGraw-Hill; 2006. Available at: http:// genetics.accessmedicine.com. Accessed March 2010.
24. Grompe M, St-Louis M, Demers SI, et al. A single mutation of the fumarylacetoacetate hydrolase gene in French Canadians with hereditary tyrosinemia type I. N Engl J Med 1994;331(6):353–7.
25. Lindstedt S, Holme E, Lock EA, et al. Treatment of hereditary tyrosinaemia type I by inhibition of 4-hydroxyphenylpyruvate dioxygenase. Lancet 1992;340(8823):813–7.
26. Weinberg AG, Mize CE, Worthen HG. The occurrence of hepatoma in the chronic form of hereditary tyrosinemia. J Pediatr 1976;88(3):434–8.
27. Kvittingen EA, Rootwelt H, Brandtzaeg P, et al. Hereditary tyrosinemia type I. Self-induced correction of the fumarylacetoacetase defect. J Clin Invest 1993;91(4): 1816–21.
28. Kvittingen EA, Rootwelt H, Berger R, et al. Self-induced correction of the genetic defect in tyrosinemia type I. J Clin Invest 1994;94(4):1657–61.
29. Demers SI, Russo P, Lettre F, et al. Frequent mutation reversion inversely correlates with clinical severity in a genetic liver disease, hereditary tyrosinemia. Hum Pathol 2003;34(12):1313–20.
30. McKiernan PJ. Nitisinone in the treatment of hereditary tyrosinaemia type 1. Drugs 2006;66(6):743–50.
31. Russo PA, Mitchell GA, Tanguay RM. Tyrosinemia: a review. Pediatr Dev Pathol 2001;4(3):212–21.
32. van Spronsen FJ, Thomasse Y, Smit GP, et al. Hereditary tyrosinemia type I: a new clinical classification with difference in prognosis on dietary treatment. Hepatology 1994;20(5):1187–91.
33. Mieles LA, Esquivel CO, Van Thiel DH, et al. Liver transplantation for tyrosinemia. A review of 10 cases from the University of Pittsburgh. Dig Dis Sci 1990;35(1): 153–7.
34. Holme E, Lindstedt S. Nontransplant treatment of tyrosinemia. Clin Liver Dis 2000; 4(4):805–14.
35. Lock EA, Ellis MK, Gaskin P, et al. From toxicological problem to therapeutic use: the discovery of the mode of action of 2-(2-nitro-4-trifluoromethylbenzoyl)-1,3-cyclohexanedione (NTBC), its toxicology and development as a drug. J Inherit Metab Dis 1998;21(5):498–506.

36. Holme E, Lindstedt S. Tyrosinaemia type I and NTBC (2-(2-nitro-4-trifluoromethyl-benzoyl)-1,3-cyclohexanedione). J Inherit Metab Dis 1998;21(5):507–17.
37. Masurel-Paulet A, Poggi-Bach J, Rolland MO, et al. NTBC treatment in tyrosinae-mia type I: long-term outcome in French patients. J Inherit Metab Dis 2008;31(1): 81–7.
38. van Spronsen FJ, Bijleveld CM, van Maldegem BT, et al. Hepatocellular carci-noma in hereditary tyrosinemia type I despite 2-(2 nitro-4-3 trifluoro- methylben-zoyl)-1, 3-cyclohexanedione treatment. J Pediatr Gastroenterol Nutr 2005;40(1): 90–3.
39. Koelink CJ, van Hasselt P, van der Ploeg A, et al. Tyrosinemia type I treated by NTBC: how does AFP predict liver cancer? Mol Genet Metab 2006;89(4):310–5.
40. Grompe M, Lindstedt S, al-Dhalimy M, et al. Pharmacological correction of neonatal lethal hepatic dysfunction in a murine model of hereditary tyrosinaemia type I. Nat Genet 1995;10(4):453–60.
41. Endo F, Tanaka Y, Tomoeda K, et al. Animal models reveal pathophysiologies of tyrosinemias. J Nutr 2003;133(6 Suppl 1):2063S–7S.
42. Jorquera R, Tanguay RM. Fumarylacetoacetate, the metabolite accumulating in hereditary tyrosinemia, activates the ERK pathway and induces mitotic abnormal-ities and genomic instability. Hum Mol Genet 2001;10(17):1741–52.
43. Prieto-Alamo MJ, Laval F. Deficient DNA-ligase activity in the metabolic disease tyrosinemia type I. Proc Natl Acad Sci U S A 1998;95(21):12614–8.
44. Orejuela D, Jorquera R, Bergeron A, et al. Hepatic stress in hereditary tyrosine-mia type 1 (HT1) activates the AKT survival pathway in the fah-/- knockout mice model. J Hepatol 2008;48(2):308–17.
45. Perlmutter DH. Pathogenesis of chronic liver injury and hepatocellular carcinoma in alpha-1-antitrypsin deficiency. Pediatr Res 2006;60(2):233–8.
46. Wu Y, Whitman I, Molmenti E, et al. A lag in intracellular degradation of mutant alpha 1-antitrypsin correlates with the liver disease phenotype in homozygous PiZZ alpha 1-antitrypsin deficiency. Proc Natl Acad Sci U S A 1994;91(19):9014–8.
47. Pan S, Huang L, McPherson J, et al. Single nucleotide polymorphism-mediated translational suppression of endoplasmic reticulum mannosidase I modifies the onset of end-stage liver disease in alpha1-antitrypsin deficiency. Hepatology 2009;50(1):275–81.
48. Eriksson S, Carlson J, Velez R. Risk of cirrhosis and primary liver cancer in alpha 1-antitrypsin deficiency. N Engl J Med 1986;314(12):736–9.
49. Dragani TA. Risk of HCC: genetic heterogeneity and complex genetics. J Hepatol 2010;52(2):252–7.
50. Elzouki AN, Eriksson S. Risk of hepatobiliary disease in adults with severe alpha 1-antitrypsin deficiency (PiZZ): is chronic viral hepatitis B or C an additional risk factor for cirrhosis and hepatocellular carcinoma? Eur J Gastroenterol Hepatol 1996;8(10):989–94.
51. Hadzic N, Quaglia A, Mieli-Vergani G. Hepatocellular carcinoma in a 12-year-old child with PiZZ alpha1-antitrypsin deficiency. Hepatology 2006;43(1):194.
52. Zhou H, Ortiz-Pallardo ME, Ko Y, et al. Is heterozygous alpha-1-antitrypsin defi-ciency type PIZ a risk factor for primary liver carcinoma? Cancer 2000;88(12): 2668–76.
53. Perlmutter DH. Alpha-1 antitrypsin deficiency. In: Suchy FJ, Sokol RJ, Balistreri WF, editors. Liver disease in children. 3rd edition. Cambridge (UK): Cambridge University Press; 2007. p. 545–71.
54. Rudnick DA, Liao Y, An JK, et al. Analyses of hepatocellular proliferation in a mouse model of alpha-1-antitrypsin deficiency. Hepatology 2004;39(4):1048–55.

55. Kowdley KV. Iron, hemochromatosis, and hepatocellular carcinoma. Gastroenterology 2004;127(5 Suppl 1):S79–86.
56. Elmberg M, Hultcrantz R, Ekbom A, et al. Cancer risk in patients with hereditary hemochromatosis and in their first-degree relatives. Gastroenterology 2003; 125(6):1733–41.
57. Wallace DF, Subramaniam VN. Co-factors in liver disease: the role of HFE-related hereditary hemochromatosis and iron. Biochim Biophys Acta 2009;1790(7): 663–70.
58. Lehmann U, Wingen LU, Brakensiek K, et al. Epigenetic defects of hepatocellular carcinoma are already found in non-neoplastic liver cells from patients with hereditary haemochromatosis. Hum Mol Genet 2007;16(11):1335–42.
59. Vautier G, Bomford AB, Portmann BC, et al. p53 mutations in British patients with hepatocellular carcinoma: clustering in genetic hemochromatosis. Gastroenterology 1999;117(1):154–60.
60. Marrogi AJ, Khan MA, van Gijssel HE, et al. Oxidative stress and p53 mutations in the carcinogenesis of iron overload-associated hepatocellular carcinoma. J Natl Cancer Inst 2001;93(21):1652–5.
61. Chou JY, Mansfield BC. Mutations in the glucose-6-phosphatase-alpha (G6PC) gene that cause type Ia glycogen storage disease. Hum Mutat 2008;29(7):921–30.
62. Kishnani PS, Koeberl D, Chen YT. Glycogen storage diseases. In: Scriver CR, Sly WS, Childs B, et al, editors. New York: McGraw-Hill; 2006. Available at: http://genetics.accessmedicine.com. Accessed March 2010.
63. Lee PJ. Glycogen storage disease type I: pathophysiology of liver adenomas. Eur J Pediatr 2002;161(Suppl 1):S46–9.
64. Rake JP, Visser G, Labrune P, et al. Glycogen storage disease type I: diagnosis, management, clinical course and outcome. Results of the European Study on Glycogen Storage Disease Type I (ESGSD I). Eur J Pediatr 2002;161(Suppl 1):S20–34.
65. Matern D, Starzl TE, Arnaout W, et al. Liver transplantation for glycogen storage disease types I, III, and IV. Eur J Pediatr 1999;158(Suppl 2):S43–8.
66. Parker P, Burr I, Slonim A, et al. Regression of hepatic adenomas in type Ia glycogen storage disease with dietary therapy. Gastroenterology 1981;81(3):534–6.
67. Kishnani PS, Chuang TP, Bali D, et al. Chromosomal and genetic alterations in human hepatocellular adenomas associated with type Ia glycogen storage disease. Hum Mol Genet 2009;18(24):4781–90.
68. Franco LM, Krishnamurthy V, Bali D, et al. Hepatocellular carcinoma in glycogen storage disease type Ia: a case series. J Inherit Metab Dis 2005;28(2):153–62.
69. Nakamura T, Ozawa T, Kawasaki T, et al. Case report: hepatocellular carcinoma in type 1a glycogen storage disease with identification of a glucose-6-phosphatase gene mutation in one family. J Gastroenterol Hepatol 1999;14(6):553–8.
70. Bianchi L. Glycogen storage disease I and hepatocellular tumours. Eur J Pediatr 1993;152(Suppl 1):S63–70.
71. Demo E, Frush D, Gottfried M, et al. Glycogen storage disease type III-hepatocellular carcinoma a long-term complication? J Hepatol 2007;46(3):492–8.
72. Labrune P, Trioche P, Duvaltier I, et al. Hepatocellular adenomas in glycogen storage disease type I and III: a series of 43 patients and review of the literature. J Pediatr Gastroenterol Nutr 1997;24(3):276–9.
73. Cosme A, Montalvo I, Sanchez J, et al. [Type III glycogen storage disease associated with hepatocellular carcinoma]. Gastroenterol Hepatol 2005;28(10):622–5 [in Spanish].
74. de Moor RA, Schweizer JJ, van Hoek B, et al. Hepatocellular carcinoma in glycogen storage disease type IV. Arch Dis Child 2000;82(6):479–80.

75. Onal IK, Turhan N, Oztas E, et al. Hepatocellular carcinoma in an adult patient with type IV glycogen storage disease. Acta Gastroenterol Belg 2009;72(3):377–8.
76. Walshe JM, Waldenstrom E, Sams V, et al. Abdominal malignancies in patients with Wilson's disease. QJM 2003;96(9):657–62.
77. Huster D, Finegold MJ, Morgan CT, et al. Consequences of copper accumulation in the livers of the Atp7b-/- (Wilson disease gene) knockout mice. Am J Pathol 2006;168(2):423–34.
78. Huster D, Purnat TD, Burkhead JL, et al. High copper selectively alters lipid metabolism and cell cycle machinery in the mouse model of Wilson disease. J Biol Chem 2007;282(11):8343–55.
79. Andant C, Puy H, Bogard C, et al. Hepatocellular carcinoma in patients with acute hepatic porphyria: frequency of occurrence and related factors. J Hepatol 2000; 32(6):933–9.
80. Scheimann AO, Strautnieks SS, Knisely AS, et al. Mutations in bile salt export pump (ABCB11) in two children with progressive familial intrahepatic cholestasis and cholangiocarcinoma. J Pediatr 2007;150(5):556–9.
81. Knisely AS, Strautnieks SS, Meier Y, et al. Hepatocellular carcinoma in ten children under five years of age with bile salt export pump deficiency. Hepatology 2006;44(2):478–86.
82. Lewis JR, Mohanty SR. Nonalcoholic fatty liver disease: a review and update. Dig Dis Sci 2010;55(3):560–78.
83. Siegel AB, Zhu AX. Metabolic syndrome and hepatocellular carcinoma: two growing epidemics with a potential link. Cancer 2009;115(24):5651–61.
84. Hashimoto E, Yatsuji S, Tobari M, et al. Hepatocellular carcinoma in patients with nonalcoholic steatohepatitis. J Gastroenterol 2009;44(Suppl 19):89–95.
85. Perlmutter DH. Alpha-1-antitrypsin deficiency. Semin Liver Dis 1998;18(3): 217–25.
86. Sveger T. Liver disease in alpha1-antitrypsin deficiency detected by screening of 200,000 infants. N Engl J Med 1976;294(24):1316–21.
87. Sveger T, Eriksson S. The liver in adolescents with alpha 1-antitrypsin deficiency. Hepatology 1995;22(2):514–7.
88. Piitulainen E, Carlson J, Ohlsson K, et al. Alpha1-antitrypsin deficiency in 26-year-old subjects: lung, liver, and protease/protease inhibitor studies. Chest 2005; 128(4):2076–81.
89. Lutsenko S. Atp7b-/- mice as a model for studies of Wilson's disease. Biochem Soc Trans 2008;36(Pt 6):1233–8.

Advances in Hepatobiliary Pathology: Update for 2010

Jay H. Lefkowitch, MD

KEYWORDS

• Hepatology • Hepatic pathology • Hepatobiliary pathology
• Liver tumors • Cholangiocarcinoma
• Primary sclerosing cholangitis

The surfeit of recent publications on liver and biliary tract diseases offers many insights with impact on liver pathology and forms the basis of this update. Liver development, viral, autoimmune and drug hepatitis, and liver tumors are among the topics surveyed. Fatty liver disease is regularly encountered by the liver pathologist because of epidemic levels of obesity and diabetes, and the issues of portal inflammation in the steatotic liver as well as the morphologic types of steatohepatitis seen in children were addressed in several very helpful studies. An authoritative overview of hepatitis D virus (the delta agent) infection by Mario Rizzetto discussed the declining prevalence of the infection since the 1970s, and provided current statistics on rates of infectivity in several European cities. For biliary disease, important topics addressed included papers on the diversity of IgG4-related hepatobiliary disorders, pre-neoplastic lesions which precede cholangiocarcinoma in primary sclerosing cholangitis, and progress in elucidating the complex network of hepatobiliary transporter proteins located within the bile canalicular membranes.

LIVER BIOPSY AND DEVELOPMENTAL BIOLOGY

Those whose routine practice involves assessing liver biopsies will find of interest the 2009 American Association for the Study of Liver Disease (AASLD) position paper on liver biopsy, which covers a broad spectrum of topics, including what constitutes an adequate specimen (lengths of 2.0, 2.5, and 3.0 cm are discussed in "optimal" terms, along with bores of 18 to 19 gauge), the type of mass lesions commonly requiring diagnosis, types of needles, indications, and contraindications.[1]

Department of Pathology, College of Physicians and Surgeons, Columbia University, 630 West 168th Street–PH 15 West, Room 1574, New York, NY 10032, USA
E-mail address: jhl3@columbia.edu

Clin Liver Dis 14 (2010) 747–762
doi:10.1016/j.cld.2010.07.007   liver.theclinics.com
1089-3261/10/$ – see front matter © 2010 Published by Elsevier Inc.

The functional heterogeneity of the liver affects myriad hepatic synthetic and metabolic activities and from the embryologic period forward the subdivision of zonal activities is maintained through many signaling processes.[2] Chief among these is the Wnt signaling pathway and its primacy in directing liver zonation was shown in an elegant study of ammonia-metabolizing enzymes in mice.[3] In these animals (and in humans), Wnt signaling and activation of β-catenin results in expression of glutamine synthetase (one of the ammonia $\rightarrow$ urea metabolic enzymes) solely in the first several layers of hepatocytes surrounding terminal venules (**Fig. 1**) (in contrast to periportal hepatocytes, which preferentially express carbamyl phosphate synthetase 1).

Advances in sinusoidal cell biology and pathobiology were the subject of an update from a recent international symposium.[4]

DRUG-INDUCED LIVER INJURY

A report on chronic outcomes of drug-induced liver injury (DILI) monitored by the Swedish Adverse Drug Reaction Advisory Committee found (for 685 patients) a low prevalence of liver morbidity and mortality after 3 to 11 years of follow-up. Cirrhosis developed in 8 (1.2%) of 685. Five patients developed positive smooth muscle or antinuclear antibody (SMA and ANA, respectively) with liver biopsy features of autoimmune hepatitis (AIH).[5] A total of 23 (3.4%) of 685 developed long-term morbidity and mortality (including prolonged abnormal serum liver tests). In those who developed complications of cirrhosis, some of the agents held responsible were amoxicillin, ranidtidine, fluconazole, hydrochlorthiazide/amilorid, and fluoxetine. Protracted DILI with eventual normalization of liver tests was most often seen in patients who developed cholestatic/mixed injury. Ramachandran and Kakar[6] provided a helpful primer on the histopathology of drug hepatotoxicity with discussion and illustrations of acute hepatitis, pure cholestasis and cholestatic hepatitis, chronic hepatitis, sinusoidal obstruction syndrome, steatohepatitis, and selective lesions, such as stellate cell hyperplasia in hypervitaminosis A.

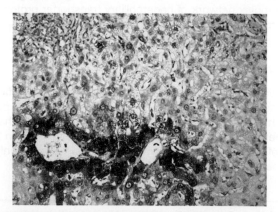

Fig. 1. Glutamine synthetase positivity in centrilobular hepatocytes. Localization of this urea cycle enzyme to the first several layers of perivenular hepatocytes is an example of the functional heterogeneity of the liver, encoded by Wnt/β-catenin signaling. (Explant liver, specific immunoperoxidase, original magnification ×100). (Topic discussed in Burke ZD, Reed KR, Phesse TJ, et al. Liver zonation occurs through a β-catenin-dependent, c-Myc-independent mechanism. Gastroenterology 2009;136:2316–24.)

The diagnostic problem of idiosyncratic DILI is its inherent unpredictability. The risk factors for DILI were reviewed recently[7] and the roles of age, gender, drug dosage, and variations in phase 1 and phase 2 drug-metabolizing/detoxifying enzymes were covered. The study reconfirmed the exclusivity of autoimmune-type DILI to women. The article further cited risk factors associated with specific agents. Cases of drug-induced AIH (DIAIH) from the Mayo Clinic showed nitrofurantoin and minocycline as the main causes and nearly all patients were female.[8] There were no significant differences in grade and stage between DIAIH and non-DIAIH or in the proportion of patients with ANA or SMA in that study. However, at baseline, 20% of "natural" AIH cases had cirrhosis, in contrast to no cases of DIAIH.

VIRAL HEPATITIS

A fascinating study in which hepatitis B virus (HBV) genotypes A2, B1, and C2 were inoculated into chimeric severe combined immunodeficiency mice containing human hepatocytes demonstrated different cytopathic differences in expression of ground-glass inclusions and immunohistochemical results for hepatitis B surface antigen (HBsAg) and hepatitis B core antigen (HBcAg) staining.[9] For example, after 22 to 25 weeks of infection , HBV/C2 animals demonstrated abundant ground-glass inclusions and fibrosis, whereas neither was seen in HBV/A2 and B1 animals. This type of study correlating HBV genotype with histologic phenotype has not yet been undertaken in humans, but would be diagnostically and pathogenetically useful for explaining the often-discordant immunohistochemical distribution of HBsAg and HBcAg in liver biopsy, explant, and postmortem tissue, as well as the mechanism(s) of the frequently varying regional positivity within hepatic lobules and/or cirrhotic nodules. An excellent review of liver biopsy in chronic hepatitis B covered the range of histopathology from acute to chronic hepatitis and cirrhosis, liver-cell dysplasia, and an overview of immunohistochemical staining for HBsAg and HBcAg.[10] The dysplastic nature of large cell liver-cell dysplasia ("large cell change") was supported by an article showing increases in Tp53 labeling, decreasing telomere length, and activation of cell cycle checkpoint markers including p21, p27, and p16.[11] However, other underlying hepatic histopathologic changes may modify large cell dysplasia, such as the presence of cholestasis (where preservation of normal cell checkpoint markers was found). Another study proposed the alternate view that large cell change represents a senescence lesion.[12] A comprehensive review on the natural course of chronic hepatitis B provided many points with relevance to liver biopsy assessment, such as the characteristic presence of minimal hepatitis seen for 1 to 3 decades (despite high levels of DNA replication) in children with perinatally acquired chronic hepatitis B.[13]

A superb update on hepatitis D virus (HDV, the delta agent) by Mario Rizzetto,[14] the principal investigator responsible for the identification of the virus 30 years ago, covers the 8 HDV genotypes and the general decline in HDV prevalence in Europe since the 1990s (but, nonetheless, with the ongoing prevalence in London of about 8.5% and in Italy of 8.1%). Therapy of HDV was also covered. The study by Schaper and colleagues[15] and an accompanying editorial[16] demonstrated the dynamic interplay of HBV and HCV viral activity in coinfected patients, with activity of both viruses found in 40.5% of patients, inactivity of both in 10.8%, activity of HDV alone (32.4%), and HBV alone in 16.2%. The latter figure contradicts the prevailing wisdom that HDV coinfection is necessarily suppressive of HBV replicative activity.

Progress in 20 years of HCV research (where at least 170 million people worldwide are symptomatically infected) was presented at a 2009 meeting at Nice and the key advances on viral entry, replication, assembly, and release, as well as the innate immune response (including roles of Toll-like receptors 3 and 8) and adaptive immunity (defect in CD8+ T cell induction), were delineated in a summary report.[17] HCV-induced oxidative stress (with production of superoxide and hydrogen peroxide) and the effects of nonstructural protein 3 (NS3) and NS5A HCV constituents on interfering with the transforming growth factor-beta (TGF-β) negative feedback loop (favoring fibrosis) were also described. A 2008 San Antonio meeting summary serves as a companion article concerning HCV research advances.[18] Liver biopsy in chronic hepatitis C has value in determining fibrosis stage to consider therapy and, according to a lengthy policy article on AASLD practice guidelines, currently should not be replaced in routine clinical practice by available noninvasive tests.[19] Increased expression of TGF-β2, vascular endothelial growth factor (VEGF) and CD34 are important in HCV-mediated hepatic angiogenesis, with a key role for HCV core protein in induction of both TGF-β2 and VEGF.[20] The possibility of occult HCV infection in individuals with negative serum HCV RNA but positive HCV antibody has been raised in a study of 66 cases meeting these serologic criteria, based on finding CD8+ T-cell portal tract infiltrates in 92% and fibrosis in 82% of the subjects with biopsies. Several investigators examined the "occult HCV infection" question with some skepticism.[21,22] HCV entry into the cell entails viral particles associating with circulating serum lipoproteins and initial attachment by binding with host cell low density lipoprotein (LDL) receptors. Exceptionally intriguing are recent data demonstrating that subsequent interactions with tight junction-associated claudin-1 and occluding proteins are also critical to viral entry.[23,24]

Several articles addressed the impact of HIV infection on the liver,[25,26] including discussions of coinfections with HBV and/or HCV. Progression of fibrosis between liver biopsies obtained over the course of 3 years occurred rapidly in a study of HIV-HCV-coinfected subjects from Spain.[27] The investigators pointing out that absent/mild lobular necroinflammation at baseline, achievement of response with HCV therapy and effective antiretroviral therapy were associated with slower progression of fibrosis.

COMMON VARIABLE IMMUNODEFICIENCY, FULMINANT HEPATITIS IN CHILDREN, AND NEONATAL HEMOCHROMATOSIS

A study of 13 liver biopsies from 10 patients with common variable immune deficiency showed mild portal tract and mild to moderate lobular lymphocytic infiltrates without plasma cells and scattered portal tract and/or lobular granulomas in 4 patients.[28] The cause of massive hepatic necrosis and submassive necrosis in infants and children was investigated in 23 patients with fulminant liver failure where 11 liver biopsies and 11 explants were available for review.[29] The etiology was determined in 36% and causes included drug reactions, AIH, mushroom poisoning, and other individual causes. The 2 basic patterns described were zonal coagulative necrosis and panlobular (nonzonal) necrosis. Central venulitis was seen in 76% of cases with panlobular necrosis and other changes described included lymphocytic infiltration of large duct/gallbladder epithelium and the presence of syncytial giant cell transformation (the latter in 18%). Ductular reaction ("neocholangiolar proliferation") was common in both patterns. The study pointed out the difficulties in establishing causation based on pathologic features in fulminant hepatitis. The investigators noted that the patients with AIH as the etiology showed a trend toward higher scores for plasma cells in both portal tracts and necrotic areas, as well as higher scores for eosinophil infiltrates in necrotic areas.

Severe necrosis of neonatal liver parenchyma with excess deposition of hepatocellular and extrahepatic iron has been termed neonatal hemochromatosis, although no known relationship to classical hereditary hemochromatosis or other primary types of genetic iron overload has been established. A recent study[30] used immunohistochemical staining for the terminal complement cascade (TCC) neoantigen that is formed after C9 polymerization with C5b-8 to form the membrane attack complex that is bound to the lipid membrane of the target cell or microbe. The TCC was localized in 100% of neonatal hemochromatosis cases to residual hepatocytes arranged in rosettes on their canalicular surfaces and to multinucleated giant hepatocytes. No staining or light staining was seen in control cases. The investigators propose that maternal IgG to an unknown alloantigen on hepatocytes crosses the placenta and activates complement with formation of the membrane attack complex. An accompanying editorial[31] put this hypothesis into perspective.

AUTOIMMUNE HEPATITIS

A review of advances in AIH[32] and the AASLD Practice Guidelines[33] provide extensive clinicopathologic data for establishing the diagnosis, including comprehensive discussions of the prevalent autoantibodies. The pathologic features are discussed, including the centrilobular histologic variant, which may be an early form of the disease that eventually transitions to (or is found in association with) the more classically described portal/periportal necroinflammatory form with lymphoplasmacytic interface hepatitis. Czaja and Manns[32] point out in their update that the autoantibody against which anti–liver-kidney microsome 1 (anti-LKM1) is formed is the cytoplasmic enzyme cytochrome monooxygenase CYP2D6, which has homologies with HCV, cytomegalovirus, and herpes simplex virus type 1, perhaps explaining why certain individuals with HCV infection (both before and after liver transplantation) develop features of AIH. Similarly, cross reactivity between HCV antigens and host-derived smooth muscle and nuclear antigens is cited as a "molecular mimicry" hypothesis behind certain cases of AIH. Atypical forms of AIH, including overlap syndromes and cases with absent serologic markers, were covered in an elaborate review.[34] A study of Swedish patients with AIH found increased hepatobiliary cancer (predominantly hepatocellular carcinoma [HCC], with one case of cholangiocarcinoma) and non-Hodgkin's lymphoma as the major malignancies.

BILIARY DISEASE

Many cholestatic disorders (particularly in infancy and childhood) are now linked to either mutations in or inhibition/reduced expression of canalicular bile salt transport proteins and recent reviews have provided insights into their variety.[35,36] The physiologic and phenotypic effects of bile canalicular transport protein mutations are diverse and relate to both the variety of the mutations and the presence of heterozygous mutations. Progressive familial inhtrahepatic cholestasis type 1 (PFIC-1) and benign recurrent intrahepatic cholestasis type 1 (BRIC-1) are examples of contrasting disorders, both related to mutation in *ATP8B1 (FIC1)*.[37] The former presents as a low/normal serum gamma glutamyl transferase bland canalicular cholestasis without giant cell transformation in the first 6 months of life associated with pruritus and later periportal fibrosis, sometimes with bile duct loss, and later cirrhosis. BRIC-1 results in episodic cholestasis, which may be triggered by release of cytokines during intermittent febrile illnesses.[38] The FIC1 protein normally serves as a flippase for movement of phosphatidylserine from the outer to the inner leaflet of the canalicular membrane, thereby maintaining an outer canalicular membrane enriched in phosphatidylcholine, sphingomyelin, and cholesterol, which serve as protection against detergent action of bile salts, and also for normal transmembrane transporter function. Instability of the mutated FIC1 protein in PFIC-1 results in complete lack of its expression on the canalicular membrane, thought to be attributable to failure of interaction with the CDC50A protein that normally translocates the protein from the endoplasmic reticulum to the canalicular membrane.[38] In contrast, FIC1 is displayed normally on the canalicular membrane in BRIC-1.[38] Loss of membrane expression of ATP8B1 recently was shown in cultured hepatocytes to produce absent or shortened F-actin filaments at the bile canalicular membrane surface, with resultant constitutive defects in formation of the apical brush border microvilli (loss of approximately 50% of microvilli on the apical membrane[39,40]). These remarkable new insights into the importance of the canalicular transport proteins in membrane stability and function have been extended into related areas, such as intrahepatic cholestasis of pregnancy (where transporter function and integrity can be affected by pregnancy-related sex hormones) and drug-induced cholestasis (where certain drugs transported across the canaliculus may selectively affect transporter proteins).[35,36] An alloimmune type of reaction against the bile salt export pump (BSEP) was described in 3 children who underwent liver transplantation for PFIC-2 (a recessive mutation in *ABCB11*, the gene encoding BSEP on canaliculi).[41] Anti-BSEP antibodies developed as a component of the graft rejection response after transplantation, phenotypically mimicking the original disease, with cholestatic episodes. Amelioration of the humoral response by immunosuppression relieved the cholestasis. The investigators discussed analogous immune responses to disease-causing mutated gene products in cardiac and renal transplant patients with Becker muscular dystrophy and Alport syndrome, respectively.

Primary biliary cirrhosis (PBC) was reviewed,[42,43] including possible roles of xenobiotics that cross-react with the lipoic acid–binding domain of the mitochondrial target 2-oxo-acid dehydrogenase and infection by the gram-negative bacterium *Novosphingobium aromaticivorous*. Altered interleukin-12 signaling may increase susceptibility to infection and increase the risk of autoimmune activity in PBC.[44] A correlative study looking at serum liver tests and liver biopsy findings in 252 patients with PBC, antimitochondrial antibody (AMA)-negative PBC, and with AIH-PBC overlap[45] found associations between increased aspartate aminotransferase (AST) and the overlap group, between increased mean AST and portal fibrosis in AMA-positive PBC, and increasing bilirubin levels in PBC related to the stage of fibrosis. The investigators also highlighted the presence of concentric periductal fibrosis in 17.7% of their PBC cases, a feature that could result in the mistaken diagnosis of primary sclerosing cholangitis (PSC). Other conspicuous findings included steatosis in 50.0% of the biopsy and lobular granulomas in 22.8% of the PBC specimens, the latter usually small, poorly defined, and consisting of histiocytes. In 2 European centers (Barcelona and Padova), there was a low prevalence of HCC in PBC (3.3%) and, of multiple risk factors assessed, advanced histologic stage was the only significant one.[46] When PBC must be distinguished from possible AIH, immunostaining for IgM and IgG shows a predominance of IgM plasma cells in the former and IgG plasma cells in the latter.[47,48]

Guidelines on the diagnosis and management of PSC were recently put forth by ASLD[49] and the European Association for the Study of the Liver,[50] with the latter document also covering the spectrum of cholestatic diseases from infancy and childhood to adulthood with several useful tables. A review of PSC[51] provided useful statistics on its incidence, proposed etiologies, the characteristics of small-duct PSC, and the development of cholangiocarcinoma in some 10% to 30% of patients with PSC. A genome-wide single nucleotide polymorphism (SNP) microarray study,[52] in addition to supporting an association with HLA, found 3 non-HLA susceptibility loci and respective gene products, which are candidates for involvement in PSC: (1) at chromosome *2q35*, G-protein-coupled bile acid receptor 1 (GPBAR1); (2) at chromosome *3p21*, macrophage stimulating 1 (MST1) (known to be associated with ulcerative colitis, Crohn disease, and inflammatory bowel disease in PSC), and in its wild-type state serving to inhibit lipopolysaccharide-induced nuclear factor kappa-beta signaling); and (3) on chromosome *13q31*, the glypican-5/glypican-6 (GPC5/GPC6) region (particularly GPC6, which is involved in susceptibility to inflammatory conditions). Given the long-term risks of cholangiocarcinoma (CCA) in PSC, surveillance for preneoplastic bile duct epithelial changes is important. The problem of surveillance is the relatively low yield seen on needle liver biopsies.[53] By taking additional sections of hilar and large intrahepatic bile ducts from explant livers with PSC, a spectrum of biliary epithelial changes was demonstrated recently[54] that further supports the proposed biliary metaplasia → dysplasia → carcinoma sequence in the development CCA. The investigators found dysplasia in 83% of PSC explants with CCA and in 36% of PSC explants without CCA. The metaplasias included mucinous, pyloric, intestinal, and pancreatic acinar types, and there were several grades of flat and papillary biliary intraepithelial neoplasia (BilIN). Identification of intestinal metaplasia in bile ducts (**Fig. 2**) appears to be the most significant finding, as it was a predictor of biliary dysplasia and was present in livers with CCA. CCA may also develop in cirrhosis attributable to alcohol and chronic hepatitis C, and a similar extensive large duct explant sampling study[55] found BilIN types 1 and 2 prominently (approximately 90%) in alcoholic and alcohol + HCV cirrhosis, but only a small number of cases (4%) with BilIN type 3.

Since the condition autoimmune pancreatitis (AIP) was described,[56] increasing diversity in extrapancreatic autoimmune IgG4 syndromes have been reported. A recent review discussed the potential overlapping features of IgG4-associated cholangitis (IAC) with PSC.[57] An assessment of PSC explants showed 23% to contain periductal IgG4+ plasma cell infiltrates.[58] Although other features of IAC (eg, obliterative phlebitis) were not seen in these PSC explants, the IgG4+ subjects had more aggressive clinical courses of their PSC and shorter duration to liver transplantation than the

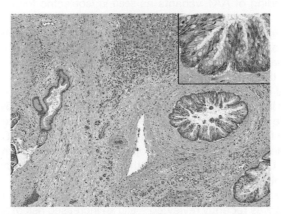

Fig. 2. Intestinal metaplasia of large bile duct epithelium. Metaplasia, dysplasia, and carcinoma may develop within the epithelium of bile ducts, and surveillance of large bile ducts such as that seen on the right in this field is important in primary sclerosing cholangitis. The duct at right shows a papillary-type epithelium with intestinal metaplasia and goblet cells (*inset*). Compare the altered duct epithelium to the normal large caliber bile duct at left (hematoxylin and eosin [H&E] stain, original magnification ×40; *inset*, original magnification ×200, explant liver).

IgG4-negative cases. Changes described in liver biopsies in IAC[59] include more than 10 IgG4+ plasma cells per high-power field, accentuation of inflammatory infiltrates around portal vein branches (rather than around bile ducts), and inflammatory nodules containing spindle-shaped fibroblasts, lymphocytes, and plasma cells. IAC was described in 2 HLA-identical siblings with ulcerative colitis[60] and an IgG4-positive histologic variant of AIH was also reported.[61] The causes and pathology of secondary sclerosing cholangitis, including discussion of ischemic cholangiopathy, biliary stricture, and infectious cholangiopathies, were reviewed.[62]

The gastrointestinal tract, pancreas, and liver of CFTR−/− pigs as models of human cystic fibrosis were examined and showed features closely resembling the "focal biliary fibrosis" seen in humans.[63] Ductular reaction was a major lesion and accompanied by mild fibrosis and intraductal aggregates of mucin and inflammatory cells as well as choleliths. The embryologic development of bile ducts from the periportal ductal plate ("bile duct tubulogenesis") involves a number of signaling factors, and Antoniou and colleagues[64] used a knockout mouse model to propose that Homolog of Hairy/Enhancer of Split-1 (HES1), a mediator of Notch signaling, is expressed by ductal pate cells near portal tracts and converts asymmetric primitive ductal structures to mature symmetric tubes that form the constitutive bile ducts. A report on the morphology of Pkd2$^{ws25/-}$ mice, an animal model generated by inducing two mutations in the *Pkd2* gene resulting in a null mutation coupled to an unstable recombinant-sensitive allele, described and illustrated the variety of cholangiocyte-lined cysts and their ultrastructurally abnormal primary cilia (shortened, with bulbous structures at their tips) in a homologous model of human autosomal dominant polycystic kidney disease (ADPKD).[65] These cysts progressively increase through continuous epithelial proliferation and apoptosis and fluid secretion, coupled to increased adjacent fibrous stroma.

METABOLIC DISEASES AND FATTY LIVER DISEASE

Overviews of alpha-1-antitrypsin (AAT) deficiency were published,[66,67] one of which illustrated the banding of AAT variants as seen in isoelectric focusing.[66] A study of AAT deficiency in explant livers where *HFE* mutational status was known[68] found a significant increase in H63D mutations, a bimodal distribution of iron accumulation of grades 1 and 3 and, overall, an increased association of high-grade (grade 3–4) iron overload in AAT-deficiency explants in association with *HFE* mutations. The investigators also suggest that individuals with HCV-cirrhosis (used as controls in their study) who show excess iron may also harbor *HFE* mutations, a useful point when considering the cause of iron overload in explant specimens. Another iron overload problem, ferroportin disease (type 4 hereditary hemochromatosis), was analyzed in a family with macrophage-type ferroportin disease and a novel mutation in the *SLC40A1* ferroportin gene.[69] Laser scanning confocal microscopy found the mutated ferroportin localized to the perinuclear Golgi region (and not to the plasma membrane where ferroportin is normally functionally active).

Fatty liver disease receives increasing coverage in publications on liver disease. Alcoholic hepatitis was recently reviewed[70] and an increased risk of nonalcoholic fatty liver disease (NAFLD) in siblings and parents of children with NAFLD was reported.[71,72] Increased hepatocellular iron and *HFE* mutations contributed a significant risk of increased fibrosis in NAFLD in an Italian study,[73] although previous data from the nonalcoholic steatohepatitis (NASH) Clinical Research Network had indicated the importance of reticuloendothelial system iron staining in the advanced fibrosis seen in NASH.[74] After liver transplantation, metabolic syndrome may contribute to

NAFLD/NASH and the prevalence of factors such as diabetes and hyperlipidemia were assessed in a review.[75]

Increased oxidative stress and gender-related variations in cytochrome P-450 enzymes were responsible for increased formation of Mallory-Denk bodies in male mice compared with females in an experimental study.[76] One specific component of NAFLD, the degree of portal tract chronic inflammation, was addressed in an important article[77] that demonstrated a range from none to mild and to "more than mild," with the latter a marker of increased histologic severity and advanced stages of fibrosis (**Fig. 3**). The diagnosis and management of pediatric NAFLD were comprehensively examined in a report that illustrated the distinctive portal tract–based "type 2" NASH pediatric lesion with chronic inflammation and periportal fibrosis.[78] However, a multicenter study found that most children with NASH had overlapping features of NASH 1 and NASH 2.[79] This study indicates the importance of careful evaluation of both centrilobular and portal/periportal regions when assessing liver specimens in children (not leastwise in adults).

A 10-year autopsy series of diabetic subjects found 12% (of 159 cases) to have diabetic hepatosclerosis (DHS), a nonzonal perisinusoidal fibrosis, and an association with diabetic nephropathy, suggesting that DHS is a hepatic form of microvascular disease.[80] Many studies now provide data linking NASH to HCC, and a study from Tokyo further demonstrated associations of older age and advanced fibrosis in NASH with HCC.[81] An important aspect of the study was the presence of only F1-F2 fibrosis in 12% of the HCC cases, indicating that in certain individuals the risk of cancer develops before late-stage NASH. Alcohol consumption[82] and iron overload[83] increase the risk of NASH progression to HCC.

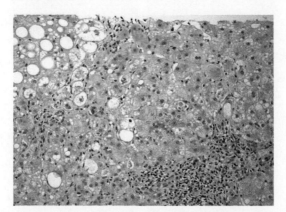

Fig. 3. Portal tract inflammation in nonalcoholic fatty liver disease. The mild macrovesicular steatosis in this case is associated with moderate chronic lymphocytic inflammation of the portal tract (*lower right*) and considerable NASH in the centrilobular region at upper left. The features of NASH seen here include the steatosis, hepatocyte ballooning, pericellular inflammation, and possible Mallory-Denk bodies in the swollen hepatocyte at upper left top. "More-than-mild" chronic portal inflammation in NAFLD correlates with worse histologic severity and advanced disease (H&E stain, original magnification ×100, needle biopsy). (Topic discussed in Brunt EM, Kleiner DE, WIlson LA, et al. Portal chronic inflammation in nonalcoholic fatty liver disease (NAFLD): a histologic marker of advanced NAFLD—clinicopathologic correlations from the Nonalcoholic Steatohepatitis Clinical Research Network. Hepatology 2009;49:809–20.)

LIVER TUMORS

Calcifying nested stromal-epithelial tumors, also known under the terms "ossifying stromal-epithelial tumor," "desmoplastic nested spindle cell tumor," and "nested stromal-epithelial tumor," are rare liver tumors with distinctive pathologic features and 9 cases were reported from the Armed Forces Institute of Pathology.[84] The tumor grows in irregular, zig-zag-like sharply circumscribed nests and islands of spindled to epithelioid cells surrounded by desmoplastic stroma (**Fig. 4**). The cases reported ranged from age 2 to 33 years and there were foci of calcifications with or without ossification within the tumor nests. All cases showed at least focal positivity for the keratin cocktail AE1/AE3/LP34; focal CD56 staining was found in 2 of 5 cases studied, and the stroma stained for smooth muscle actin and vimentin. Immunohistochemistry provides useful information in distinguishing among several benign tumors. In liver-cell adenomas, lesional hepatocytes may show considerable positivity with cytokeratin 7 immunostaining (**Fig. 5**), as demonstrated in a very helpful study that also examined CD34 and neuronal cell adhesion molecule comparative immunostain results for adenoma and focal nodular hyperplasia.[85] Immunostaining for glutamine synthetase shows maplike large areas (often surrounding veins, but not near fibrous septa containing arteries and ductules) in focal nodular hyperplasia.[86] In adenomas, the staining

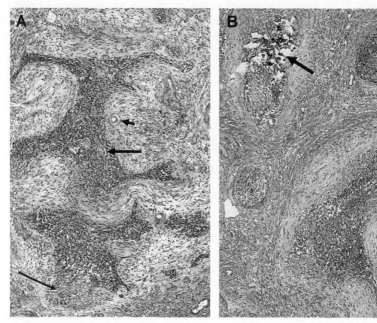

Fig. 4. Calcifying nested stromal-epithelial tumor. This unusual neoplasm features a prominent stromal component in combination with irregular islands of epithelioid and/or spindled cells. (*A*) Irregular, zig-zag pattern islands of spindled cells are present and often are adjacent to bile duct structures (*short arrow*) or contain developing bile duct structures (*long arrow*). More epithelioid, plump tumor cells may be evident (*thin arrow at bottom*). (*B*) Nests of epithelioid/spindle cells may show calcifications (*arrow*) (*A* and *B*, H&E stain, original magnification ×40, explant liver). (Topic discussed in Makhlouf HR, Abdul-AL HM, Wang G, et al. Calcifying nested stromal-epithelial tumors of the liver. A clinicopathologic, immunohistochemical, and molecular genetic study of 9 cases with a long-term follow-up. Am J Surg Pathol 2009;33:976–83.)

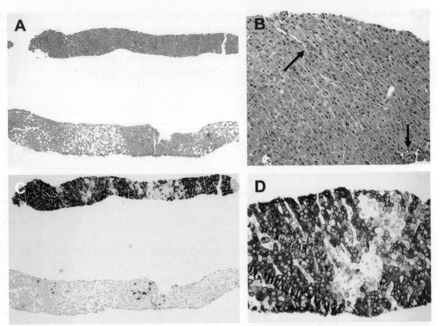

Fig. 5. Cytokeratin 7 immunohistochemistry in liver-cell adenoma. (*A*) Needle biopsy from one of several liver masses contained 2 discordant liver cores: the core with steatosis at bottom was normal and contained normal portal tracts, whereas the homogeneous benign-appearing liver tissue in the core at top was liver-cell adenoma. (*B*) Thickened plates of hepatocytes with interspersed isolated vessels (*arrows*) were present in the lesion. Note the absence of fat and atypia. (*C*) Cytokeratin 7 immunostain shows marked differences in staining of the biopsy cores, with only focal staining of a few bile ductular structures in the fatty liver below, and diffuse staining of the lesional adenomatous tissue at top. (*D*) The adenoma shows many cells positive with cytokeratin 7, whereas a few of the larger, more mature hepatocytes have lost the positivity of the lesional tissue (*A* and *B*: H&E stain; *C* and *D*: specific immunoperoxidase; original magnifications, *A* and *C*: ×25, *B* and *D*: ×100). (Topic discussed in Ahmad I, Iyer A, Marginean CE, et al. Diagnostic use of cytokeratins, CD34, and neuronal cell adhesion molecule staining in focal nodular hyperplasia and hepatic adenoma. Hum Pathol 2009;40:726–34.)

was diffuse and not maplike. Because HCC may histologically show a "clear-cell" pattern resembling renal cell carcinoma, and because HCC and renal cell carcinoma share other staining features (eg, negativity with immunostains for cytokeratins 7 and 20, PAS positivity, loss of glycogen with diastase pretreatment), the immunostain positivity of renal cell carcinoma for PAX8 can be a tie-breaker in difficult cases.[87]

SUMMARY

New publications have provided extensive information that affects liver histopathology, including articles on the morphologic changes in chronic hepatitis B and C, large cell liver-cell dysplasia, and immunostaining for cytokeratin 7 and CD34 in the evaluation of hepatic adenomas and focal nodular hyperplasia. More extensive sampling of large bile ducts and hilar ducts from primary sclerosing cholangitis explants allowed identification of several types of bile duct epithelial metaplasia (with intestinal metaplasia associated with increased risk of dysplasia and cholangio-carcinoma). In children with NAFLD, careful examination of centrilobular and portal/periportal regions is advisable to recognize and discriminate types 1 and 2 NASH. IgG4-related liver and biliary diseases and neonatal hemochromatosis are among other conditions that received attention in recently surveyed articles.

REFERENCES

1. Rockey DC, Caldwell SH, Goodman ZD, et al. Liver biopsy. Hepatology 2009;49: 1017–44.
2. Lemaigre FP. Mechanisms of liver development: concepts for understanding liver disorders and design of novel therapies. Gastroenterology 2009;137:62–79.
3. Burke ZD, Reed KR, Phesse TJ, et al. Liver zonation occurs through a b-catenin-dependent, c-Myc-independent mechanism. Gastroenterology 2009;136: 2316–24.
4. Smedsrod B, LeCouteur D, Ikejima K, et al. Hepatic sinusoidal cells in health and disease: update from the 14th International Symposium. Liver Int 2009;29:490–9.
5. Björnsson E, Davidsdottir L. The long-term follow-up after idiosyncratic drug-induced liver injury with jaundice. J Hepatol 2009;50:511–7.
6. Ramachandran R, Kakar S. Histological patterns in drug-induced liver disease. J Clin Pathol 2009;62:481–92.
7. Chalasani N, Björnsson E. Risk factors for idiosyncratic drug-induced injury. Gastroenterology 2010;138:2246–59.
8. Björnsson E, Talwalkar J, Treeprasertsuk S, et al. Drug-induced autoimmune hepatitis: clinical characteristics and prognosis. Hepatology 2010;51:2040–8.
9. Sugiyama M, Tanaka Y, Kurbanov F, et al. Direct cytopathic effects of particular hepatitis B virus genotypes in severe combined immunodeficiency transgenic with urokinase-type plasminogen activator mouse with human hepatocytes. Gastroenterology 2009;136:652–62.
10. Mani H, Kleiner DE. Liver biopsy findings in chronic hepatitis B. Hepatology 2009; 49:S61–71.
11. Kim H, Oh B-K, Roncalli M, et al. Large liver cell change in hepatitis B virus-related liver cirrhosis. Hepatology 2009;50:752–62.
12. Ikeda H, Sasaki M, Sato Y, et al. Large cell change of hepatocytes in chronic viral hepatitis represents a senescent-related lesion. Hum Pathol 2009;40:1774–82.
13. Fattovich G, Bortolotti F, Donato F. Natural history of chronic hepatitis B: special emphasis on disease progression and prognostic factors. J Hepatol 2008;48: 335–52.
14. Rizzetto M. Hepatitis D: thirty years after. J Hepatol 2009;50:104–1050.
15. Schaper M, Rodriguez-Frias F, Jardi R, et al. Quantitative longitudinal evaluations of hepatitis delta virus RNA and hepatitis B virus DNA shows a dynamic, complex replicative profile in chronic hepatitis B and D. J Hepatol 2010;52:658–64.
16. Wedemeyer H. Re-emerging interest in hepatitis delta: new insights into the dynamic interplay between HBV and HDV. J Hepatol 2010;52:627–9.
17. Pawlotsky J-M, Cocquerel L, Durantel D, et al. HCV research 20 years after discovery: a summary of the 16th International Symposium on hepatitis C virus and related viruses. Gastroenterology 2010;138:6–12.
18. Lanford RE, Evans MJ, Lohmann V, et al. The accelerating pace of HCV research: a summary of the 15th international symposium on hepatitis C virus and related viruses. Gastroenterology 2009;136:9–16.

19. Ghany MG, Strader DB, Thomas DL, et al. Diagnosis, management, and treatment of hepatitis C: an update. Hepatology 2009;49:1335–74.
20. Hassan M, Selimovic D, Ghozlan H, et al. Hepatitis C virus core protein triggers hepatic angiogenesis by a mechanism including multiple pathways. Hepatology 2009;49:1469–82.
21. Welker M-W, Zeuzem S. Occult hepatitis C: how convincing are the current data? Hepatology 2009;49:665–75.
22. Pham TNQ, Coffin CS, Michalak TI. Occult hepatitis C virus infection: what does it mean? Liver Int 2010;30:502–11.
23. Ploss A, Evans MJ, Gaysinskaya VA, et al. Human occludin is a hepatitis C virus entry factor required for infection of mouse cells. Nature 2009;457:882–6.
24. Liu S, Yang W, Shen L, et al. Tight junction proteins claudin-1 and occludin control hepatitis C virus entry and are downregulated during infection to prevent superinfection. J Virol 2009;83:2011–4.
25. Sulkowski MS. Viral hepatitis and HIV coinfection. J Hepatol 2008;48:353–67.
26. Sherman KE, Soriano V, Chung RT. Human immunodeficiency virus and liver disease: conference proceedings. Hepatology 2010;51:1046–54.
27. Macías J, Berenguer J, Japón MA, et al. Fast fibrosis progression between repeated liver biopsies in patients coinfected with human immunodeficiency virus/hepatitis C virus. Hepatology 2009;50:1056–63.
28. Daniels JA, Torbenson M, Vivekanandan P, et al. Hepatitis in common variable immunodeficiency. Hum Pathol 2009;40:484–8.
29. Kirsch R, Yap J, Roberts EA, et al. Clinicopathologic spectrum of massive and submassive hepatic necrosis in infants and children. Hum Pathol 2009;40:516–26.
30. Pan X, Kelly S, Melin-ALdana H, et al. Novel mechanism of fetal hepatocyte injury in congenital alloimmune hepatitis involves the terminal complement cascade. Hepatology 2010;51:2061–8.
31. Knisely AS, Vergani D. "Neonatal hemochromatosis": a re-vision. Hepatology 2010;51:1888–90.
32. Czaja AJ, Manns MP. Advances in the diagnosis, pathogenesis, and management of autoimmune hepatitis. Gastroenterology 2010;139:58–72.
33. Manns MP, Czaja AJ, Gorham JD, et al. Diagnosis and management of autoimmune hepatitis. Hepatology 2010;51:2193–213.
34. Czaja AJ, Bayraktar Y. Non-classical phenotypes of autoimmune hepatitis and advances in diagnosis and treatment. World J Gastroenterol 2009;15:2314–28.
35. Wagner M, Zollner G, Trauner M. New molecular insights into the mechanisms of cholestasis. J Hepatol 2009;51:565–80.
36. Stapelbroek JM, van Erpecum KJ, Klomp LWJ, et al. Liver disease associated with canalicular transport defects: current and future therapies. J Hepatol 2010;52:258–71.
37. Paulusma CC, Elferink RPJO, Jansen PLM. Progressive familial intrahepatic cholestasis type 1. Semin Liver Dis 2010;30:117–24.
38. Folmer DE, van der Mark VA, Ho-Mok KS, et al. Differential effects of progressive familial intrahepatic cholestasis type 1 and benign recurrent intrahepatic cholestasis type 1 mutations on canalicular localization of ATP8B1. Hepatology 2009;50:1597–605.
39. Verhulst PM, van der Velden LM, Oorschot V, et al. A flippase-independent function of ATP8B1, the protein affected in familial intrahepatic cholestasis type 1, is required for apical protein expression and microvillus formation in polarized epithelial cells. Hepatology 2010;51:2049–60.

40. Dawson PA. Liver disease without flipping: new functions of ATP8B1, the protein affected in familial intrahepatic cholestasis type 1. Hepatology 2010;51:1885–7.
41. Jara P, Hierro L, Martínez-Fernández P, et al. Recurrence of bile salt export pump deficiency after liver transplantation. N Engl J Med 2009;361:1359–67.
42. Poupon R. Primary biliary cirrhosis: a 2010 update. J Hepatol 2010;52:745–58.
43. Selmi C, Zuin M, Gershwin ME. The unfinished business of primary biliary cirrhosis. J Hepatol 2008;49:451–60.
44. Hirschfield GM, Liu X, Xu C, et al. Primary biliary cirrhosis associated with HLA, IL12A, and IL12RB2 variants. N Engl J Med 2009;360:2544–55.
45. Drebber U, Mueller JJM, Klein E, et al. Liver biopsy in primary biliary cirrhosis: clinicopathological data and stage. Pathol Int 2009;59:546–54.
46. Cavazza A, Caballería L, Floreani A. Incidence, risk factors, and survival of hepatocellular carcinoma in primary biliary cirrhosis: comparative analysis from two centers. Hepatology 2009;50:1162–8.
47. Daniels JA, Torbenson M, Anders RA, et al. Immunostaining of plasma cells in primary biliary cirrhosis. Am J Clin Pathol 2009;131:243–9.
48. Moreira RK, Revetta F, Koehler E, et al. Diagnostic utility of IgG and IgM immunohistochemistry in autoimmune liver disease. World J Gastroenterol 2010;16:453–7.
49. Chapman R, Fevery J, Kalloo A, et al. Diagnosis and management of primary sclerosing cholangitis. Hepatology 2010;51:660–78.
50. European Association for the Study of the Liver. EASL clinical practice guidelines: management of cholestatic liver diseases. J Hepatol 2009;51:237–67.
51. Maggs JRL, Chapman RW. An update on primary sclerosing cholangitis. Curr Opin Gastroenterol 2008;24:377–83.
52. Karlsen TH, Franke A, Melum E, et al. Genome-wide association analysis in primary sclerosing cholangitis. Gastroenterology 2010;138:1102–11.
53. Fleming KA, Boberg KM, Glaumann H, et al. Biliary dysplasia as a marker of cholangiocarcinoma in primary sclerosing cholangitis. J Hepatol 2001;34:360–5.
54. Lewis JT, Talwalkar JA, Rosen CB, et al. Precancerous bile duct pathology in end-stage primary sclerosing cholangitis, with and without cholangiocarcinoma. Am J Surg Pathol 2010;34:27–34.
55. Wu T-T, Levy M, Correa AM, et al. Biliary intraepithelial neoplasia in patients without chronic biliary disease. Analysis of liver explants with alcoholic cirrhosis, hepatitis C infection, and noncirrhotic liver diseases. Cancer 2009;115:4564–75.
56. Yoshida K, Toki F, Takeuchi T, et al. Chronic pancreatitis caused by an autoimmune abnormality. Proposal of the concept of autoimmune pancreatitis. Dig Dis Sci 1995;40:1561–8.
57. Webster GJM, Pereira SP, Chapman RW. Autoimmune pancreatitis/IgG4-associated cholangitis and primary sclerosing cholangitis—overlapping or separate diseases? J Hepatol 2009;51:398–402.
58. Zhang L, Lewis JT, Abraham SC, et al. IgG4+ plasma cell infiltrates in liver explants with primary sclerosing cholangitis. Am J Surg Pathol 2010;34:88–94.
59. Deshpande V, Sainani NI, Chung RT, et al. IgG4-associated cholangitis: a comparative histological and immunophenotypic study with primary sclerosing cholangitis on liver biopsy material. Mod Pathol 2009;22:1287–95.
60. Dastis SN, Latinne D, Sempoux C, et al. Ulcerative colitis associated with IgG4 cholangitis: similar features in two HLA identical siblings. J Hepatol 2009;51:601–5.
61. Chung H, Watanabe T, Kudo M, et al. Identification and characterization of IgG4-associated autoimmune hepatitis. Liver Int 2010;30:222–31.

62. Ruemmele P, Hofstaedter F, Gelbmann CM. Secondary sclerosing cholangitis. Nat Rev Gastroenterol Hepatol 2009;6:287–95.
63. Meyerholz DK, Stoltz DA, Pezzulo AA, et al. Pathology of gastrointestinal organs in a porcine model of cystic fibrosis. Am J Pathol 2010;176:1377–89.
64. Antoniou A, Raynaud P, Cordi S, et al. Intrahepatic bile ducts develop according to a new mode of tubulogenesis regulated by the transcription factor SOX9. Gastroenterology 2009;136:2325–33.
65. Stroope A, Radtke B, Huang B, et al. Hepato-renal pathology in Pkd2^ws25/- mice, an animal model of autosomal dominant polycystic kidney disease. Am J Pathol 2010;176:1282–91.
66. Kalsheker NA. α1-antitrypsin deficiency: best clinical practice. J Clin Pathol 2009; 62:865–9.
67. Silverman EK, Sandhaus RA. Alpha-1-antitrypsin deficiency. N Engl J Med 2009; 360:2749–57.
68. Lam M, Torbenson M, Yeh MM, et al. HFE mutations in α-1-antitrypsin deficiency: an examination of cirrhotic explants. Mod Pathol 2010;23:637–43.
69. Griffiths WJH, Mayr R, McFarlane I, et al. Clinical presentation and molecular pathophysiology of autosomal dominant hemochromatosis caused by a novel ferroportin mutation. Hepatology 2010;51:788–95.
70. Lucey MR, Mathurin P, Morgan TR. Medical progress: alcoholic hepatitis. N Engl J Med 2009;360:2758–69.
71. Schwimmer JB, Celedon MA, Lavine JE, et al. Heritability of nonalcoholic fatty liver disease. Gastroenterology 2009;136:1585–92.
72. Speliotes EK. Genetics of common obesity and nonalcoholic fatty liver disease. Gastroenterology 2009;136:1492–5.
73. Valenti L, Fracanzani AL, Bugianesi E, et al. HFE genotype, parenchymal iron accumulation, and liver fibrosis in patients with nonalcoholic fatty liver disease. Gastroenterology 2010;138:905–12.
74. Kowdley KV. The role of iron in nonalcoholic fatty liver disease: the story continues. Gastroenterology 2010;138:817–9.
75. Watt KDS, Charlton MR. Metabolic syndrome and liver transplantation: a review and guide to management. J Hepatol 2010;53:199–206.
76. Hanada S, Snider NT, Brunt EM, et al. Gender dimorphic formation of mouse Mallory-Denk bodies and the role of xenobiotic metabolism and oxidative stress. Gastroenterology 2010;138:1607–17.
77. Brunt EM, Kleiner DE, Wilson LA, et al. Portal chronic inflammation in nonalcoholic fatty liver disease (NAFLD): a histologic marker of advanced NAFLD—clinicopathologic correlations from the Nonalcoholic Steatohepatitis Clinical Research Network. Hepatology 2009;49:809–20.
78. Loomba R, Sirlin CB, Schwimmer JB, et al. Advances in pediatric nonalcoholic fatty liver disease. Hepatology 2009;50:1282–93.
79. Carter-Kent C, Yerian LM, Brunt EM, et al. Nonalcoholic steatohepatitis in children: a multicenter clinicopathological study. Hepatology 2009;50:1113–20.
80. Chen G, Brunt EM. Diabetic hepatosclerosis: a 10-year autopsy series. Liver Int 2009;29:1044–50.
81. Hashimoto E, Yatsuji S, Tobari M, et al. Hepatocellular carcinoma in patients with nonalcoholic steatohepatitis. J Gastroenterol 2009;44(Suppl XIX):89–95.
82. Ascha MS, Hanouneh IA, Lopez R, et al. The incidence and risk factors of hepatocellular carcinoma in patients with nonalcoholic steatohepatitis. Hepatology 2010;51:1972–8.

83. Pietrangelo A. Iron in NASH, chronic liver diseases and HCC: how much iron is too much? J Hepatol 2009;50:249–51.

84. Makhlouf HR, Abdul-Al HM, Wang G, et al. Calcifying nested stromal-epithelial tumors of the liver. A clinicopathologic, immunohistochemical, and molecular genetic study of 9 cases with a long-term follow-up. Am J Surg Pathol 2009;33: 976–83.

85. Ahmad I, Iyer A, Marginean CE, et al. Diagnostic use of cytokeratins, CD34, and neuronal cell adhesion molecule staining in focal nodular hyperplasia and hepatic adenoma. Hum Pathol 2009;40:726–34.

86. Bioulac-Sage P, Laumonier H, Rullier A, et al. Over-expression of glutamine synthetase in focal nodular hyperplasia: a novel easy diagnostic tool in surgical pathology. Liver Int 2009;29:459–65.

87. Tong G-X, Yu WM, Beaubier NT, et al. Expression of PAX8 in normal and neoplastic renal tissues: an immunohistochemical study. Mod Pathol 2009;22: 1218–27.

Index

Note: Page numbers of article titles are in **boldface** type.

A

AAT deficiency. See *α₁-Antitrypsin (AAT) deficiency.*
Acidophil bodies, in NAFLD, 596
Adenocarcinoma, metastatic, of liver, diagnosis of, immunohistochemistry in, 693
Adenoma(s)
    hepatocellular
        diagnosis of, immunohistochemistry in, 695
        update on, 721–725
    multiple, update on, 725
    telangiectatic hepatocytic, diagnosis of, immunohistochemistry in, 695–696
Adenomatosis, liver, update on, 725
AIH. See *Autoimmune hepatitis (AIH).*
Alcoholic steatohepatitis (ASH), NASH vs., 597
Allograft(s), liver, pathology of, problematic areas in, 672–674
Angiomyolipoma(s)
    hepatic, diagnosis of, immunohistochemistry in, 696–697
    update on, 726–727
Angiosarcoma, diagnosis of, immunohistochemistry in, 698
α₁-Antitrypsin (AAT) deficiency, in children, 735–737
Apoptosis, in NAFLD, 596
ASH. See *Alcoholic steatohepatitis (ASH).*
Autoimmune hepatitis (AIH)
    acute, histology of, 578–582
    advances in, 751
    as part of overlap syndrome, 586–587
    chronic "grumbling," 583–584
    diagnostic scoring systems for, overview of, 577–578
    duct injury in, 582
    fulminant, histology of, 582–583
    HCV and, 568
    histology of, **577–590**
        acute AIH, 578–582
        cryptogenic chronic hepatitis, 584
        cryptogenic cirrhosis, 585
        fulminant AIH, 582–583
    posttreatment care, 584

B

Benign and recurrent intrahepatic cholestasis (BRIC), to PFIC, 623–626
Bile, formation of, inaccessibility of, in trafficking and transporter disorders in infants
    and children with cholestasis, 619–620

Clin Liver Dis 14 (2010) 763–771
doi:10.1016/S1089-3261(10)00132-7
1089-3261/10/$ – see front matter © 2010 Elsevier Inc. All rights reserved.

liver.theclinics.com

Bile duct lesions, in HCV, 566
Bile salt handling, in infants and children with cholestasis, 620–621
Biliary disease, advances in, 751–754
Biopsy(ies), liver. See *Liver biopsy.*
BRIC. See *Benign and recurrent intrahepatic cholestasis (BRIC).*
Byler disease, 622–623

C

Carcinogenesis, hepatic progenitor cells in, 711–713
CD34, in hepatocellular carcinoma diagnosis, 692
Centrilobular necrosis, passive congestion and, 643–644
Chemotherapy
    OX-based, for CRLM, SOS diagnosis and, 661–662
    SOS related to, effect on CRLM, 659–661
Children
    AAT deficiency in, 735–737
    cholestasis in, trafficking and transporter disorders in, **619–633.** See also
        Cholestasis, in infancy and childhood, trafficking and transporter disorders in.
    GSD-I in, 737–738
    GSD-II in, 738
    GSD-IV in, 738
    hepatic neoplasia and metabolic diseases in, **731–746**
    hereditary hemochromatosis in, 737
    hereditary tyrosinemia in, 733–735
    Wilson disease in, 740
Cholangiocarcinoma, diagnosis of, immunohistochemistry in, 693–695
Cholestasis
    FXR sequence variation and, 627
    in infancy and childhood
        classes of, 621
        familial hypercholanemia, 627–628
        secondary intrahepatic cholestasis, variability in and predisposition to, 622
        trafficking and transporter disorders in, **619–633**
            bile salt handling in, 620–621
            Byler disease, 622–623
            Dubin-Johnson syndrome, 626
            inaccessibility of bile formation, 619–620
            MDR3 deficiency, 626–627
            primary intrahepatic cholestasis, 622
    intrahepatic. See *Intrahepatic cholestasis.*
    low-GGT, 622–623
Chronic "grumbling" AIH, 583–584
Cirrhosis
    cryptogenic, histology of, 585
    intrahepatic blood flow in, obstruction to, pathophysiology of, 641–642
    NAFLD and, 597–598
    primary biliary, hepatic granulomas and, 608–609
Colorectal liver metastases (CRLMs), chemotherapy-associated SOS effects on, 659–661
Colorectal metastases, hepatic, chemotherapy-associated SOS effects on, 659–661
Common variable immunodeficiency, advances in, 750–751

CRLMs. See *Colorectal liver metastases (CRLMs)*.
Cryptogenic chronic hepatitis, histology of, 584
Cryptogenic cirrhosis, histology of, 585
Cystadenoma(s), hepatobiliary, diagnosis of, immunohistochemistry in, 698
Cytokeratin, in metastatic adenocarcinoma of liver diagnosis, 693

D

Developmental biology, liver biopsy and, advances in, 747–748
Drug(s)
    hepatic granulomas and, 613
    liver injury related to, advances in, 748–749
Dubin-Johnson syndrome, 626

E

Epithelioid hemangioendothelioma, diagnosis of, immunohistochemistry in, 697

F

Familial hypercholanemia, 627–628
FARSIGHT, 678–680
Fatty liver disease, advances in, 754–755
FCH. See *Fibrosing cholestatic hepatitis (FCH)*.
Fibrosing cholestatic hepatitis (FCH), 569
Fibrosis(es), NAFLD and, 597–598
Focal nodular hyperplasias
    diagnosis of, immunohistochemistry in, 695
    update on, 719–721
Foreign bodies, hepatic granulomas and, 613
Fulminant hepatitis, advances in, 750–751
FXR sequence variation, cholestasis and, 627

G

Glycogen storage disease (GSD)
    type I, in children, 737–738
    type II, in children, 738
    type IV, in children, 738
Glycogenated nuclei, in NAFLD, 596–597
Glypican-3, in hepatocellular carcinoma diagnosis, 689–691
Granuloma(s), hepatic, **605–617**
    biology of, 605–606
    described, 605
    drugs and, 613
    foreign bodies and, 613
    incidence of, trends in, 606–608
    infectious diseases and, 611–613
    neoplasia and, 613–615
    noninfectious immunologic diseases and, 608–611
    PBC and, 608–609
    sarcoidosis and, 609–610
GSD. See *Glycogen storage disease (GSD)*.

H

HBV. See *Hepatitis, B.*
HCV. See *Hepatitis, C.*
HDV. See *Hepatitis, D.*
Hemangioendothelioma, epithelioid, diagnosis of, immunohistochemistry in, 697
Hemangioma(s), update on, 725
Hemochromatosis
    hereditary, in children, 737
    neonatal, advances in, 750–751
Hepatic angiomyolipoma, diagnosis of, immunohistochemistry in, 696–697
Hepatic artery compromise, 638
Hepatic granulomas, **605–617.** See also *Granuloma(s), hepatic.*
Hepatic neoplasia, in children, **731–746**
Hepatic progenitor cells, **705–718**
    activation of, mechanisms of, 709–711
    described, 706–709
    in carcinogenesis, 711–713
Hepatic vein thrombosis, 645–646
Hepatic venous outflow obstruction, 645–647
Hepatitis
    autoimmune. See *Autoimmune hepatitis (AIH).*
    B
        chronic
            clinical course of, 561
            clinical diagnosis of, 561
            described, 560–561
            diagnosis of, practical approach to, 569
            histologic features of, 561–564
            immune-active phase of, 563
            immune-inactive phase of, 563–564
            immune-tolerant phase of, 562
            pathology of, **555–564**
                immunohistochemical staining patterns in, 564
            prevalence of, 560
        coinfection with HDV, HIV, and HCV, 564
    C
        chronic, **564–569**
            described, 564–565
            diagnosis of, practical approach to, 569
            fibrosis/architectural changes in, 568
            inflammation/degree of injury in, 568
            pathology of, **555–575**
            prevalence of, 564
        HBV coinfection with, 564
        overlap syndrome of, 568
        with autoimmune features, 569
    chronic
        architectural changes in, 559
        cryptogenic, histology of, 584
        defined, 555

diagnosis of, approach to, 555–556
features of, 559–560
grading and staging of, scoring systems for, 556–560
lobular changes in, 558
necroinflammation in, grade of, 556
portal changes in, 556–558
D, HBV coinfection with, 564
fibrosing cholestatic, 569
fulminant, advances in, 750–751
pathology of, chronic
bile duct lesions in, 566
clinical course of, 565–566
diagnosis of, 565
lymphoid follicles and aggregates in, 566–567
pathology of, histopathologic features of, 566–568
steatosis in, 567
peliosis, 644–645
viral, advances in, 749–750
Hepatobiliary cystadenomas, diagnosis of, immunohistochemistry in, 698
Hepatobiliary pathology, advances in, **747–762**
AIH, 751
biliary disease, 751–754
common variable immunodeficiency, 750–751
drug-induced liver injury, 748–749
fatty liver disease, 754–755
fulminant hepatitis, 750–751
liver biopsy, developmental biology and, 747–748
liver tumors, 756–757
metabolic diseases, 754–755
neonatal hemochromatosis, 750–751
viral hepatitis, 749–750
Hepatocellular adenomas
diagnosis of, immunohistochemistry in, 695
update on, 721–725
Hepatocellular carcinoma, diagnosis of, immunohistochemistry in
CD34, 692
glypican-3, 689–691
hepatocyte paraffin 1, 687–689
polyclonal carcinoembryonic antigen, 691–692
Hepatocellular carcinoma–cholangiocarcinoma, diagnosis of, immunohistochemistry
in, 695
Hepatocellular tumors, update on, 719–725
focal nodular hyperplasias, 719–721
hepatocellular adenomas, 721–725
liver adenomatosis, 725
multiple adenomas, 725
Hepatocyte(s), stem cell properties of, 706
Hepatocyte ballooning, in NAFLD, 593–595
Hepatocyte paraffin 1, in hepatocellular carcinoma diagnosis, 687–689
Hereditary hemochromatosis, in children, 737

Hereditary tyrosinemia, in children, 733–735
HIV, HBV coinfection with, 564
Hypercholanemia, familial, 627–628
Hyperplasia(s)
    focal nodular
        diagnosis of, immunohistochemistry in, 695
        update on, 719–721
    nodular, 647–648
Hypertension, idiopathic portal, 640–641

I

Idiopathic portal hypertension, 640–641
Immunohistochemistry, in liver tumors, **687–703.** See also *Liver tumors, immunohistochemistry in.*
Infant(s), cholestasis in, trafficking and transporter disorders in, **619–633.** See also *Cholestasis, in infancy and childhood, trafficking and transporter disorders in.*
Infectious diseases, hepatic granulomas and, 611–613
Inferior vena cava thrombosis, 645–646
Inflammation
    lobular, in NAFLD, 595
    portal, in NAFLD, 595
Intrahepatic cholestasis
    benign and recurrent, to PFIC, 623–626
    immunohistochemical studies in, 629
    low-GGT, trafficking of polarity defects and, 628–629
    primary, in infancy and childhood, 622
    progressive familial, BRIC to, 623–626
Iron, in NAFLD, 596–597

L

Lipogranuloma(s), in NAFLD, 596–597
Liver
    anatomy of, 627, 635
    microanatomy of, 637–648
    vascular disorders of, **635–650.** See also *Vascular disorders, of liver.*
Liver adenomatosis, update on, 725
Liver allograft, pathology of, problematic areas in, 672–674
Liver allograft biopsy, **669–685**
    interpretation of, limitations of, 669–671
Liver biopsy, **669–685**
    developmental biology and, advances in, 747–748
    histopathologic examination of, strengths of, 671–672
    in NAFLD/NASH, drawbacks of, 599–600
    interpretation of, limitations of, 669–671
    pathology of
        microscopic
            challenges related to, 680–681
            FARSIGHT in, 678–680
            limitation of, multiplex tissue staining for, 674–678
            tissue evaluation tools using image analysis software in, 678–680

uses of, 680–681
   problematic areas in, 672–674
Liver injury, drug-induced, advances in, 748–749
Liver metastases, colorectal, chemotherapy-associated SOS effects on, 659–661
Liver tumors
   advances in, 756–757
   benign
      angiomyolipomas, 726–727
      update on, **719–729**
         focal nodular hyperplasias, 719–721
         hemangiomas, 725
         hepatocellular adenomas, 721–725
         hepatocellular tumors, 719–725
         liver adenomatosis, 725
         multiple adenomas, 725
   immunohistochemistry in, **687–703.** See also specific tumor types,
      e.g., *Hepatocellular carcinoma.*
      angiosarcoma, 698
      cholangiocarcinoma, 693–695
      combined hepatocellular carcinoma–cholangiocarcinoma, 695
      epithelioid hemangioendothelioma, 697
      focal nodular hyperplasia, 695
      hepatic angiomyolipoma, 696–697
      hepatobiliary cystadenomas, 698
      hepatocellular adenoma, 695
      hepatocellular carcinoma, 687–692
      lymphangioma, 697
      metastatic adenocarcinoma, 693
      telangiectatic hepatocytic adenoma, 695–696
Lobular inflammation, in NAFLD, 595
Low gamma-glutamyl transpeptidase (GGT) cholestasis, 622–623
Low gamma-glutamyl transpeptidase (GGT) intrahepatic cholestasis, trafficking
   of polarity defects and, 628–629
Lymphangioma, diagnosis of, immunohistochemistry in, 697

M

Mallory-Denk bodies (MDBs), in NAFLD, 595–596
MDBs. See *Mallory-Denk bodies (MDBs).*
MDR3 deficiency, 626–627
Metabolic diseases
   advances in, 754–755
   in children, hepatic involvement in, **731–746**
Metastatic adenocarcinoma, of liver, diagnosis of, immunohistochemistry in, 693
Microgranuloma(s), in NAFLD, 596–597
MOC-31, in metastatic adenocarcinoma of liver diagnosis, 693
Multiplex tissue staining
   imaging solutions for, 675–678
   in light microscopic pathology, 674–675

N

NAFLD. See *Nonalcoholic fatty liver disease (NFALD).*

NASH. See *Nonalcoholic steatohepatitis (NASH)*.
Neonatal hemochromatosis, advances in, 750–751
Neoplasia(s)
    hepatic, in children, **731–746**
    hepatic granulomas and, 613–615
Nodular hyperplasias, 647–648
Nonalcoholic fatty liver disease (NFALD), **591–604**
    acidophil bodies in, 596
    apoptosis in, 596
    ASH vs., 597
    cirrhosis and, 597–598
    described, 591–592
    fibrosis and, 597–598
    hepatocyte ballooning in, 593–595
    histopathologic lesions of, grading and staging of, 598–599
    iron in, 596–597
    lipogranulomas in, 596–597
    liver biopsy in, drawbacks of, 599–600
    lobular inflammation in, 595
    MDBs in, 595–596
    microgranulomas in, 596–597
    morphology of, 592
    NASH vs. ASH, 597
    portal inflammation in, 595
    progenitor cells in, 598
    steatosis in, 592–593
Nonalcoholic steatohepatitis (NASH), in NAFLD, glycogenated nuclei in, 596–597
Noninfectious immunologic diseases, hepatic granulomas and, 608–611

O

Overlap syndrome
    AIH as part of, 586–587
    of HCV, 568
OX-based chemotherapy, for CRLM, SOS diagnosis and, 661–662

P

PBC. See *Primary biliary cirrhosis (PBC)*.
Peliosis hepatitis, 644–645
PFIC. See *Progressive familial intrahepatic cholestasis (PFIC)*.
Polyclonal carcinoembryonic antigen, in hepatocellular carcinoma diagnosis, 691–692
Portal inflammation, in NAFLD, 595
Portal vein obstruction/thrombosis, 638–640
Primary biliary cirrhosis (PBC), hepatic granulomas and, 608–609
Primary intrahepatic cholestasis, in infancy and childhood, 622
Progenitor cells, in NASH, 598
Progressive familial intrahepatic cholestasis (PFIC), BRIC to, 623–626

S

Sarcoidosis, hepatic granulomas and, 609–610

Scoring systems, for grading and staging of chronic hepatitis, 556–560
Sinusoid(s), physical occlusion of, 642–643
Sinusoidal obstruction syndrome (SOS), 646–647, **651–668**
   causes of, 651–652
   chemotherapy-associated, effect on hepatic colorectal metastases, 659–661
   described, 651
   diagnosis of, OX-based chemotherapy for CRLM and, 661–662
   normal sinusoids and, 654–657
   pathogenesis of, 654–659
      in animal models, 657–658
      in humans, 659
   pathologic lesions of, 652–654
   postoperative complications of, prevention of, 662–664
SOS. See *Sinusoidal obstruction syndrome (SOS)*.
Steatohepatitis, alcoholic, NASH vs., 597
Steatosis
   in HCV, 567
   in NAFLD, 592–593
Stem cell(s)
   described, 705–706
   hepatocytes with properties of, 706

T

Telangiectatic hepatocytic adenoma, diagnosis of, immunohistochemistry in, 695–696
Thrombosis(es)
   hepatic vein, 645–646
   inferior vena cava, 645–646
Trafficking disorders, in cholestasis in infants and children, **619–633**. See also *Cholestasis, in infancy and childhood, trafficking and transporter disorders in.*
Transporter disorders, in cholestasis in infants and children, **619–633**. See also *Cholestasis, in infancy and childhood, trafficking and transporter disorders in.*
Tumor(s), liver. See *Liver tumors.*
Tyrosinemia, hereditary, in children, 733–735

V

Vascular disorders, of liver, **635–650**
   anatomy related to, 627, 635
   classification of, 636
   hepatic artery compromise, 638
   hepatic venous outflow obstruction, 645–647
   idiopathic portal hypertension, 640–641
   impaired blood flow into, 638–641
   impaired blood flow through, 641–645
   microanatomy related to, 637–648
   portal vein obstruction and thrombosis, 638–640
Venoocclusive disease, 646–647
Viral hepatitis, advances in, 749–750

W

Wilson disease, in children, 740

United States Postal Service
Statement of Ownership, Management, and Circulation
(All Periodicals Publications Except Requestor Publications)

1. Publication Title	2. Publication Number	3. Filing Date
Clinics in Liver Disease	0 1 6 - 7 5 4	9/15/10

4. Issue Frequency	5. Number of Issues Published Annually	6. Annual Subscription Price
Feb, May, Aug, Nov	4	$235.00

7. Complete Mailing Address of Known Office of Publication (Not printer) (Street, city, county, state, and ZIP+4®)

Elsevier Inc.
360 Park Avenue South
New York, NY 10010-1710

Contact Person
Stephen Bushing
Telephone (Include area code)
215-239-3688

8. Complete Mailing Address of Headquarters or General Business Office of Publisher (Not printer)

Elsevier Inc., 360 Park Avenue South, New York, NY 10010-1710

9. Full Names and Complete Mailing Addresses of Publisher, Editor, and Managing Editor (Do not leave blank)

Publisher (Name and complete mailing address)

Kim Murphy, Elsevier, Inc., 1600 John F. Kennedy Blvd. Suite 1800, Philadelphia, PA 19103-2899

Editor (Name and complete mailing address)

Kerry Holland, Elsevier, Inc., 1600 John F. Kennedy Blvd. Suite 1800, Philadelphia, PA 19103-2899

Managing Editor (Name and complete mailing address)

Catherine Bewick, Elsevier, Inc., 1600 John F. Kennedy Blvd. Suite 1800, Philadelphia, PA 19103-2899

10. Owner (Do not leave blank. If the publication is owned by a corporation, give the name and address of the corporation immediately followed by the names and addresses of all stockholders owning or holding 1 percent or more of the total amount of stock. If not owned by a corporation, give the names and addresses of the individual owners. If owned by a partnership or other unincorporated firm, give its name and address as well as those of each individual owner. If the publication is published by a nonprofit organization, give its name and address.)

Full Name	Complete Mailing Address
Wholly owned subsidiary of	4520 East-West Highway
Reed/Elsevier, US holdings	Bethesda, MD 20814

11. Known Bondholders, Mortgagees, and Other Security Holders Owning or Holding 1 Percent or More of Total Amount of Bonds, Mortgages, or Other Securities. If none, check box ▶ ☐ None

Full Name	Complete Mailing Address
N/A	

12. Tax Status (For completion by nonprofit organizations authorized to mail at nonprofit rates) (Check one)
The purpose, function, and nonprofit status of this organization and the exempt status for federal income tax purposes:
☐ Has Not Changed During Preceding 12 Months
☐ Has Changed During Preceding 12 Months (Publisher must submit explanation of change with this statement)

PS Form 3526, September 2007 (Page 1 of 3 (Instructions Page 3)) PSN 7530-01-000-9931 PRIVACY NOTICE: See our Privacy policy in www.usps.com

13. Publication Title	14. Issue Date for Circulation Data Below
Clinics in Liver Disease	August 2010

15. Extent and Nature of Circulation			Average No. Copies Each Issue During Preceding 12 Months	No. Copies of Single Issue Published Nearest to Filing Date
a. Total Number of Copies (Net press run)			863	887
b. Paid Circulation (By Mail and Outside the Mail)	(1)	Mailed Outside-County Paid Subscriptions Stated on PS Form 3541. (Include paid distribution above nominal rate, advertiser's proof copies, and exchange copies)	268	243
	(2)	Mailed In-County Paid Subscriptions Stated on PS Form 3541 (Include paid distribution above nominal rate, advertiser's proof copies, and exchange copies)		
	(3)	Paid Distribution Outside the Mails Including Sales Through Dealers and Carriers, Street Vendors, Counter Sales, and Other Paid Distribution Outside USPS®	155	156
	(4)	Paid Distribution by Other Classes Mailed Through the USPS (e.g. First-Class Mail®)		
c. Total Paid Distribution (Sum of 15b (1), (2), (3), and (4))			423	399
d. Free or Nominal Rate Distribution (By Mail and Outside the Mail)	(1)	Free or Nominal Rate Outside-County Copies Included on PS Form 3541	79	69
	(2)	Free or Nominal Rate In-County Copies Included on PS Form 3541		
	(3)	Free or Nominal Rate Copies Mailed at Other Classes Through the USPS (e.g. First-Class Mail)		
	(4)	Free or Nominal Rate Distribution Outside the Mail (Carriers or other means)		
e. Total Free or Nominal Rate Distribution (Sum of 15d (1), (2), (3) and (4))		▶	79	69
f. Total Distribution (Sum of 15c and 15e)		▶	502	468
g. Copies not Distributed (See instructions to publishers #4 (page #3))		▶	361	419
h. Total (Sum of 15f and g)		▶	863	887
i. Percent Paid (15c divided by 15f times 100)			84.26%	85.26%

16. Publication of Statement of Ownership
☐ If the publication is a general publication, publication of this statement is required. Will be printed
in the November 2010 issue of this publication.
☐ Publication not required.

17. Signature and Title of Editor, Publisher, Business Manager, or Owner

Stephen R. Bushing Date

Stephen R. Bushing – Fulfillment/Inventory Specialist September 15, 2010

I certify that all information furnished on this form is true and complete. I understand that anyone who furnishes false or misleading information on this form or who omits material or information requested on the form may be subject to criminal sanctions (including fines and imprisonment) and/or civil sanctions (including civil penalties).

PS Form 3526, September 2007 (Page 2 of 3)

Moving?

Make sure your subscription moves with you!

To notify us of your new address, find your **Clinics Account Number** (located on your mailing label above your name), and contact customer service at:

Email: journalscustomerservice-usa@elsevier.com

800-654-2452 (subscribers in the U.S. & Canada)
314-447-8871 (subscribers outside of the U.S. & Canada)

Fax number: 314-447-8029

Elsevier Health Sciences Division
Subscription Customer Service
3251 Riverport Lane
Maryland Heights, MO 63043

*To ensure uninterrupted delivery of your subscription, please notify us at least 4 weeks in advance of move.

Printed and bound by CPI Group (UK) Ltd, Croydon, CR0 4YY

03/10/2024

01040459-0004

1